Quick Reference to Ob-Gyn Procedures

Quick Reference to *OB-GYN Procedures*

Second Edition

Hugh R.K. Barber, M.D.
Clinical Professor of Obstetrics and Gynecology
Cornell University Medical College; and
Director of Obstetrics and Gynecology
Lenox Hill Hospital
New York, New York

David H. Fields, M.D.
Assistant Adjunct Obstetrician/Gynecologist
Lenox Hill Hospital
New York, New York

Sherwin A. Kaufman, M.D.
Attending Obstetrician/Gynecologist
and Director in Fertility Clinic
Lenox Hill Hospital
New York, New York

J. B. Lippincott Company
Philadelphia • Toronto

Second Edition

ISBN 0-397-50423-3

Library of Congress Catalog Card Number 79-20474

Printed in the United States of America

1 3 5 4 2

Library of Congress Cataloging in Publication Data

Barber, Hugh R K 1918–
Quick reference to ob-gyn procedures.

Includes index.
1. Obstetrics—Handbooks, manuals, etc. 2. Gynecology—Handbooks, manuals, etc. I. Fields, David H., joint author. II. Kaufman, Sherwin A., joint author. III. Title. [DNLM: 1. Genital diseases, Female. 2. Obstetrics. 3. Pregnancy complications. WP100.3 B234q]
RG110.B37 1979 618'.02'02 79-20474
ISBN 0-397-50423-3

To our wives, Mary Louise Barber, Claire Kaufman, and Ailene Fields, for their patience and help.

To [illegible] Mary Louise Barber, Clyde [illegible]
[illegible] for their patience [illegible]

Preface

The warm reception given to the first edition of *Quick Reference to Ob-Gyn Procedures,* which presented material using a new outline format, attests to the success of our endeavors. It stimulated us to review our efforts for an even more successful second edition. We have kept the same format that was used in the first edition, but there was a need to update the material and to include additional chapters. This has been the chief goal of this revision.

Since the publication of the first edition in 1969, the field of obstetrics and gynecology has made rapid and explosive advances. The fields of reproductive endocrinology and immunology, genetics, maternal-fetal medicine, oncology, the control of Rh sensitization, and the ability to create life in a test tube have literally created a new specialty. These staggering advances have challenged the imagination of students and have served to recruit them into the field of obstetrics and gynecology. The potential for contributions has made obstetrics and gynecology one of the most exciting specialties in the field of medicine today.

The volume of material, the changing concepts, and the almost daily additions to the literature make it difficult for the busy clinician to read the literature and organize and incorporate it into the everyday practice of medicine. The *Quick Reference* attempts to do this. We have tried to make each chapter concise without being superficial. The format should provide an overall review that can serve as a framework upon which new knowledge may be placed and then used in clinical practice. The book is not designed for originality, but rather to present the basics, as well as updated material, in a readable format. It is truly the physician's assistant for giving patient care and is designed to save the doctor time, without sacrificing the quality of care given to the patient. We have attempted to bring the art and science of medicine together for the benefit of the patient and to lighten the work of the busy physician. The book qualifies as an outline for each physician's continuing medical education.

We are grateful for the suggestions made by students, residents, practicing physicians, and our colleagues. The house staff at Lenox Hill Hospital has, as a group, made very helpful suggestions to us.

Other members of the Lenox Hill Hospital staff have also been most helpful. We would like to particularly thank the library staff, especially Chief Librarian Shirley Dansker, who has been extremely helpful in researching new material that we have incorporated into the book. Penelope Dell has been most helpful to Dr. David Fields in the preparation of his chapters.

As always, we are most grateful to Marcia Miller, who has played a key role in helping us to complete this book. Her typing skill has only been surpassed by her able editorial assistance and dedication above and beyond her routine work. Her superb efforts have played a significant, if not major, role in bringing this second edition to fruition.

To J. B. Lippincott Company, a division of Harper & Row, we want to express our appreciation for the opportunity to update *Quick Reference to Ob-Gyn Procedures*. We want to express our thanks to Mr. Stuart Freeman, Editor-in-Chief, Medical Books Division, for his encouragement in undertaking this revision and for the help he has given us.

We are most appreciative to the many doctors who have taken time from their busy practices to thank us for the help that the first edition of this book has provided them. It has made our work on this edition even more worthwhile.

We are especially grateful to our wives for their help, encouragement, and patience. It has truly been a team effort.

Hugh R. K. Barber, M.D.

Contents

Quick Reference to Ob-Gyn Procedures

1. Infertility

Sherwin A. Kaufman, M.D.

DEFINITIONS

1. *Infertility* is the inability to achieve pregnancy and carry through to live birth; thus, a woman who has had only miscarriages may be considered infertile. *Primary infertility* means that pregnancy has never taken place, while *secondary infertility* denotes that one or more previous conceptions have occurred.

2. *Sterility*, though technically synonymous with infertility, implies that some absolute factor precludes conception; this could be temporary (previous tubal ligation) or permanent (previous hysterectomy). In general, the term infertility is preferable to sterility because it has a less ominous connotation.

3. A couple is considered infertile if pregnancy has not occurred after 1 year of coitus without contraception. Normally, 75 per cent of women conceive during the first 6 months, and 85 per cent conceive in the first year. Therefore, if a couple has been trying to conceive for 1 year (or an older couple for 6 months), it is time to begin a workup.

BASIC PRINCIPLES

1. It is estimated that between 15 and 20 per cent of couples are either unable to initiate a pregnancy or carry to term.

2. This means that approximately 6 million couples in the U.S. are involuntarily childless, which makes infertility a common medical problem.

3. Management of infertility requires an organized plan of study, particularly because in the majority of couples, more than one cause is found.

4. The various tests for infertility to be described are related to the basic prerequisites for fertility, which are as follows:

a. The male gonads must produce sperm of reasonable quantity and quality.

b. There must be no obstruction in the male genital tract.

c. The ejaculate must have access to the cervix.

d. The endocervical mucus must be favorable for sperm survival.

e. The tubes must be patent to allow for ascent of sperm and descent of the ovum.

f. The ovaries must produce and release normal ova.

g. There must be no obstruction between the ovaries and the fimbriated end of the tubes.

h. The endometrium must be physiologically capable of permitting normal implantation of the fertilized ovum and continued embryonic growth.

Causes of Infertility

1. In the majority of cases, there are multiple causes for infertility.

2. About 40 per cent of infertility problems relate to the husband (male factor) in whole or in part.

3. In the female, the most common causes of infertility, in order of frequency, relate to ovulation disturbances, tubal problems, and cervical factors; the last two are especially common in secondary infertility.

4. Less frequently, the cause is related to the uterine corpus, metabolic factors, or immunological problems.

5. In some, no etiological factors are

discernible despite complete investigation. However, this is another way of saying that the causes remain elusive.

6. Contrary to popular belief, psychological or emotional factors are actually an infrequent cause of infertility in those desiring a child. Any psychosomatic aspects are generally the result of the frustration owing to barren marriage.

Doctor-Patient Relationship

1. Infertility is the only "illness" that involves two people. The physician must appreciate the sensitivities and frustrations of the couple.

2. It is wise to enlist the husband's cooperation by having him present at the first interview and by explaining that infertility is considered a bilateral problem.

3. The terms "fault"and "blame" have no place in the management of infertility.

4. A well organized and systematic approach yields the best results. It saves time, and the rate of ultimate success is high.

5. The physician should outline the nature, scope, and purpose of the tests contemplated, the time involved (3 to 6 months), and the costs.

6. If necessary, the gynecologist should utilize the services of a urologist, endocrinologist, and psychologist or psychiatrist.

7. The doctor's purpose is to first determine why the couple is infertile, then what treatment is indicated and the prognosis.

8. It is encouraging to note that from 50 to 70 per cent of infertility patients can be helped.

INFERTILITY INVESTIGATION OF THE HUSBAND

Investigation of the male should be first or relatively early in the study. Detailed history and physical examination are of obvious importance when the semen quality is subnormal.

History

1. Past History

a. *Previous Marriage.* Fertility or infertility

b. *Previous Studies.* Previous infertility tests or treatments

c. *Medical.* Anomalies, variocele, venereal disease, orchitis (e.g., mumps), chronic illness, obesity, endocrine disorders, allergies, drugs, recent febrile illness. (A recent flu, for example,can severely depress sperm quality for several weeks)

d. *Surgical.* Variococelectomy, herniorrhaphy, hydrocelectomy, genital injuries

e. *Occupational.* Radiographs; chemicals (exposure to metals as in painting or printing); thermal factors: possible sources of excessive heat include febrile illness, prolonged or frequent hot baths, and tight scrotal supports. (*Note*: the deleterious effects of hyperthermia or viral illness—other than mumps orchitis—is completely dissipated after 3 months.) The ordinary pressures of life and work do not generally affect sperm quality; however, extreme stress can have a deleterious effect on male fertility and sexual functioning.

2. Present History

a. *Type of Problem.* Duration of infertility

b. *Habits.* Marijuana may depress the sperm count and can also cause chromosomal anomalies that can lead to genetic damage. Heavy tobacco smoking may cause some depression of sperm production, but no well controlled studies have been reported. Excessive use of alcohol may contribute to liver damage with resultant depression of sperm production. In addition, potency may be adversely affected by excessive use of alcohol or other drugs.

c. *Sexual History.* If the couple

normally has intercourse two to three times a week it is unnecessary (and counterproductive) to belabor the question of timing. Only if intercourse is relatively infrequent is there merit in discussing the most fertile days in the wife's cycle (which can be quite variable). However, when the frequency of spontaneous coitus is very low, the reasons for the lack of desire (or response), or potency problems, should be explored. Here the unsatisfactory sexual relationship takes precedence over the infertility problem; solving the former may well solve the latter.

Physical Examination

1. The presence of varicocele may be significant. In addition, congenital disorders such as hypospadias, testicular atrophy, cryptorchidism, or absence of vas deferens must be ruled out.
2. In the general physical examination, special attention must be given to secondary sexual characteristics, poor nutrition, and evidence of any endocrinopathy.

Diagnostic Procedures

1. Semen Analysis
   a. The period of abstinence should correspond to the couple's usual coital frequency in order to obtain a representative sample.
   b. The semen should be collected in a clean, dry glass or plastic wide-mouthed container by masturbation or coitus interruptus. A condom should not be used, but a commercially prepared plastic sheath with perforation is available for devout Catholics.
   c. Examine within 3 hours of collection, preferably within 2 hours.
   d. The normal standards against which to measure the semen are as follows:
      (1) Liquefaction: usually complete in 5 to 20 minutes
      (2) Volume: averages between 2 and 5 ml.
      (3) Sperm count: a minimum of 20 to 40 million per ml.
      (4) Motility at room temperature: Examination of several fields is done under high dry magnification. The numbers per high power field (HPF) roughly correspond to millions per ml. At least 60 per cent of the sperm should have vigorous, progressive motion at initial examination. (Subsequent examinations in vitro are of no clinical significance.)
      (5) Morphology: A simple stain is mixing a drop of semen with a drop of 1-per-cent aqueous gentian violet. At least 60 per cent should be normal (oval) forms.
2. Urologic examination, especially for varicocele, if semen analysis is subnormal
3. Testicular biopsy when indicated. (Regarding azoospermia, the absence of fructose in the semen suggests congenital absence of vas deferens.)
4. Endocrine evaluation of pituitary, adrenal, and testicular function
5. Sex chromatin and chromosome analysis when indicated

INFERTILITY INVESTIGATION OF THE WIFE

The importance of a detailed history cannot be overemphasized.

History

1. Past History

a. *Previous Marriage.* Fertility or infertility

b. *Medical.* Serious illnesses, endocrine disorders, psychiatric history

c. *Gynecological.* Menstrual irregularities, methods of contraception (e.g., IUD, Pill), pelvic inflammatory disease, possible endometriosis, venereal disease

d. *Surgical.* Pelvic operations, ruptured appendix

e. *Obstetrical.* Abortions (spontaneous or induced), deliveries, postpartum or postabortal complications

f. *Previous Studies.* Previous infertility tests and treatments

2. Present History

a. *Marital History.* Years married and duration of infertility

b. *Sexual History.* Coital frequency, and whether natural or "scheduled," use of lubricants, and postcoital habits such as arising immediately or douching

c. *Social Habits.* Excessive smoking or drinking, use of drugs or other medications

d. *Psychosomatic Evaluation*

Physical Examination

1. General physical examination
2. Gynecological examination

Diagnostic Procedures

1. Routine Pap smears, urinalysis, blood count, serology, sedimentation rate
2. Thyroid evaluation. T_3 and T_4
3. Basal body temperatures (BBT)
4. Tubal insufflation (Rubin test)
5. Hysterosalpingogram
6. Postcoital examinations (Sims-Huhner test), including evaluation of cervical mucus
7. Endometrial biopsy

Additional Studies That May Be Necessary

1. Serum progesterone by radioimmunoassay to establish occurrence of ovulation and to appraise adequacy of corpus-lutem function
2. Adrenal function studies. 17-ketosteroids, 17-hydroxysteroids, pregnanetriol, dexamethasone suppression test. (See Chap. 24).
3. Pituitary gonadotropins (serum FSH and LH) by radioimmunoassay to rule out hypopituitarism (decreased value) or premature menopause (elevated)
4. Metopirone test of pituitary reserve
5. Glucose tolerance test
6. Skull film, for visualization of sella turcica, and visual field examination to rule out pituitary tumor in amenorrheic or oligomenorrheic patients, combined with serum prolactin level (galactorrhea)
7. Progesterone withdrawal test (100 mg. progesterone in oil I.M.) in amenorrhea, to establish presence of endogenous estrogen and to demonstrate integrity of the endometrium
8. Sex chromatin test (Barr) to rule out chromosomal anomaly
9. In-vitro test of sperm-cervical mucus compatibility; determination of antisperm antibodies
10. Endoscopy, either culdoscopy or laparoscopy, to rule out endometriosis, tubal strictures or obstruction, peritubal or peri-ovarian adhesions, Stein-Leventhal syndrome (polycystic ovaries), ovarian dysgenesis

Determination of Ovulation

1. Evidence of Ovulation. Most indices of ovulation depend upon the elaboration of progesterone by the corpus luteum. Although they are not absolute evidence that ovulation has occurred, they are sufficient for practical, clinical purposes. The only direct evidence that ovulation has taken place is: (1) visualization of the ovulation process at laparotomy or endoscopy, and (2) occurrence of pregnancy.

2. Methods for the Detection of Ovulation

a. *Basal Body Temperature (BBT).* A biphasic curve suggests ovulation. Progesterone is thermogenic, causing the typical elevation during the second half of the cycle.

b. *Cervical Mucus Changes.* Progesterone causes changes in the mucus, from profuse, clear, and watery to scant, cloudy, and viscous, and causes a gradual disappearance of microscopic ferning when the mucus is allowed to dry.

c. *Endometrial biopsy,* for secretory changes, including "dating" of the endometrium according to the number of days past ovulation

d. *Serum progestone* by radioimmunoassay, to establish the occurrence of ovulation and ascertain the adequacy of corpus-luteum function

e. *Endoscopy,* seeing a corpus luteum or corpus hemorrhagicum

Evaluation of Tubal Function

1. Purpose of Tubal-Function Tests. Tubal-function tests may be therapeutic as well as diagnostic, inasmuch as they may overcome minor degrees of phimosis, agglutination, or obstruction. Partial or complete tubal obstruction may be caused by pelvic inflammatory disease resulting from a wide variety of bacteria, including gonorrhea, postabortal or postpartum infections, or tuberculosis. Obstruction may also be caused by adhesions resulting from endometriosis, appendicitis, or bleeding caused by a ruptured follicle or corpus luteum. Obstruction may, of course, be the expected result of tubal ligation or cauterization for sterilization.

2. Methods for Determining the State of the Tubes

a. *Tubal Insufflation.* For tubal patency

(1) The instrument should supply a constant source of carbon dioxide (never oxygen, which can cause air embolism). There should be a flowmeter, pressure gauge, and kymograph for recording pressure oscillations, believed related to tubal peristalsis.

(2) Under continuous observation, pressure may be permitted to a maximum of 200 to 250 mm. Hg if necessary. If gas is passing through, however, about 80 to 100 ml. CO_2 are allowed to enter.

(3) The most frequent source of error is failure to secure a leakproof application of the cervical cannula; proper countertraction with a tenaculum on the cervix is helpful.

(4) Contraindications of Tubal Insufflation Test

(a) Local (vaginal) or pelvic infection. A white count and sedimentation rate are helpful to clarify, particularly if there is a history of previous infection

(b) Uterine bleeding

(c) If the patient has had a spontaneous or induced abortion within the preceding 2 months

(d) If there is any possibility of a pregnancy having been initiated. (The test is normally done a few days after a normal menstrual period, not only to avoid this possibility but because there is least pelvic congestion at this time of cycle.)

(5) Evaluation of the Tubal Insufflation Test

(a) If normal patency is present there is usually an initial rise in pressure up to 80 to 120 mm. Hg, with a sudden drop to a lower level as gas passes into the peritoneal cavity.

(b) When either blockage or tubal (cornual) spasm is present, the kymograph shows a steady rise to 250 mm.; this maximum pressure should not be exceeded.

(c) Passage of CO_2 into the peritoneal cavity is confirmed by the presence of pain in one or both shoulders after the test, when the patient sits up. Without such pain, whether immediate or delayed, there is no proof that gas went through.

(d) If there is no passage (i.e., maximum pressure required throughout and no shoulder pain following) owing to spasm or obstruction, the test should be repeated at another time, preceded by a sedative or tranquilizer.

(e) In essence, a positive test shows only that there is a free communication between the uterine cannula and the peritoneal cavity. It does not show that both tubes are patent because the same result can be obtained with one patent tube as with two. Most important, it does not show if the tubes (though patent) are physiologically *normal.* Tubes may be partially occluded, or be bound down by adhesions and unable to pick up or transport an expelled ovum, and yet show a "normal" Rubin test.

(f) Conversely, if the test is consistently negative, it does not mean that the tubes are necessarily occluded. A hysterosalpinogram should be done.

b. *Hysterosalpingogram*

(1) A radiograph of the uterine cavity and tubes is not competitive with a Rubin test. Each has its own value and is capable of revealing things that the other may not. A Rubin test remains a good screening procedure and can prove immediately that at least one tube is open, which is of great reassurance to the anxious patient.

(2) A hysterosalpingogram is helpful in clarifying a questionable or abnormal tubal insufflation test. Some physicians prefer to use the radiograph alone, omitting the Rubin test.

(3) However, a hysterosalpingogram has its own limitations. It can indicate that dye passed through both tubes, but one cannot be certain from this information that the tubes are anatomically normal, because dye can pass through partially strictured or adherent tubes as well.

(4) Nevertheless, the radiograph can provide further information:

(a) Determination of the site of tubal obstruction if it exists

(b) Delineation of suspected adhesions in the event of pooling of dye near the fimbriated ends

(c) Detection of uterine malformations (anomalies), submucous leiomyomata, endometrial polyps, synechiae

(d) Delineation of cervical canal, as in incompetent cervix, cervical stenosis, isthmic synechiae

(e) Capability of overcoming minor obstructions from the force of hydrostatic pressure employed

(5) Contraindications. The same as for tubal insufflation

(6) Technique

(a) As with a Rubin test, it is performed 3 to 5 days after cessation of menses.

(b) Either an oil medium or a water-soluble medium may be used. For evaluation of tubal and peritoneal factors an oil medium is preferable. With water-soluble media, tubal outline is often overshadowed by rapid spillover into the pelvis. Rapid absorption precludes obtaining a 24-hour film, which is often necessary to rule out tubal spasm and to establish normal dispersion of dye, indicating the probable absence of significant pelvic adhesions.

(c) A sterile technique is used, and the same instruments are used as for the tubal insufflation test. A scout film is taken first. The cannula must be emptied of air by filling it with dye before insertion. The guard at the tip of the cannula is tightened so that the tip enters the external cervical os for a distance of 1 cm., in order to get a picture of the cervical canal. Fractional amounts (0.5 to 2 ml.) are injected and the film is taken and developed after each instillation. Attachment of a television screen during the procedure is helpful. In instances of uterine flexion, it is important to apply traction in order to straighten out the uterus.

(d) If cornual or fimbrial blockage is seen, a 24-hour film is necessary before a final interpretaiton can be made. However, shifting the patient's position from side to side or, better still, allowing her to sit up and bounce up and down a few times usually permits adequate dispersion of the dye, making the 24-hour film unnecessary in many cases.

(e) As stated, the Rubin test and salpingography are not competitive tests, in that each can give information the other cannot. Moreover, it has been amply demonstrated that both these procedures can reveal "normal" tubes, which are later shown to be pathological at endoscopic examination. Therefore, no firm conclusions should be drawn from either procedure. It should also be kept in mind that both of these procedures, although primarily diagnostic, may be therapeutic in clearing out minor degrees of phimosis and agglutination.

c. *Endoscopy:* culdoscopy or laparoscopy. *Culdoscopy* is the direct visualization of the pelvic organs through the vagina. *Laparoscopy* is the direct visualization of the pelvic organs through the abdomen.

(1) INDICATIONS FOR ENDOSCOPY

(a) Endoscopy is the definitive method for ruling out suspected or unsuspected tubal pathology, peri-adnexal adhesions, endometriosis, polycystic or other ovarian disease, abnormalities in uterine contour in the infertile patient.

(b) Endoscopy is an essential prerequisite to any tubal plastic or ovarian (wedge) procedure for infertility.

(c) An integral part of the procedure is tubal perfusion of indigo-carmine dye (chromotubation) under direct vision through the endoscope. Unlike the Rubin test or salpingography, this clarifies whether dye is passing through freely or whether there is phimosis, agglutination, occlusion, or adhesions. Moreover, in an operating-room setting, much more pressure can be exerted, which may be therapeutic in overcoming lesser degrees of phimosis and agglutination.

(2) CONTRAINDICATIONS TO CULDOSCOPY

(a) Fixed retroverted uterus or other mass in the cul-de-sac

(b) Acute pelvic infection

(c) Orthopaedic or other disorder that precludes placing the patient in the knee-chest position

(3) TECHNIQUE OF CULDOSCOPY

(a) Best performed in a hospital operating room

(b) Preoperative Preparation. Low enema the night prior to surgery and perineal prep only. Benadryl 50 mg. I.M., 1 hour before surgery.

(c) Proper placement in the knee-chest position is of paramount importance for satisfactory examination. Padded shoulder braces should be used to prevent movement.

(d) Sterile technique is used throughout.

(e) The following combination has been found most satisfactory in the prevention of discomfort: (a) local infiltration of the uterosacral ligaments with 2 ml. of 1-per-cent lidocaine without adrenalin on each side; (b) Demerol 50 mg. to 100 mg. and diazepam (Valium) 2.5 to 5 mg. given intravenously, very slowly. The dosages should be individualized according to the amount of patient anxiety.

(f) The actual technique of cul-de-sac puncture and visualization cannot be learned by description but should be taught in the operating room. A cervical cannula is also positioned in order to instill dilute indigo-carmine dye under direct vision. This is an integral part of the procedure.

(g) A fractional D and C is easily performed at the end of the procedure without requiring any change in the patient's position. This will rule out cervical or uterine pathology.

(h) After culdoscopy, it is important, for later comfort, to expel the air that has entered the abdomen by the sucking in of negative pressure. As much air as possible is expelled by abdominal pressure as the patient assumes the prone position, while the cannula is still in place. The puncture site in the cul-de-sac requires no stitches, as a rule. The patient may feel sleepy the rest of the day but is usually quite comfortable except, perhaps, in the upright position. Some shoulder pain may remain. She may have diet as tolerated, be ambulated ad lib, and go home the following morning.

(4) INDICATIONS FOR LAPAROSCOPY

(a) For infertility patients, the indications are the same as those described under culdoscopy.

(5) CONTRAINDICATIONS OF LAPAROSCOPY

(a) Previous abdominal or pelvic surgery where intestinal adhesions are suspected near the parietal peritoneum

(b) When general anesthesia is contraindicated and thus cannot supplement local if needed

(c) Extreme obesity (relative)

(6) TECHNIQUE OF LAPAROSCOPY

(a) Patient is in a modified dorsal-lithotomy position

(b) After examination under anesthesia, a fractional D and C is performed, followed by insertion of a special cannula into the cervix, which can be attached to a tenaculum already on the anterior cervical lip.

(c) Dilute, sterile indigo-carmine dye in a 20 ml. syringe is attached to the cannula for instillation during the subsequent laparoscopy. The cannula is also useful in moving the uterus into different positions.

(d) With the patient now in the supine position, the laparoscopy may now proceed. As with culdoscopy, the technique cannot be learned from description but must be carefully taught in the operating room. In this procedure, about 3 L. of suitable gas are first instilled into the abdominal cavity to distend it, then the laparoscope is thrust through the enlarged opening at the lower margin of the umbilicus.

(e) Numerous complications of laparoscopy have been documented, often proportional to the experience of the operator. These include minor problems such as hematoma of the abdominal wall and subcutaneous emphysema (especially in obese patients) or, more serious, the perforation of a viscus or vessel. Anesthetic complications may also occur and emphasize the need for an experienced anesthetist.

d. *Comparison Between Culdoscopy and Laparoscopy*

(1) Choice is usually the operator's preference, according to his or her own experience.

(2) General visibility may be somewhat better at laparoscopy, especially a view of the cul-de-sac.

(3) The position at laparoscopy is more convenient in the event that laparotomy is to be performed immediately after the procedure.

(4) Culdoscopy has the significant advantage of no risk from general anesthesia because none is employed.

(5) The puncture site of culdoscopy (cul-de-sac) is far less risky than the abdominal puncture site at laparoscopy.

(6) In over 20,000 culdoscopic examinations reported over the past 20 years in the world literature, there have been no deaths. Even complications are rare.

e. *Hysteroscopy.* The endoscopic visualization of the uterine cavity, it has had a renewed interest in recent years.

(1) Indications for this procedure for infertility (e.g., detection of uterine polyps, submucous myomas, synechiae, and septal defects) are limited in that most of these diagnoses can easily be made with other, more familiar procedures.

(2) The procedure is not without complications for the inexperienced operator.

Endometrial Biopsy

1. Purposes

a. Provision of evidence of the occurrence of ovulation

b. Evaluation of the adequacy of endometrial maturation ("dating") in preparation for ovum implantation

c. Ruling out unsuspected endometrial pathology such as chronic endometritis or tuberculosis

2. Contraindications

a. Acute pelvic inflammatory disease

b. Possible pregnancy

3. Procedure

a. The ideal time for an endometrial biopsy is about a week after presumptive ovulation (Day 20) because this is when implantation is thought to be taking place. Large surveys have shown that the risk of interrupting a pregnancy is extremely small. If either the doctor or the patient is concerned about this, the patient can abstain or use precautions that cycle, or the biopsy may be deferred until there is a premenstrual basal-temperature drop, or even until the first day of the menstrual cycle.

b. When there is a suspected inadequate luteal phase (character of the BBT), then it is best to take it 7 to 8 days postovulatory for more precise "dating." If the histologic dating differs from the chronologic by more than 2 days, a luteal-phase defect is suggested.

c. An endometrial biopsy can be an extremely uncomfortable procedure, particularly in the nulligravida. The use of an extra-thin, malleable curette, which some instrument companies make, is appreciated by the patient.

Evaluation of Cervical Mucus

Certain physical and chemical characteristics of cervical mucus change according to the phase of the menstrual cycle, reflecting the effects of estrogen and progesterone. The endocervical glands are stimulated by estrogen and inhibited by progesterone. During ovulation, the cervical mucus becomes most favorable for sperm penetration. Under estrogenic influence the mucus changes from scant, viscous, and acidic to profuse, watery, and alkaline.

1. Parameters for the Evaluation of Cervical Mucus

a. *Spinnbarkeit or Stretchability.* At ovulation may be 10 to 15 cm. in length.

b. *Fern Phenomenon.* Under estrogenic influence, cervical mucus forms a fern pattern when allowed to dry on a slide. After ovulation, under the influence of progesterone, the fern pattern gradually disappears.

c. *Leukocytes.* Very few (0 to 4 per HPF) at ovulation time. Greater numbers at midcycle suggest endocervicitis, though they may be present in greater quantity normally at other times of the cycle.

d. *pH.* maximum alkalinity at the time of ovulation

2. Postcoital Test (Sims-Huhner test)

a. *Purpose*

It provides information regarding the quality and quantity of cervical mucus, the degree and quality of sperm penetration into the cervical canal, and (indirectly) coital technique.

b. *Timing of the Test*

(1) Ideal at ovulation time, but because this is not precisely known, especially in advance, it is best performed on alternate days during a typical ovulatory phase (e.g., days 10, 12, 14). Once the basal temperature has risen for 2 days or more, ovulation is presumed to have occurred, and there is no purpose in repeating the test. (The last drop before the sustained rise is ideal.)

(2) The optimal time interval between coitus and examination is unsettled, probably because surveys using widely varying intervals have reported comparable results. It would seem reasonable to suggest an interval within 12 hours, preferably within 6 hours. The longer interval would accommodate couples who are not "morning" people as far as intercourse is concerned, so that they may have coitus the night before.

(3) When there is a moot question as to whether the semen is being properly deposited in the vagina, the husband's semen may be artificially placed against the cervix, and the patient is asked to return in several hours for the same test.

c. *Instructions to Patient*

(1) Intercourse under normal conditions within 12 hours preceding the office visit

(2) No precoital lubricants

(3) No postcoital douching

d. *Procedure*

(1) The speculum must be dry.

(2) Samples aspirated from posterior vaginal fornix, external cervical os, mid cervical canal, and from area of internal os should be separated. The external cervix is wiped before taking the last two samples.

(3) Observer should note the volume of mucus, also color, *spinnbarkeit*, and viscosity. A portion is allowed to dry for evaluation of ferning. The remaining samples are separately examined under high dry magnification for spermatozoa and cellular content.

d. *Evaluation*

(1) It must be stressed that results are interpreted in light of (1) quality of cervical mucus, (2) sperm quality, and (3) relation to time of ovulation. If it turns out that the same test done 2 to 4 days later is closer to ovulation, then the initial findings are discarded in favor of those closest to midcycle. Thus interpretation may be retrospective.

(2) There is no unanimity of opinion regarding the minimum qualifications of a good postcoital test. However, it would be reasonable to say that if there are 5 to 20 actively motile sperm per high power field in the low- and midcanal samples (there may be fewer at the internal os level), then the result is favorable.

(3) It should be emphasized that a single observation, even at midcycle, is not necessarily conclusive; several cycles should be similarly studied to see if this is a consistent pattern (when poor). On the other hand, if the initial results are excellent, there is no purpose in repeating the test at a more favorable time of cycle because it would only be expected to be even better.

(4) The vaginal-pool sample should expectedly show only dead sperm because vaginal secretions are hostile to sperm motility. The only purpose in viewing this sample is in the event the endocervical sample shows no sperm at all. That finding would suggest extreme oligospermia (or azoospermia) or faulty coital technique.

(5) A consistently fair-to-poor result in cervical samples may be caused by (*1*) poor sperm quality (a semen analysis would clarify this), (*2*) poor quality of cervical mucus ("hostile mucus"), (*3*) poor timing of the test in relation to ovulation, (*4*) a combination of these. Poor quality of cervical mucus may be caused by (*1*) endocervicitis, or (*2*) poor estrogen production.

MANAGEMENT OF THE MALE

General Measures

1. Adequate sleep, rest, diet, and exercise
2. Avoidance of excessive use of alcohol and tobacco
3. Relief of emotional tension
4. Avoidance of regimented coitus as long as spontaneous exposures average two to three times a week
5. Weight reduction in obesity
6. Treatment of chronic illness or metabolic disorder
7. Avoidance of excessive or prolonged heat to scrotum
8. A patient with azoospermia, significant oligospermia, or poor motility should have a urological consultation. The following tests are indicated: urinary gonadotropins assay, 17-ketosteroids,

thyroid function, and testicular biopsy in certain cases. Testicular failure is suggested by high urinary gonadotropins and low 17-ketosteroids.

9. Varicocele should be excluded. In subnormal specimens, varicocelectomy is particularly helpful in improving motility and reducing immature and tapering sperm forms. Some studies report a 75-per-cent-improvement rate and a pregnancy rate of 45 per cent. Careful selection of patient is stressed.

10. A patient with abnormal external genitals or poorly developed secondary sex characteristics warrants chromosomal study to rule out Klinefelter's syndrome (seminiferous tubule dysgenesis). Eunuchoidism, gynecomastia, and elevated urinary gonadotropins are variable findings with this syndrome. The cardinal finding is the characteristic histology, showing hyalinization of the seminiferous tubules and Leydig-cell clumping.

Treatment of Azoospermia

1. A patient with azoospermia but with normal-appearing testes and normal spermatogenesis on testicular biopsy may have an obstruction of the distal epididymis or proximal vas deferens. Vasoepididymostomy may be considered.

2. Consideration of artifical insemination with donor semen (therapeutic donor insemination, A.I.D.)

Treatment of Oligospermia

1. With *demonstrable* thyroid deficiency, the use of triiodothyronine (Cytomel) is justified. Too often, thyroid therapy is given on a purely empirical basis and has not been documented to be of value.

2. The use of clomiphene citrate (Clomid) for oligospermia has been generally disappointing, some showing an early increase in sperm count followed by a decline during continuation of the treatment. Actually, the use of Clomid in the oligospermic male must at present be considered experimental, as it has not yet been approved by the FDA. There are ongoing studies to determine if Clomid may be of some value in men with diminished FSH, 17-ketosteroid, or testosterone secretions.

3. Similar disappointing results have been found after the experimental use of human menopausal gonadotropin (Pergonal).

4. Injections of human chorionic gonadotropin (HCG) have been reported, in some cases, to increase sperm motility. The usual dosage is 2,500 to 3,000 I.U. given I.M. every 5 days. Some have employed HCG empirically in patients with idiopathic oligospermia and after varicocelectomy in patients who had preoperative counts below 10 million per ml. Some improvement in semen quality was noted about 3 months after completion of a series of injections of 4,000 I.U., twice weekly for 10 weeks. A more constant result was an increase of libido.

5. The so-called testosterone-rebound phenomenon has had a long and generally disappointing history and fell into disuse because some oligospermic men became permanently azoospermic as a result of therapy. In addition, methyltestosterone was shown to be hepatotoxic. However, another oral androgen, fluoxymesterone (Halotestin) has more recently been tried in doses of 10 mg., twice daily for 6 weeks, with reported improvement in sperm motility for at least a limited time after cessation of therapy. The sperm count should nevertheless be watched carefully because some patients may develop spermatogenic depression even at this dosage level.

6. Cortisone therapy has proved generally unsuccessful and should probably be reserved for suppression of the adrenal cortex in those patients with oligospermia secondary to the adrenogenital syndrome.

7. Arginine, an amino acid, has re-

ceived some attention but has been a generally ineffective approach for the treatment of poor semen quality.

8. *Split-Ejaculate Technique for Homologous Artifical Insemination (A.I.H.).* This is based on the fact that in 90 per cent of males, the first portion of the ejaculate contains at least 75 per cent of all the sperm and also those of best quality. (In 5 per cent of males, there is no difference between the first portion and the remainder of the ejaculate, and in another 5 per cent, the findings are reversed.) Utilizing this knowledge, insemination of the superior portion of the husband's ejaculate into the cervix of the wife during her most fertile day or days may be of value in cases of oligospermia, hypomotility, or in couples with repeatedly poor postcoital tests who do not respond to the usual measures. This method is the quickest way of obtaining instant improvement in sperm quality and utilizing it to advantage.

9. The technique of freezing and storing subnormal sperm, then combining several samples for insemination, has proven to be unrewarding.

MANAGEMENT OF THE FEMALE

Ovarian Factor

Major factors to be considered include ovulation defects, endometriosis, periovarian adhesions, and an inadequate luteal phase.

1. Ovulation Defects

a. General defects include: nutritional, metabolic disorders (hypopituitarism, hypothyroidism, hyperthyroidism, diabetes mellitus, adrenogenital syndrome, Cushing's disease), chronic illness, neurogenic disorders, psychogenic disorders, and specific ovarian disorders (polycystic ovarian disease, ovarian dysgenesis, ovarian tumors)

b. Because failure of ovulation (anovulation), faulty ovulation, or infrequent ovulation (oligo-ovulation) can be the result of deficiencies in other endocrine organs, the pituitary, thyroid, and adrenal glands must be investigated. Psychosomatic factors should also be considered, particularly in women who have had a normal menstrual history prior to deciding to conceive.

c. Pituitary, thyroid, and adrenal dysfunctions are treated as indicated (see Chap. 24).

d. Polycystic or sclerocystic ovaries (Stein-Leventhal Syndrome) should be treated with: Clomiphene citrate (Clomid), the nonhormonal drug of choice, starting with 5 mg. daily for 5 days, from the fifth day of the cycle. It may be necessary to gradually increase the dosage up to 200 mg. daily, but, in all instances, there should be careful monitoring by pelvic examination to make sure that overstimulation (cystic enlargement) of the ovaries does not occur. Ovulation is presumed if the basal temperature graph becomes normally biphasic, if the endometrial biopsy shows secretory endometrium, or if there is significant urinary or plasma progesterone. It is definitely confirmed if the patient becomes pregnant. If clomiphene fails in such cases, after several months of trial, then wedge resection of the ovaries may be considered, preceded by endoscopy to confirm the diagnosis of sclerocystic ovaries.

e. Patients with demonstrable pituitary-gonadotrophic (FSH) failure, normal ovaries, and no other causes for infertility may be candidates for Pergonal (human menopausal gonadotropin) in combination with HCG. With dosages and frequent monitoring carefully worked out on an individualized basis, a high percentage of patients will ovulate with such therapy. However, the medication is expensive, the incidence of multiple births can be high, and potential side effects include cystic enlargement of the ovaries including rupture, ascites, and hydrothorax. Such side effects can be minimized by careful patient selection, preliminary evaluation of ovarian function, utilization of minimal effective doses, and frequent examination of the patient during and after each cycle of treatment.

2. Endometriosis

a. The ovary is the most common site of external endometriosis.

b. Endometriosis is associated with infertility in 30 to 40 per cent of patients even when lesions are minimal with no gross anatomical changes, for reasons that are obscure.

c. The more obvious cases of infertility associated with endometriosis are caused by interference with tubo-ovarian motility and disturbance in ovum pickup, related to demonstrable adhesions around the tubes and ovaries.

d. Endometriosis should be considered in all patients with a "normal" infertility investigation. The diagnosis is confirmed by direct visual endoscopic examination.

e. The diagnosis of endometriosis is suggested in patients with menstrual irregularities, progressive dysmenorrhea, dyspareunia, fixed retroverted uterus, and nodularity of the uterosacral ligaments. However, a patient may also have a normal menstrual history and pelvic findings, yet have fairly extensive endometriosis. As stated, endoscopy is the only way to establish the diagnosis with certainty.

f. The treatment of endometriosis associated with infertility is varied and depends upon the patient's age, the extent of the disease process, and the presence and degree of other symptoms. The use of progestational steroids (e.g., Enovid-E in sufficient daily dosage to prevent menstruation and breakthrough bleeding) to induce pseudopregnancy provides good symptomatic relief and has a salutary effect upon the disease process. Instead of steroids, one may employ a mildly androgenic, newer preparation, danazol (Danocrine) daily in the same manner to induce pseudopregnancy. Since this drug, unlike the steroids, is neither estrogenic nor progestational, it has not been implicated in thromboembolic complications. Minor side effects are common, however, and the drug is expensive. Whichever drug is used, it requires many months to obtain a beneficial effect, during which time the patient, of course, remains infertile. More often, endoscopy will demonstrate tubal or peritubal problems associated with the disorder and, if all other factors are normal, laparotomy is useful not only to correct the tubal abnormalities but to excise any major implants. Some employ progestational steroids or danazol prior to such contemplated surgery, others afterward, and still others rely on surgery alone if the endometriosis is not too extensive (though its effects on the tubes may be considerable). Each patient must, therefore, be individually considered.

3. Peri-ovarian Adhesions

a. They may result from pelvic inflammatory disease, appendicitis, endometriosis, previous surgery, or from the process of monthly rupture of the ovarian follicle.

b. Peri-ovarian adhesions diminish fertility either by blocking the extrusion of the ovum or by interfering with the pickup of the ovum by the tube.

c. Such adhesions often involve the tube, uterus, lateral pelvic wall, or intestine.

d. The diagnosis is confirmed by endoscopy.

e. Treatment consists of:

(1) Lysis of adhesions

(2) Suspension of the uterus, if it is retroverted, brings the tubes and ovaries forward and may be of value in preventing new adhesions.

(3) Corticosteroids such as dexamethasone are used by some during the operation and postoperatively, in the

hope that future adhesions will be minimized.

4. Inadequate Luteal Phase

a. The condition usually results from inadequate progesterone production by the corpus luteum and has been associated with both infertility and early miscarriage.

b. In turn, it is believed to give insufficient hormonal support to the endometrium, which then cannot properly support nidation.

c. The diagnosis is suspected from studies of the basal temperature graph (short, 8- to 10-day luteal phase), endometrial biopsy (off phase, by dating), urinary or blood progesterone excretion (relatively low), and cervical mucus changes plus vaginal smears to determine whether estrogen stimulation is adequate.

d. *Treatment* of inadequate luteal phase is often difficult but essentially depends upon the specific hormone deficiency involved.

(1) General constitutional measures should not be overlooked (i.e., nutritional deficiencies, emotional tension, or metabolic disease).

(2) Low-dosage estrogen (e.g., 0.1 mg. stilbestrol or 0.02 mg. ethinyl estradiol) during the first half of the cycle is ordinarily not enough to interfere with ovulation but is aimed at maintaining a normal follicular-phase endometrium in preparation for the oncoming progestational stimulation by the corpus luteum.

(3) For progesterone deficiency, the synthetic compounds are prone to give unusual endometrial responses. Although difficult to obtain unless specially made up, pure progesterone (25 mg., vaginal suppositories) twice daily during the second half of the cycle is more physiological.

(4) Although understandably not comfortable or practical, chorionic gonadotropin (HCG) can be used to stimulate endogenous progesterone secretion from the normal corpus luteum. A dosage of 3,000 to 4,000 I.U. every third day from the twelfth (i.e., pre-ovulatory) day to the twenty-fourth day, a total of five injections, has been recommended.

Tubal Factor

1. Function of the Fallopian Tubes

a. Permit ascent of spermatozoa to site of fertilization

b. Pick up ovum and transport it to the site of fertilization

c. Nurture zygote as it is transformed into a blastocyst, during transport to the uterine cavity

2. Etiology of Abnormal Function of the Tubes

a. Alteration in ovum pickup (e.g., hydrosalpinx, fimbrial occlusion or phimosis, peritubal adhesions)

b. Damaged cilia secondary to endosalpingitis, interfering with normal ovum transport

c. Midportion or cornual occlusion of tubes secondary to inflammation or a sterilization procedure

d. Restriction of normal tubal motility (e.g., peritubal adhesions secondary to pelvic inflammatory disease, endometriosis, appendicitis, or previous pelvic surgery)

3. Classification of Tubal Pathology

a. *Peritubal Adhesions.* Related to perisalpingitis or peritonitis

b. *Fimbrial End Obstruction.* The result of endosalpingitis or perisalpingitis

c. *Middle-Third Obstruction.* Generally the result of tubal sterilization

d. *Cornual Obstruction.* This may result from salpingitis isthmica nodosa, endosalpingitis, adenomyosis, or pressure from myomata.

4. Classification of Operative Techniques

a. *Fimbriolysis.* Separation of agglutinated fimbria that are otherwise grossly fairly normal

b. *Salpingolysis.* Lysis of peritubal adhesions

c. *Salpingostomy.* The creation of a new ostium or opening

d. *Resection and anastomosis* of midtubal obstruction

e. *Tubal implantation* for cornual obstruction

5. Tubal Plastic Surgery

a. Assuming that the rest of the diagnostic infertility workup is normal, the prognosis for conception and live birth after tubal surgery will depend on the type and extent of pathology, the type of surgery performed, the skill of the surgeon, and the postoperative care.

b. The couple should be thoroughly enlightened regarding the statistical possibilities of conception following tuboplasties. The only criterion for success is term live birth. Because tuboplasty is a last-resort procedure for damaged tubes, the true success rate is not notably high—30 to 40 per cent term live births is considered acceptable, and, with some tubal disease, pregnancy rates are considerably lower. When only periadnexal adhesions are present, the rate may be as high as 60 per cent within 3 years of surgery. In general, the results with distal tubal disease are not as good because there is usually more tubal destruction; in proximal disease, the rest of the tube is often basically normal. When both proximal and distal occlusions are present in both tubes, the prognosis is so poor that tubal surgery should probably not be considered. Also, tubal surgery is generally not considered in women approaching age 40 because of the lessened fertility owing to age alone. The possibility of an ectopic pregnancy should also be mentioned.

c. In general, pregnancy rates are roughly one-half the patency rates in long-term follow-up.

d. Statistically, the peak success rate occurs relatively late—between 12 to 24 months after the surgery. The reason for this long lapse in time is not precisely known, but it is believed to represent the long healing time and recanalization apparently needed.

6. Surgical Technique

a. For simple dilatation and phimosis, the use of a pediatric (#8) Foley catheter, or the thinner Fogarty catheter may often be used to advantage by delicately swelling and deflating the inner "bolus" in order to exert equal, atraumatic pressure in all directions.

b. In those instances where the agglutinated fimbriated folds require it, a better ostium may be created by everting the tip of several folds to the serosal surface of the tube with very thin (e.g., 5-0 chromic) sutures.

c. The value of different types of prostheses has been controversial for years. Unfortunately, comparison of results has been difficult or impossible because of the variability in etiology, extent of tubal damage, and different techniques used. Many surgeons use no prostheses at all with distal disease, while others use polyethylene, Silastic, or Teflon in various shapes.

d. Microsurgery is an interesting new technique requiring elaborate, expensive apparatus and considerable experience. However, it shows promise and would be the procedure of choice, for example, in end-to-end anastomosis of tubes that have been previously ligated. (Tubes that have been sterilized by coagulation are often too damaged for salvage.) Whether or not the results with microsurgery for tubal disease in general will prove superior to conventional techniques (which often use 4–6× magnifying glasses) remains to be seen.

7. Postoperative Care

a. Because even a slight infection would probably negate the benefits of surgery, it would seem advisable to use prophylactic broad-spectrum antibiotics for about a week postoperatively.

b. There is no unanimity of opinion regarding the parenteral use of dexamethasone (Decadron), ostensibly to minimize postoperative adhesions. Some use it intraperitoneally at the conclusion of surgery, while others give it (or oral prednisone) for several days postoperatively.

c. Some utilize hydrotubation during the proliferative phase of the cycle (e.g., 30 mg. hydrocortisone sodium succinate (Solu-Cortef) and 5 mg. streptomycin sulfate, diluted with sterile saline to 15 ml. which may be followed by carbon dioxide insufflation). Others prefer to leave the tubes alone postoperatively. As stated, it is difficult to assess, not to mention compare, the results obtained by different investigators because of the general lack of meaningful classification of procedures relative to the precise pathology present.

d. Whether or not postoperative hydrotubations are done, it is common to perform a hysterosalpingogram about 3 to 6 months following surgery if pregnancy has not intervened.

8. New Research. An entirely new approach for women with hopelessly damaged tubes is the much publicized in vitro fertilization and reimplantation technique of Drs. Steptoe and Edwards in England. It is to be hoped that further work along these lines will enable women with very serious problems to become pregnant.

Uterine Factor (Corpus)

1. Leiomyomata Uteri

a. Most uterine fibroids do not prevent conception.

b. Although the spontaneous miscarriage rate is higher in women with myomata, it is difficult to prove a cause-and-effect relationship.

c. Submucous fibroids, diagnosed by hysterography or hysteroscopy, may interfere with implantation or may cause cornual occlusion.

d. If a thorough investigation reveals no other cause for the infertility, and if the myomata are of sufficient size and strategically located (submucous or cornual), myomectomy may be considered.

e. Postoperatively, contraception is advisable for at least 3 months to allow for complete healing.

f. If the endometrial cavity was entered during the operative procedure, subsequent pregnancy is likely to be delivered by elective cesarean section.

2. Retroversion

a. A movable retroversion is common, and does not have a causative role per se in infertility.

b. A fixed retroversion is often associated with infertility, not from the position of the uterus but from the underlying cause of the fixation (e.g., pelvic inflammatory disease or endometriosis).

c. A fixed retroversion noted at laparotomy for pathology of the corpus, tubes, or ovaries in an infertile patient may be treated by uterine suspension. This minimizes further peri-adnexal adhesions and permits the uterus to rise out of the pelvis should pregnancy occur.

3. Anomalies

a. Uterine anomalies are related to varying degrees of failure of fusion of the Müllerian ducts.

b. The three most common anomalies are uterus didelphys, bicornuate uterus, and septate uterus (not to be confused with a slight arcuate tendency, which is common).

c. It is the septate type that is most often associated with secondary infertility. Primary infertility is rarely associated with uterine anomalies.

d. Even if there is a history of repeated miscarriages or premature births with a uterine anomaly present, it is still important to rule out metabolic, endocrine, and genetic causes before attempting surgical reconstruction.

e. The diagnosis is generally made on hysterography, using both lateral and oblique views while pulling down on the cervix.

f. As stated, it is the septate uterus

that is usually associated with secondary infertility. With this anomaly, bimanual examination reveals one uterus, while the radiograph shows two cavities.

g. The three procedures used for septate uterus are wedge excision of the septum, a vertical incision without removal of the septum, and the classical Strassman operation, which fuses the two halves.

h. A high percentage of patients who undergo a unification operation carry subsequent pregnancies to term.

4. Traumatic Intrauterine Synechiae (Asherman Syndrome)

a. A significant number of these cases are probably undiagnosed.

b. Synechiae may occur in the corpus alone, in the cervix, or in both.

c. They are usually related to postpartum or postabortal curettage.

d. *Symptoms*. Amenorrhea or hypomenorrhea, dysmenorrhea, infertility, or habitual abortion

e. *Diagnosis*. By hysterography, probing the cervix or corpus, or by hysteroscopy (direct visualization)

f. *Treatment*

(1) *Cervical or isthmic synechiae* sometimes respond to gentle, gradual dilatation of the cervix.

(2) *Uterine (corpus) synechiae* can be gently lysed with thin sounds, preferably under hysteroscopic visualization during the proliferative phase.

(3) *Postoperative Treatment*. Antibiotics and an intrauterine device such as a tipless, inflated Foley catheter, which projects slightly into the vagina, is advisable for 1 or 2 weeks. Postoperative administration of estrogen for the same length of time will help to proliferate the endometrium. The use of progesterone cyclically will help shed the endometrium at intervals.

(4) *Prognosis*. Most reported series give a generally unfavorable prognosis regarding term pregnancy. Repeated surgery is often required. The prognosis is particularly poor when intrauterine synechiae are associated with amenorrhea from destruction of the endometrium.

5. Endometrial Polyps, Hyperplasia. The diagnosis of endometrial polyps can be made on hysterography or hysteroscopy. Treatment is by uterine curettage, particularly with the use of polyp forceps, or by direct removal during hysteroscopy. Hyperplasia is generally the result of unopposed estrogen stimulation, as with anovulation, and treatment is directed to correcting the cause.

Cervical Factor

The problems to be considered are (1) failure in sperm deposition or ascent, (2) poor or hostile cervical mucus, and (3) local cervical pathology.

1. Improvement in Coital Techniques. In history taking, inquiry should be made regarding coital techniques. It is surprising how many women will jump up immediately after intercourse and even douche. While this may not totally prevent conception, it is at least a deterrent that the couple may be unaware of. Others use large amounts of lubricating jelly, which can act as a sperm barrier.

2. Poor or hostile cervical mucus may be caused by:

a. Endocervicitis from inflammation, with destruction of endocervical glands and resultant alteration in mucus quality

b. Inadequate estrogenic stimulation of the cervical glands. This may also be combined with endocervicitis.

c. Immunological problems: reaction of sperm antigen with antibody in the cervical mucus or in the serum

3. Treatment of These Conditions

a. Endocervicitis may be treated with antibiotics, electrocautery (gentle), or cryosurgery. When the condition is chronic and does not respond well to therapeutic measures, the area may be "bypassed" by artificial insemination with the husband's semen to the level of the internal os (A.I.H.).

b. Inadequate estrogenic stimulation is often remedied by administering small doses of estrogen (e.g., stilbestrol, 0.1 mg., or ethinyl estradiol, 0.02 mg. daily) for the first 2 weeks of the menstrual cycle. This dose does not generally interfere with ovulation, but, if there is a tendency for it to inhibit ovulation, the dose may be further reduced (e.g., every other day, or by restricting medication to days five to twelve). If endocervicitis is also present, local antibiotic therapy may be given as well, and there is often a marked improvement in the postcoital test following a few cycles of such measures.

c. Although many studies and reports have appeared for more than a decade, the basic question of whether circulating antibodies in the female interfere with or prevent conception remains unanswered. Because of inconclusive results and different interpretations, the role of immunology in infertility remains controversial. The common test employed is the sperm agglutination test, which relates the husband's sperm against the wife's serum. If such a test is strongly positive (in the absence of other causes for infertility), the recommended treatment is the use of a condom for about 6 months to prevent sperm contact. This also necessitates avoiding semen exposure through oral-genital or anal contact. When repeat agglutinating antibody reaction disappears or becomes minimal, the couple is permitted unprotected intercourse around the time of ovulation, to minimize overall exposure. Because pregnancies have been reported following such a regime, it is worth trying. It should be added that there is ongoing research in the field that may eventually clarify this vexing problem, as well as sperm *immobilizing* antibodies in men, for which there is no specific treatment at present.

4. Local Cervical Pathology

a. *Endocervical polyps* should be twisted off or excised, and the base lightly cauterized to minimize regrowth. Sometimes a prolapsed endometrial polyp (or even submucous myoma) is mistaken for an endocervical polyp. Thus, when the polyp is large, with a broad base, the extent of which cannot be easily determined at office examination, excision is best performed in the hospital. However, the common variety of small endocervical polyp is easily removed in the office and is almost invariably benign.

b. *Cervical stenosis,* whether congenital (rare) or after overly vigorous cauterizations or frequent cervical infections, is suspected when there is an inability to pass a small probe (e.g., when attempting to do an endometrial biopsy). Treatment is by gentle, careful sounding, beginning with very thin (2 mm.) graduated sounds. Paracervical infiltration with 1-per-cent lidocaine is often helpful to facilitate dilatation as well as reduce discomfort. One should be mindful that with an acute flexion of the uterus, the internal os may normally be difficult to bypass unless there is strong traction on the tenaculum to straighten the uterus. In rare instances, when the stenosis does not respond to any of the above procedures or maneuvers, dilatation may have to be done under anesthesia in the operating room.

c. *Cervical erosions* (often eversions) are not generally associated with infertility; in any event, the postcoital test will clarify. If there is interference, it is more likely the result of the associated endocervicitis. As mentioned under that heading, the treatment of endocervicitis must be most gentle in order not to destroy or scar the canal. Electrocautery, for example, should be done only in stages at intervals of 4 to 8 weeks, using a nasal-tip cautery in one or two areas only. This permits normal endocervical tissue to grow in gradually and does not compromise the whole canal.

d. *Hypoestrinism and synechiae* have been discussed on pages 17 and 18.

e. *Incompetent Cervix.* The typical history is that of repeated, painless abortions during the second trimester, usually preceded by bulging amniotic membranes. Diagnosis in the nonpregnant state is suggested by the ability to pass a #9 Hegar dilator easily through the internal os. Hysterography, which should be performed during the secretory phase (when the cervical canal width is smallest), may also be suggestive if the isthmic width is 8 mm. or more. Whenever incompetent cervix is suspected, weekly bimanual examinations are performed to note if there is any gradual dilatation of the internal cervical os. In carefully selected cases, once the diagnosis is made, and there are signs of cervical widening during pregnancy, operative cerclage of the internal os by one of several methods has been successfully employed.

2. Maternal Adaptations To Pregnancy

David H. Fields, M.D.

BASIC PRINCIPLES

1. Pregnancy results in great changes in the functions of most of the body's organ systems.

2. These changes are manifested as alterations in normal values of both physical examination and laboratory testing, and result in maternal symptoms which would be considered pathologic outside of pregnancy. See Table 2-1.

The normal ranges for many laboratory values are altered by pregnancy. Below is a list of the most commonly used tests, how they are altered by pregnancy, and why, if it is known.

3. These changes are caused by

a. Alterations in maternal endocrine function

b. Superimposition of fetal and placental endocrine function

c. Fetal metabolic and physical demands

So that the physican may properly evaluate maternal complaints and phys-

Table 2-1. **Laboratory Interpretation**

Test	*Alteration in Limits of Normal*	*Mechanism*
Hematology		
Hemoglobin	Decreased to 10 g./100 ml.	Hemodilution secondary to increased blood volume
Hematocrit	Decreased to 30%	
WBC count	Increased up to 15,000/cu. mm.	? Increased corticosteroids
Erythrocyte sedimentation rate	Increased up to 40 mm./hr.	Increased fibrinogen; hemodilution
Blood Chemistry		
Potassium	Decreased to 3 mEq./L.	Respiratory alkalosis
Sodium, Chloride	No change	———
BUN	Decreased to 5–10 mg./100 ml.	Increased GFR; hemodilution
Creatinine	Decreased to 0.3–0.8 mg./100 ml.	Increased GFR; hemodilution
Creatinine clearance	Increased to 150 ml./min.	Increased GFR; hemodilution
Albumin	Decreased to 2.5–3.0 g./100 ml.	
Fasting blood sugar	Upper limit decreased to 90 mg./100 ml.	Increased insulin
2-hr. postprandial sugar	Upper limit increased to 145 mg./100 ml.	HPL, estrogen
Alkaline phosphatase	Increased up to twice normal	Placental production
T_4	Increased up to 16 g./100 ml.	Estrogen effect causing increased thyroid-binding globulin
T_3 resin uptake	Decreased up to 30%	
Thyroid-binding globulin	Increased up to 30%	
Free thyroxine	No change	
Free thyroxine index	No change	

ical and laboratory data during pregnancy, these changes will be reviewed system by system.

GENITAL SYSTEM

The female reproductive tract is the most intimately involved with pregnancy, and the changes it undergoes are most familiar to physicans and patient alike. Therefore, patient complaints referable to these organs are usually ascribed to pregnancy rather than disease, and rightly so.

Uterus

1. The uterus enlarges almost 1,000 times in volume and 30 times in weight, to a 1-Kg. organ with a capacity of approximately 5 L. It enlarges steadily throughout pregnancy to occupy most of the abdominal cavity. The pressure it exerts is responsible for changes in the gastrointestinal, respiratory, cardiovascular, and urinary systems (see specific areas).

2. The blood flow to the uterus increases 60 times, to approximately 600 ml. per minute (about 10 per cent of cardiac output) at term, and is accomodated by huge increases in the size of the uterine and ovarian vessels.

Vagina and Cervix

Many pregnant women experience a large increase in vaginal discharge usually secondary to increased cervical secretion caused by high estrogen levels. Unless a specific pathogen (Trichomonas vaginalis, Candida albicans, Hemophilus vaginalis) can be identified, treatment is usually unrewarding and unnecessary.

Ovaries

The corpus luteum usually begins to regress by the eighth week of pregnancy, and the ovaries become largely inactive because placental estrogen and progesterone production inhibits pituitary gonadotropins. Any ovarian cyst which persists into the second trimester should be treated surgically (see ovarian tumors).

Any ovarian cyst discovered at cesarean section should be resected and treated appropriately. Frequently the ovaries at term will be covered with a pink frothy material which is decidual reaction secondary to high progesterone levels. This is not pathological and may cover the tubes as well.

Breasts

1. Both acinar and ductal breast growth are greatly accelerated by steadily increasing production of estrogen, progesterone, and prolactin throughout pregnancy. Because of the rapid growth in size, the overlying skin may develop striae. In addition, the areola (like all pigmented skin in pregnancy) becomes darker and the nipple itself increases in erectile capacity.

2. In spite of the very high prolactin levels near term, lactation does not occur until after delivery, most likely because placental progesterone prevents prolactin from stimulating the production of lactalbumin.

ENDOCRINE SYSTEM

The hormonal changes associated with pregnancy are attributable to the production of huge amounts of placental estrogen and progesterone, as well as other placental hormones. In addition, the fetus contributes several hormones to the maternal circulation. Finally, the maternal endocrine system responds to the placental and fetal systems by altering its hormonal output.

Placental Hormones

All are thought to be made by the syntrophoblast.

1. Estrogen. Placental estrogen production increases steadily throughout pregnancy, so that at term, maternal estrogen levels are 100 times nonpregnant values. Most of this is estriol; however estradiol levels themselves are also increased 10 times. These high estrogen levels have far-reaching effects (see below).

2. Progesterone. The placenta produces even more progesterone than estrogen, so that near term, it is producing approximately 250 mg. daily. One major maternal effect of this is a generalized decrease in smooth muscle tone and a natiuretic, diuretic effect (see below).

3. Human Chorionic Gonadotropin. This is detectable in maternal serum several days after conception. Its measurement is the basis of all pregnancy tests. Peaking at about 60 days of gestation, its major function seems to be maintenance of the corpus luteum, although it may also play a role in placental immunology.

4. Human Placental Lactogen (Placental Growth Hormone, Human Chorionic Somatomammotropin, HPL). This also steadily increases throughout pregnancy so that daily production near term may be as much as 2 g. HPL's major effects seem to be like those of growth hormone. It also, via its diabetogenic effects, leads to compensatory increase in maternal insulin levels.

Maternal Hormones

1. Pituitary. The gland itself enlarges significantly during pregnancy (rarely enough to cause symptoms), mostly because increased estrogen levels stimulate increased production of prolactin by acidophilic cells.

a. *Gonadotropins.* Follicle-stimulating hormone and luteinizing hormone are maintained at very low levels throughout pregnancy by negative feedback of placental estrogen and progesterone.

b. *Prolactin (see above).* Produced in increasingly large amounts throughout pregnancy, secondary to high estrogen levels, it causes increased breast growth. Lactation is blocked by progesterone until after placental expulsion.

c. *Somatotrophic Hormone (Growth Hormone).* Present at very low levels throughout pregnancy, it probably is suppressed by very high levels of its placental counterpart, HPL.

d. *Thyroid-stimulating hormone, adrenocorticotrophic hormone* and *melanocyte-stimulating hormone* are largely unaffected by pregnancy.

2. Thyroid Hormone. The gland hypertrophies significantly during pregnancy. Although production of thyroxin (T_4) is increased, free T_4 levels are essentially unchanged. This is because there is an increase in thyroid-binding globulin prompted by high estrogen levels.

3. Adrenal Hormones

a. There is a large increase in bound cortisol secondary to an increase in estrogen-mediated levels of transcortin, the cortisol-binding hormone. Free cortisol may be slightly increased.

b. Aldosterone, renin, and angiotensin tend to increase intravascular volume. These are all increased in normal pregancy, although angiotensin sensitivity (vasospasm) is decreased. Increase is probably secondary to the natiuretic effect of the large amounts of progesterone produced, and to the relative lack of vascular reactivity to angiotensin.

4. Insulin. The beta cells of the Islets of Langerhans undergo significant hypertrophy and insulin levels are increased in pregnancy, both fasting and non-fasting. Many of the hormones of pregnancy, including estrogen, progesterone, and human placental lactogen, tend to increase insulin needs.

5. Parathormone. Although there may be some increase in the size of the parathyroid glands, their function seems to be largely unchanged during pregnancy.

CARDIOVASCULAR SYSTEM

Many physiologic effects of pregnancy duplicate otherwise pathological conditions. Basic to the cardiovascular changes are an increase in circulating blood volume by up to 50 per cent and in cardiac output by 30 to 40 per cent. In addition, in the second half of pregnancy, the large uterus serves as a functional obstruction to venous return. The following complaints and abnormal physical findings simulating heart disease may occur:

Complaints

1. Dyspnea, either at rest or on exertion, is probably secondary to the hyperventilatory drive of progesterone, or perhaps secondary to the large uterus raising the diaphragm
2. Palpitations, etiology unknown
3. Orthopnea, secondary to large intra-abdominal mass
4. Orthostatic hypotension, secondary vascular pooling

Abnormal Physical Findings

1. Heart rate increase of 10 beats per minute
2. PMI of heart pushed laterally by the growing uterus
3. Apparent increase in cardiothoracic ratio on radiograph to more than one-half
4. Systolic murmurs secondary to increased cardiac output are found in almost all pregnant women
5. Diastolic murmurs, evanescent, usually pathologic
6. Third-heart sound, etiology unknown
7. Lower extremity edema, secondary to partial venous obstruction by a large uterus
8. Lower-extremity and trunk varicosities, secondary to increased venous pressure

RESPIRATORY SYSTEM

The major respiratory changes are an increased tidal volume and minute ventilation (secondary to progesterone drive and metabolic demand) in the face of decreased diaphragmatic excursion (secondary to the enlarging uterus). Dyspnea is a very common complaint and may be due to the slight respiratory alkalosis induced by high levels of progesterone.

URINARY SYSTEM

Renal

1. The glomerular filtration rate (GFR) and renal plasma flow (RPF) are increased up to 50 per cent, secondary to increased cardiac output.
2. Mild hydronephrosis and hydroureter occur (right more than left), most likely secondary to decreased muscle tone and pressure from the enlarging uterus.

Bladder

1. Urinary frequency secondary to stretching by the enlarged uterus
2. Stress incontinence in the second half of pregnancy is secondary to changes in the urethro-vesicle angle when the bladder is pulled up to become an intra-abdominal organ.

GASTROINTESTINAL SYSTEM

Most of the gastrointestinal changes are secondary to the effect of an enlarging intra-abdominal mass (uterus).

1. Heartburn and Belching. Secondary to changes in position of the stomach and reflux of stomach acid into the lower esophagus. Stomach acid production in fact decreases and ulcers are less common.

2. Nausea and Vomiting of the First Trimester. Probably secondary to human chorionic gonadotropin

3. Ptyalism. The cause of excess salivation is controversial and may be a failure to swallow rather than excess production.

4. Pica. Although abnormal cravings in diet may be signs of nutritional failure, some feel they are more likely cultural aspects of pregnancy.

5. Hemorrhoids. Secondary to increased venous pressure in the lower body secondary to the pressure of the uterus on the vena cava.

6. Constipation. Frequent and may be due to increased progesterone levels resulting in decreased gastrointestinal motility.

SKELETAL SYSTEM

1. The enlarging uterus increases the normal lordosis and probably contributes to frequent backaches.

2. Demineralization of the bones (but not the teeth) may occur in severely calcium-deficient women.

3. The joints, especially of the pelvis, may become more mobile and slight pubic separation may occur.

3. Ectopic Pregnancy

Hugh R. K. Barber, M.D.

DEFINITION

1. Ectopic pregnancy is one in which the products of conception are developing outside the uterus. By far the commonest site is the fallopian tube.

2. Combined heterotopic pregnancy is characterized by the existence of simultaneous intrauterine and extrauterine pregnancies.

3. Cornual pregnancy is gestation that has developed in a rudimentary horn of the uterus (rudimentary horn pregnancy).

BASIC PRINCIPLES

1. Ectopic pregnancy is second only to toxemias of pregnancy as a cause of maternal death. In view of the role of ectopic pregnancy as a cause of maternal death (6 per cent), there is no substitute for awareness of the possibility of ectopic pregnancy.

2. Any woman of childbearing age, with an acute abdominal pain or with anemia out of proportion to external blood loss, should be considered to have an ectopic until it is ruled out.

3. It is better to operate and be wrong in the diagnosis of ectopic pregnancy than to lose a patient by not operating.

4. Laparoscopic examination is very helpful in making the diagnosis.

5. Primary ectopics: when the process continues at the site of original nidation.

6. Secondary ectopics: when the initial nidation is changed either by rupture or by continued development at a secondary site in the abdomen.

7. Ectopic pregnancies are manifested in two forms:

a. Acute: intraperitoneal hemorrhage, acute pain, and shock.

b. Chronic: obscure symptomatology, less pain, and absence of shock.

8. Ectopic implantation must be regarded as fortuitous; but there are some recognized predisposing factors:

a. Preceding tumor or pelvic inflammation with residual chronic infection and distortion by adhesions.

b. Migration of ovum across the pelvic cavity to the fallopian tube on the side opposite to the follicle from which ovulation occurred.

c. Congenital abnormality of the tube such as hypoplasia, elongation, diverticula. Diverticula are occasionally seen and, in theory, present a cul-de-sac in which the ovum may lodge.

9. The rising ratio of extrauterine to intrauterine pregnancies is traceable to changing mores of sexually active young people, the rising incidence of venereal disease, and the effectiveness of modern antibiotic therapy in preventing total tubal occlusion after salpingitis.

10. The increasing use of the IUD has had a remarkable influence on the oc-

Relative Incidence of Tubal Ectopic Pregnancies

Ampullar	42 per cent
Isthmic	28 per cent
Interstitial	13 per cent
Fimbrial	7 per cent
Ovarian	less than 1 per cent
Cervical Peritoneal	Very rare

currence of extrauterine pregnancies. There are reports showing that when extrauterine pregnancy occurs in the IUD users, a high percentage are ovarian ectopics. It seems clear that the IUD affords good protection from intrauterine implanation but has little effect on the occurrence of extrauterine pregnancies. Consequently, the ratio of extrauterine to intrauterine pregnancy is destined to increase with increased use of an IUD.

11. Among patients taking progesterone-only oral contraceptives, studies in this country and abroad show a proportionately high incidence of ectopic pregnancies (4.1 per cent).

12. Induced abortion appears to be associated with an increased risk of ectopic pregnancy. The mechanism of this complication seems quite clear: subclinical endometritis associated with induced abortion produces secondary perisalpingitis and peritubal adhesions leading to partial oviduct obstruction. Because there is no decidual membrane in tubal mucosa, and no submucosa, the ovum rapidly burrows through the mucosa and embeds in the muscular wall of the tube, opening up maternal blood vessels and causing necrosis and the proliferation of connective tissue.

13. The uterus may enlarge in the first 3 months of an ectopic pregnancy. The uterine decidua grows abundantly and when the ovum or embryo dies, bleeding occurs as the decidua degenerates. Rarely it is expelled entirely as a decidua cast, and it is replaced within a few weeks (perhaps before clinical diagnosis) by normal endometrium.

14. Arias-Stella reaction is an atypical glandular proliferation of the endometrium associated with ectopic pregnancy. A decidual cast containing no villi may be expelled.

15. Signs and symptoms include amenorrhea, pain, and vaginal bleeding which may present as spotting. The urge to have a bowel movement, and fainting in the bathroom ("bathroom sign") are almost diagnostic of ectopic pregnancy. Unfortunately, these signs and symptoms are often obscure and a high degree of suspicion is required in their evaluation.

16. The differential diagnosis must include salpingitis, abortion, appendicitis, torsion of pedicle of ovarian cyst, rupture of corpus luteum or follicular cyst, lateral displacement of a gravid uterus.

17. The diagnostic measures include a careful history and physical examination. A thorough abdominal examination as well as pelvic and rectal examinations must be carried out. In addition: immunologic and biologic pregnancy tests, culdocentesis, colpotomy, culdoscopy, laparoscopy, and ultrasonography.

18. There is no substitute for the carefully elicited history and the physical examination followed by surgical abdominal exploration if suspicion is high. Always take a careful history and always think of ectopic pregnancy!

19. Bolt's sign is characterized by severe tenderness when the examiner lifts the uterine cervix. It is a sign associated with ruptured tubal pregnancy.

ECTOPIC TUBAL PREGNANCY

Basic Principles

Ectopic tubal pregnancy is a difficult diagnosis to make. Few present with the classical signs and symptoms. It should always be considered as a possibility in patients with salpingitis, threatened abortion, appendicitis, torsion of ovarian cyst or rupture of corpus luteum or follicular cyst, infertility of 3 or more years, and a history of previous ectopic pregnancies. The tubes should be carefully examined when any cyst is excised from the ovary. The three most common signs and symptoms are: abdominal pain, vaginal bleeding or spotting, and amenorrhea.

Ampullar Pregnancy

1. Ampullar pregnancy is an ectopic pregnancy in the ampullar portion of the fallopian tube. It is the commonest site of implantation.

2. It generally ends in tubal abortion if it is within 1 cm. from the fimbriated end of the tube. There is a trickle of bleeding into the peritoneal cavity, and this may collect as a clot in the pouch of Douglas. It is then called a hematocele.

3. These ectopics may be situated 1 to 4 cm. from the fimbriated end of the tube and rupture in 8 to 12 weeks. This may occur spontaneously or from pressure (such as straining at stool, coitus, or pelvic examination) and occurs at about 8 to 12 weeks. Hemorrhage may be severe.

4. Sometimes rupture is retroperitoneal between the leaves of the broad ligament—broad ligament hematoma. Hemorrhage in this site is more likely to be controlled.

Isthmic Pregnancy

1. Isthmic pregnancy is an ectopic gestation in the narrow portion of the tube. It follows the ampullary ectopics as the next most common ectopic. It occurs in the middle-third of the tube.

2. Rupture usually occurs at 8 weeks and the hemorrhage is severe and often accompanied by shock. It is rarely diagnosed prior to rupture.

Interstitial Pregnancy

1. Interstitial pregnancy is a pregnancy in the interstitial portion of the fallopian tube (angular pregnancy, tubouterine pregnancy) and lies within the uterus and is 1 to 3 cm. in length.

2. It is rare but very dangerous because it ends in rupture of the uterine muscle with severe hemorrhage. It may rupture into the peritoneal cavity or into the upper part of the uterus.

Management

1. The cardinal principle in the management of ectopic pregnancy is to institute treatment immediately after the diagnosis is made or suspected.

2. Examination under anesthesia and D and C, if uterine bleeding is heavy and intrauterine pregnancy has not been ruled out.

3. Laparoscopic examination has been a major advance in early diagnosis in patients with suspected unruptured ectopic pregnancy.

4. Culdoscopy or colpotomy if the patient is not in shock and the diagnosis is obscure

5. Laparotomy. The basic treatment is salpingectomy, but if the other tube is compromised and the affected tube salvageable, salpingostomy may be attempted.

Preoperative Orders

1. Nothing per os, no catharsis or enemas
2. CBC, hematocrit every 4 hours, erythrocyte sedimentation rate, urinalysis, blood volume
3. Type and crossmatch 1,500 ml. of whole blood.
4. Complete bed rest
5. Radioreceptor assay test
6. Infusion 1,000 ml. with 5-per-cent glucose and water. Use a large No. 16 or No. 18 needle.
7. If the vein is not available, do an immediate cutdown.
8. If shock is present, treat it but do not delay surgery.
9. Check vital signs every 15 minutes.
10. Notify the O.R. staff and anesthetist as soon as the diagnosis is suspected.
11. Culdocentesis
12. Abdominal and perineal preparation
13. Preoperative medication: Demerol, 50 mg. and atropine, 0.4 mg. This is given one-half hour before surgery.

Postoperative Orders

1. Nothing per os until bowel sounds indicate normal peristalsis beyond 24 hours of the operation
2. Fluid balance sheet (measure of fluid intake and output and record)
3. Replacement of blood loss
4. Hematocrit 12, 24, and 48 hours postoperative
5. Replacement of fluids and electrolytes as indicated
6. Vital signs every 30 minutes for 6 hours
7. Monitoring of primary urinary output on an hourly basis. An output of 40 ml. per hour indicates adequate tissue perfusion.
8. Demerol, 75 mg., every 3 hours p.r.n. for pain
9. Seconal, 100 mg., I.M. every hour of sleep p.r.n. for sleep
10. Compazine, 10 mg., I.M. every 6 hours p.r.n. for nausea

ECTOPIC OVARIAN PREGNANCY

Basic Principles

1. Primary ovarian pregnancy is a rare form of ectopic pregnancy in which impregnation of the ovum by the speratozoon occurs before the former is extruded from the ovary.
2. The association of IUD and ovarian pregnancy has been reported several times.
3. Ovarian pregnancy is probably not an uncommon entity as previously reported. It may be overlooked clinically in unexplained cases of hematoperitoneum or because it is of too little interest to warrant publication.
4. These pregnancies frequently rupture before the end of the third month and almost never reach viability.
5. Their preoperative diagnosis is impossible because the clinical signs and symptoms are the same as those of tubal pregnancy.
6. At operation ovarian pregnancy resembles a ruptured ovarian cyst, and diagnosis is made on histological examination if placental and fetal elements cannot be identified.
7. For a valid diagnosis of this rare form of ectopic pregnancy the postulates of Spiegelberg are mandatory:
   a. The tube, including the fimbria, must be intact, and clearly separate from the ovary.
   b. The gestation sac must occupy the normal position of the ovary.
   c. The sac must be connected to the uterus by the ovarian ligament.
   d. Ovarian tissue should be demonstrable in the walls of the sac.
8. Ovarian pregnancies may become abdominal pregnancies if the fetus survives and reimplants after rupture.
9. Secondary ovarian pregnancy is a rare form of ectopic pregnancy in which the blastocyst implants on the surface of the ovary.

Management

Depends on how much ovary is destroyed, the number of children the patient has, and her age.

ECTOPIC CERVICAL PREGNANCY

Cervical pregnancy is gestation that develops when the fertilized ovum becomes implanted in the cervical canal of the uterus.

Basic Principles

1. Are extremely rare. The responsible physician usually does not entertain the diagnosis because it is so rare.
2. The bleeding is profuse and the patients usually go into shock.
3. Usually the physician makes a diagnosis of incomplete abortion. When an attempt is made to remove the products of conception that present at the os, the bleeding becomes profuse.

Criteria for Diagnosis

1. There must be cervical glands opposite placental attachment.
2. The attachment of the placenta to the cervix must be intimate.
3. Fetal elements are not recovered from the corpus of the uterus.
4. The whole placenta is implanted below the internal os of the cervix.
5. Cervical pregnancy should be suspected in patients with first trimester painless vaginal bleeding with a large ballooning cystic-like cervix that feels flush with the vault and has a firm uterus sitting on top.
6. Early abortion fortunately is the rule, but occasionally cervical pregnancies continue for more than 16 weeks.
7. These patients have profuse hemorrhage and shock and hemostasis is a problem.

Management

1. Finger curettage and tight cervical packing is the preferred mode of treatment.
2. If the therapy proves inadequate, ligation of the descending cervical branches of the uterine artery may be indicated.
3. If bleeding cannot be controlled, a total hysterectomy may be necessary.
4. Delayed hemorrhage may occur as late as 6 weeks after evacuation of the cervical pregnancy.
5. The preoperative and postoperative orders are the same as those for tubal pregnancy.

ABDOMINAL PREGNANCY

Abdominal pregnancy is gestation occurring within the peritoneal cavity (intraperitoneal pregnancy).

Primary Abdominal Pregnancy

Is growth of the fetus and placenta within the peritoneal cavity. Fertilization and embryonic growth occur before entrance into the fallopian tube. It is a rare condition.

Secondary Abdominal Pregnancy

Is a pregnancy that develops in the abdominal cavity following tubal abortion or rupture. The fetus may continue to grow until term or become macerated, skeletonized, or mummified.

Basic principles

1. Unlike other ectopic pregnancies, frequently approach term.
2. Abdominal pregnancy is very rare.
3. Most abdominal pregnancies begin initially as ectopic tubal pregnancies that are expelled from the tube and implant elsewhere in the pelvis; or implantation occurs primarily in the peritoneum.
4. The ovum may be expelled intra- or retroperitoneally. The trophoblast develops its connection with the nearest blood supply (usually on the broad ligament and back of the uterus); and/or in the retroperitoneal situation, the proximity of great vessels will increase the risk of hemorrhage.
5. For the first 6 weeks the history is similar to that of tubal ectopic pregnancy, but after a few months gastrointestinal and genitourinary symptoms develop.

Clinical Features

1. There is a history of threatened abortion with irregular bleeding.
2. Continued abdominal discomfort is felt and fetal movements are painful.
3. Fetal abnormality is common and fetal mortality is high. Fetal death may be followed by suppuration with abscess pointing into bowel or bladder, by calcification and lithopedion formation.
4. The suggestive symptoms and signs are the following:
   a. Painful fetal movements
   b. Palpable fetal parts in the cul-de-sac

c. Absence of Braxton-Hicks contractions

d. Abnormal presentation and abdominally palpable fetal parts

e. A pelvic mass (uterus) may be felt separately from the fetal mass

5. Diagnosis is difficult; Palpation is unreliable even when fetal limbs are easily felt.

a. X-ray findings should show a fetus in an abnormal position in the abdominal cavity, absence of the uterine and placental shadows in the normal position, unusual clarity of the fetus and fetal parts, unchanged position of the fetus on serial studies, presence of pelvic or lower abdominal mass, close proximity of the fetus to the anterior abdominal wall, fetal parts that overlie the maternal vertebral column.

b. Hysterography and aortography confirm the diagnosis.

c. Serial sonographic studies may be helpful and eliminate x-ray exposure.

d. The fetus will be "small for dates."

e. Estriol excretion levels will be below normal.

Management

1. Many physicians advocate early treatment after the diagnosis is made.
2. The chief risk in continuing pregnancy is hemorrhage, and very few babies survive beyond 36 weeks because of placental insufficiency.
3. The fetus is removed, the cord is tied, and the abdomen closed.
4. No attempt is made to detach the placenta. The absence of a contractile uterus leaves no means of controlling hemorrhage.

Preoperative Orders

1. CBC and hematocrit. Urinalysis, ESR. Blood sugar, urea, and creatinine.
2. Standing and reclining, A.P. and lateral radiograph of the abdomen
3. Chest radiograph and EKG
4. Uterogram in cases in which it is indicated
5. Fetal electrocardiogram
6. Type and crossmatch 4,000 ml. of whole blood.
7. Cantor tube through the pylorus
8. Foley catheter
9. N.P.O. 12 hours preoperative
10. Intestinal preparation with Neomycin
11. Abdominal and perineal preparation
12. Infusion 1,000 ml. 5-per-cent glucose/water with a No. 18 or a No. 16 needle at two sites

Surgery

1. Great care is exercised in opening the abdomen.
2. The incision should not be made near the placenta if it can be avoided.
3. Remove the fetus gingerly and steady the insertion of the placenta.
4. Do not separate the placenta unless it is attached to an organ to which the blood supply can be controlled.
5. Do not pull on the cord.
6. Do not remove the placenta from bowel or mesentery.
7. Ligate the cord at its insertion and leave the placenta in situ.
8. Close the abdomen without drainage.

Postoperative Orders

The postoperative orders are the same as those for tubal pregnancy.

4. Antepartum Care

David H. Fields, M.D.

DEFINITION

Care for the pregnant woman instituted upon the diagnosis of pregnancy and continued until delivery. Its aim is to safeguard the health of the mother and fetus and smooth the transition to parenthood.

BASIC PRINCIPLES

1. Pregnancy is not a disease. It is, however, a physiologic process which places increasingly severe metabolic and nutritional demands on the mother as gestation advances. These demands must be met to insure a healthy outcome for both mother and infant. Because they become progressively more severe, they are best satisfied in advance, rather than by playing catch-up throughout the pregnancy.

2. A safe and satisfying pregnancy requires not only maternal physical adjustments, but also mental and psychic preparation on the part of both parents.

3. The cornerstones of good antepartum care are:

a. Good nutrition

b. Early detection and treatment of illness

c. Adjustment to physical limitations of pregnancy if any

d. Education of prospective parents to normal and abnormal events of pregnancy

e. Avoidance of substances harmful to the fetus

All of these can best be achieved by the maintenance of open communication between the woman and her obstetrician.

THE INITIAL VISIT

This should be as early in pregnancy as possible and should include a complete history, physical examination, and laboratory screen, to establish as many baseline parameters as possible.

Essentials of History

1. Information regarding this pregnancy, including date and character of last menstrual period, and normal frequency of menstruation

2. Previous ostetric history, including weight, condition, timing, and type of previous deliveries

3. Medical history, especially diabetes, hypertension, cardiovascular disease

4. Surgical history, especially abdominal or uterine surgery

5. Medications used during this pregnancy (including alcohol, tobacco, marijuana)

6. Any problems encountered during this or previous pregnancy

Essentials of Physical Examination

1. General examination with special emphasis on:

a. Weight, height, blood pressure

b. Heart murmurs, breasts

c. Lower extremity edema or varices

d. Pelvic examination (While many physicians gauge pelvic architecture on the first visit, it may be preferable to defer this to the third trimester when both the patient and her perineum are more relaxed.)

Laboratory Screening

1. Hemoglobin, hematocrit (as well as red blood cell indices, if available)
2. Clean-catch urinalysis—for sugar, acetone, protein, and microscopic exam
3. Blood type and Rh identification, with antibody screening
4. Papanicoulau smear
5. Serologic test for syphilis (VDRL, STS)
6. Cervical culture for gonorrhea
7. Tine test for tuberculosis; if positive, chest radiograph with abdominal shield to rule out pulmonary tuberculosis
8. Rubella and Toxoplasma gondii antibody tests. Many physicians have begun to do routine screening for susceptibility to these teratogenic agents. Both are preferably done before conception, since exposure, if susceptible, is most serious in the first trimester.

Advice to the Prenatal Patient at the First Visit

1. Diet. A normal diet consisting of meats, eggs, milk, vegetables should be encouraged for the woman of normal prepregnancy weight. The following requirements should be met:

a. Kilocalories. Approximately 2,400, as three good meals per day

b. Protein. Supplied by meat or fish daily, eggs several times per week, and 1 quart of milk daily

c. Minerals

(1) All basic minerals except iron may be met by adequate vegetable, fruit, and milk intake.

(2) Iron must be supplied as ferrous sulfate (or gluconate or fumarate) tablets at least once daily.

(3) Many physicians recommended prenatal vitamins, all of which have supplementary minerals, including calcium.

(4) If the patient cannot drink adequate amounts of milk, her needs may be met by calcium supplement of 1 to 2 g. daily.

d. Vitamins

(1) All vitamin needs are met by adequate vegetable and fruit intake, but are usually supplied in extra amounts by any of the prenatal vitamins.

(2) In addition, many physicians prescribe supplementary folic acid (0.5 to 1.0 mg daily), although the need for this has not been proven.

2. Weight Gain

a. Normal pregnancy is associated with a minimum 20-pound weight gain.

(1) 11 pounds: intrauterine contents

(2) 7 pounds: uterus, breasts, intravascular volume

(3) 2 pounds: extravascular fluid retention

b. Weight gains from 20 to 30 pounds are associated with optimal fetal growth and minimal maternal complications.

c. Weight gain greater than 30 to 35 pounds is associated with an increase in maternal morbidity, especially abnormal glucose tolerance, and with difficulty losing the extra fat after delivery.

d. Obese women should still gain the minimum 20 pounds, with all attempts at dieting strictly watched for the development of ketosis.

3. Activity

a. Unless there is a risk of premature labor (e.g., twins), the normal pregnant woman may carry out virtually any activity with which she is comfortable. She should not undertake new and dangerous sports (e.g., water skiing or sky diving).

b. She may continue to work at her job until she cannot easily physicially perform it, as long as it does not involve specifically dangerous conditions (i.e., radiation). Many women remain at work until they go into labor.

c. There are no restrictions on travel, with the understanding that the woman should not sit in positions that compromise lower extremity circulation for long periods of time. She should move about every 1 or 2 hours.

4. Sexual Intercourse

a. Coitus may be unrestricted in normal pregnancy as long as the cervix is not significantly dilated. It should be forbidden in pregnancies complicated by vaginal bleeding, ruptured membranes, or premature labor.

b. Under no circumstances should air be blown into the vagina if cunnilingus is performed. This has resulted in fatal air embolus.

c. Although its significance is unknown, fetal bradycardia has been reported after orgasm, presumably secondary to uterine contraction. Perhaps orgasm should be advised against in pregnancies at high risk for fetal distress.

5. Drug Use

a. All drug use should be cleared in advance with the obstetrician. Currently, alcohol, tobacco, and marijuana are all suspect in more than minimal amounts and the physician should probably discourage more than occasional use.

b. Any prescription item should be researched and its benefits weighed against its potential hazards. A good reference for this is the Physician's Desk Reference, which is very wary of drug use in pregnancy.

6. Clothing

a. Common sense should dictate comfortable clothes. The only real caveats are:

(1) Constriction of venous return below the waist, most commonly caused by tight girdles or socks (stockings) with elastic tops and

(2) High-heeled shoes

b. Adequate support of the breasts with a brassiere usually adds to maternal comfort.

7. Hygiene

a. Normal hygiene is encouraged.

b. Tub baths and showers are acceptable as long as the mother is not at risk of falling.

c. Douching should be avoided unless specifically indicated for medication delivery. If necessary, it must be performed gently and carefully.

d. Dental care should be sought early in pregnancy. All necessary work may be done with local anesthesia.

8. Prepared Childbirth Classes

a. These are now readily available throughout the country and should be attended by every patient whether or not she intends to have "prepared childbirth."

b. The preparation given and the knowledge gained about labor and delivery will serve to decrease anxiety, cutting down on intrapartum medication in almost all cases.

c. The exercises and toning in preparation for labor will make labor easier for most women.

d. The involvement of the husband in the pregnancy and delivery will usually serve to make both a more enjoyable "family experience" and may result in a smoother transition to the postpartum period.

9. Warning Signs

Certain symptoms or signs may be of grave importance. The pregnant woman should be encouraged to report any of the following:

a. Vaginal bleeding
b. Leakage of fluid from the vagina
c. Blurring of vision
d. Persistent headache or dizziness
e. Fever or chills
f. Abdominal pain
g. Recurrent vomiting
h. Swelling of hands or face

Follow-up Visits

1. The normal ostetric patient should be seen at least at 4-weekly intervals from the first visit until approximately 32 weeks gestation. Many physicians see their patients monthly until 26 weeks, then at 3-week intervals until 32 weeks. From 32 to 36 weeks, visits should be biweekly, and after 36 weeks, weekly.

2. The following information should be obtained at every visit: weight, blood

pressure, urine sugar and protein, uterine size, fetal lie and heart rate, if possible, after 20 weeks gestation.

3. Unless there is a specific contraindication, vaginal examination for cervical dilatation and presenting part should be performed weekly from the thirty-sixth week.

4. Pelvic architecture, if not evaluated previously, should be thoroughly examined at the thirty-sixth week.

5. The following laboratory work should be routinely obtained after the first visit in normal pregnancy.

a. Hemoglobin/hematocrit, at least once in the second and third trimester, each

b. Repeat type, Rh and antibody screen—at 20 to 24 weeks and at 36 weeks gestation

c. Serologic test for syphilis (VDRL, STS), in the third trimester

d. Cervical culture for gonorrhea, in the third trimester

Special Diagnostic Studies

Any special diagnostic studies may be performed as long as they do not require the administration of medication or exposure to radiation. If either of these is necessary, the benefits must be weighed against the risks.

1. Radiographic Studies With the exception of x-ray pelvimetry and the single flat plate of the abdomen to determine fetal lie, x-ray studies for obstetric indications have been largely supplanted by ultrasonography which may be used to document fetal death, fetal maturity, fetal abnormality, and placental location.

2. Chest Radiography. Provides minimal radiation, especially when performed with an abdominal shield. It should be obtained in cases of suspected pulmonary tuberculosis (all positive Tine tests), as well as on suspicion of pneumonia.

3. Radiographic Contrast Studies. Intravenous pyelograms, barium enemas, upper GI series can usually be postponed until the postpartum period. If the need to know is great enough, all can be performed with less than 10 rads of exposure by keeping the number of films and fluoroscopy to a minimum.

4. Radioactive Scanning. (lung, liver, thyroid) should be avoided unless the situation is life-threatening.

5. Ultrasonography Has been in use for over 15 years and is so far considered safe. The indications for its use expand almost daily and currently include placental localization, determination of fetal size, age, lie, growth patterns, and detection of fetal abnormalities.

Commonly Encountered Problems in Antepartum Care

1. Nausea and Vomiting

Possibly a reaction to high levels of human chorionic gonadotropin, this is essentially a problem of the first trimester. So-called morning sickness is probably the most commonly encountered side effect of pregnancy and is covered in great detail in Chapter 5.

2. Fatigue

Another common complaint, extreme tiredness is also a first and early second trimester problem. If anemia or chronic disease is not present, the physician should explain the need for extra rest during pregnancy.

3. Ptyalism

a. When excessive salivation occurs, the most reasonable approach is to reassure the patient that it is harmless. Attempts at treatment with anticholinergic agents such as Propantheline are usually unsuccessful.

b. Some investigators have suggested that ptyalism is actually failure to swallow, rather than increased salivary gland production.

4. Pica

a. Although the ingestion of bizarre substances (most commonly clay or starch) is probably more a social custom than anything else, investigation of the diet for a specific deficiency should be made.

b. It is rarely a problem unless huge quantities of the particular substance are eaten.

5. Heartburn

a. This is due to reflux of gastric acid into the esophagus secondary to upward pressure on the stomach by the growing uterus. It is probably made worse by the decreased gastric motility of pregnancy.

b. Tremendous relief is obtained with antacids, which should be of the magnesium or aluminum salt types. Amphojel and Gelusil are constipating, while milk of magnesia, Maalox, and Mylanta have the opposite effect.

c. Sodium bicarbonate antacids should be avoided because of the large sodium load which may be involved.

6. Constipation

a. This frequent complaint is best treated by diets high in fiber, fluid intake, and cathartic substances (prunes, raisins), combined with retraining of bowel habits.

b. If necessary, commercial cathartics and stool softeners may be used.

c. It is not a problem unless the stool is especially hard and bowel movements become painful.

7. Hemorrhoids

a. These inevitable results of pregnancy are made worse by constipation and eased by soft, regular bowel movements without straining.

b. Surgical treatment during pregnancy is only indicated for acutely thrombosed hemorrhoids, and then should usually be limited to clot evacuation under local anesthesia.

c. Hemorrhoidectomy is not indicated since they regress spontaneously postpartum and recur with the next pregnancy.

8. Lower extremity varicosities

a. Like hemorrhoids, these are due to increased venous pressure from the growing uterus.

b. Treatment is almost always conservative, consisting of support elastic stockings (perferably the pantyhose type) and elevation of the legs while sitting or lying.

9. Excessive Vaginal Discharge

a. The key to treatment of leukorrhea during pregnancy is identical to that outside of pregnancy: identification of the causative organism.

b. This is best done by a wet mount preparation in saline to check for trichomonads and "clue cells" (Hemophilus vaginalis) followed by a 10% KOH or NaOH preparation to detect candidiasis.

c. If the above are not revealing or if therapy is unsuccessful, cultures for Candida albicans (on Nickerson's medium), H. vaginalis (standard "culturette"), and gonorrhea (Thayer-Martin medium, Transgro) may be performed. Trichomonads are best identified on Pap smear.

d. Therapy should be directed toward a specific etiology:

(1) *Candida*: Nystatin (Mycostatin) suppositories b.i.d. × 2 weeks; miconazole (Monistat) cream O.D. × 1 week; clotrimazole (Gyne-Lotrimin) suppositories, O.D. × 1 week; painting with 1-per-cent gentian violet solution

(2) *H. vaginalis*: sulfa cream (Sultrin, AVC) b.i.d. × 1 week; ampicillin (P.O.) 500 mg. every 6 hrs. × 1 week

(3) *Trichomonas*: Although metronidazole (Flagyl) is the drug of choice for this, it is contraindicated in first-trimester pregnancy. It should probably be reserved during later gestation for cases which MUST be treated and do not respond to local povidone iodine (Betadine) application or other creams. If metronidazole is used, the dosage is 250 mg. t.i.d. × 7 days.

10. Abdominal Cramping

a. This is common in the third and fourth months of pregnancy as the uterus rises out of the pelvis, and is commonly ascribed to the "round ligament syndrome."

b. It can be distinguished from urinary and gastrointestinal problems by careful history, examination, and urinalysis.

c. Benign in nature, it usually responds well to mild bed rest and local application of heat.

11. Backache

a. Usually caused by the exaggerated lordosis of pregnancy, low back pain responds well to relief of the strain.

b. If conservative measures do not afford relief, orthopaedic consultation should be sought.

12. Headaches

a. Very common in early pregnancy, these should respond well to simple analgesia.

b. If they persist beyond the first few weeks of gestation, are not relieved by aspirin, or are accompanied by neurologic symptoms, they should be thoroughly investigated.

13. Edema

a. Swelling of the feet or legs during the course of the day is normal for pregnancy. The swelling responds well to elevation.

b. Swelling of the face or hands is less likely normal and preeclampsia should be suspected.

c. Diuretics and salt restriction are not indicated for simple edema of pregnancy since it is a hydrostatic phenomenon.

5. Nausea and Vomiting of Pregnancy

Hugh R. K. Barber, M.D.

BASIC PRINCIPLES

1. Nausea and vomiting is probably the most common disorder seen in the first 12 weeks of pregnancy. It is estimated that about one-half of all pregnant women have some nausea or vomiting, but of this group, only about one-half need any treatment at all.

2. Treatment can usually be given on an ambulatory basis. However, about one gravida in 300 requires hospitalization.

3. The criteria for hospitalizing a patient with vomiting of pregnancy are:

   a. Acetone or diacetic acid in urine
   b. Weight loss of 5 per cent or over
   c. Pulse of 120
   d. Elevated temperature with signs of dehydration
   e. Elevated specific gravity of the urine in the presence of low urinary output

4. It is important to be certain of the diagnosis. Marked vomiting in early pregnancy may be associated with twins or a hydatidiform mole. More serious problems such as hepatitis, diabetic acidosis, or acute porphyria may be mistaken for vomiting of pregnancy.

5. The average case of vomiting in pregnancy presents a picture of electrolyte and water imbalance not unlike that seen in the nonpregnant patient. Although the hydrochloric-acid content is reduced below nonpregnant values, there is still enough loss of chlorides in the early phases of vomiting to lead to hypochloremic alkalosis. Vomiting leads to starvation with the initiation of ketosis. It is not uncommon to have hypochloremic alkalosis and ketosis coexisting in the early stage of vomiting.

6. If therapy is not instituted, dehydration becomes marked, and there is a reduction in the extracellular fluid with a drop in glomerular filtration. The urine output drops, the specific gravity of the urine is increased, and sulfates and phosphates accumulate in the extracellular space. The resultant acidosis represents a very serious problem, which demands prompt and intelligent therapy.

MANAGEMENT

1. The basic fluid and electrolyte requirements are:

   1,000 ml. of 5% glucose and water
   1,000 ml. of 5% glucose and water
   500 ml. of 5% glucose and saline

2. To this should be added the replacement of fluid and electrolytes lost in vomitus. Inasmuch as the vomiting is almost entirely gastric, it can be replaced in the ratio of two-thirds 5-per-cent glucose and saline and one-third 5-per-cent glucose and water. This replacement is satisfactory, even though the gastric juice in a pregnant patient usually contains less hydrochloric acid than is seen in the normal nonpregnant patient.

3. As soon as the urinary output is improved to about 1,000 ml. per day, it is important to replace the daily requirement of KCl (30 to 40 mEq.) plus another 20 mEq. of KCl for each 1,000 ml. of vomitus that is replaced.

4. The use of amino acids has very little place in the therapy of the patient with acute vomiting of pregnancy and

may, in itself, cause vomiting. Because the enzyme systems concerned with the utilization of the amino acids are functioning poorly, the amino acids are often excreted in the same concentration as they are infused. The liver in the pregnant patient with acute vomiting may have central necrosis and resemble the hepatic lesions in starvation. Liver insufficiency is not conducive to the utilization of infused amino acids.

5. Severe cases present a real challenge to the institution of intelligent therapy. The problem of acidosis occurring as a late phase of vomiting of pregnancy may be accompanied by some degree of liver insufficiency, and attempts to correct acidosis with sodium lactate is to be discouraged. The poorly functioning liver is unable to adequately metabolize the lactate, and it accumulates in the extracellular space. In situations of this kind, the use of sodium bicarbonate is preferred. When sodium bicarbonate is given, the bicarbonate ion (HCO_3^-) dissociates, and the CO_2 is blown off by the lungs, while the sodium ion remains in the extracellular space and carries out its functions as a cation.

6. The problem of ammonium toxicity has not been investigated in cases of vomiting of pregnancy. Whether present research in the field of ammonium toxicity will find any application in evaluating these problems remains to be determined. However, certain of these cases have some liver insufficiency, and it has been shown that ammonium toxicity is frequently associated with liver insufficiency. Sodium glutamate can be substituted for sodium bicarbonate in these cases. The rationale behind this plan is that the glutamate reacts with ammonium to form the easily metabolized glutamine, while the sodium combines with the metabolically available carbon dioxide to form sodium bicarbonate. Sodium glutamate is given in 30-to 40-g. doses and is added to the glucose-and-water solution.

7. In summary, the fluid regimen to be used in severe cases of vomiting of pregnancy is as follows:

a. 1,500 to 2,000 ml. 5-per-cent glucose and water. Five-per-cent glucose and water may be used as all or part of the infusion in order to increase the caloric intake.

b. 500 ml. 5-per-cent glucose and saline

c. Replacement of the vomitus (replace as two-thirds 5-per-cent glucose and saline, and one-third 5-per-cent glucose and water)

d. 30 to 40 mEq. of potassium chloride (only after the urinary output is 1,000 ml. a day)

e. 20 mEq. potassium chloride for each 1,000 ml. of vomitus replaced

f. 44 to 88 mEq. of sodium bicarbonate in cases of marked acidosis (run frequent EKG determinations so that any dangerous fall in potassium can be detected)

g. 30 to 40 g. of sodium glutamate in glucose and water (if liver insufficiency or ammonium toxicity is present)

8. The total infusion should be divided into a morning and late afternoon infusion. This cuts down the period of starvation between the end of one infusion and the start of the next. Because the body can only utilize 0.5 g. of glucose per Kg. of body weight, it is wise to run the infusion slowly. This means that the body can only utilize about 30 to 50 g. of glucose per hour. If the infusion is run at a more rapid rate, dehydration may result secondary to the osmotic diuresis.

9. There are very few indications for the use of clysis in these cases. However, the opinion has been that it may serve a purpose as part of the therapy. This must be accepted with reservations, because the use of clysis only serves to aggravate the existing water-and-electrolyte imbalance. A glucose-and-water clysis is accompanied by a transient transfer of electrolytes from the blood and interstitial fluid into the pool formed

by the clysis. A state of equilibrium must be established between this pool and the extracellular fluid before absorption can take place. This further decreases (temporarily) an already depleted extracellular fluid with the production of hypotension and, not uncommonly, a fall in the urinary output. If a clysis is used, the only safe clysis is one containing 2.5-per-cent glucose with 0.45-per-cent sodium chloride, and even this is far from ideal.

10. The above regimen is concerned only with the replacement of fluids and electrolytes. In treatment these cases, the standard regimen, which includes sedation, vitamins, psychotherapy, and antiemetics, should be employed.

a. Sedation and antiemetics:

(1) Phenobarbital 30 to 60 mg., P.O., I.M., b.i.d. or t.i.d.

(2) Bendectin tablets, 2 at bedtime if patient is able to tolerate per-os medication. Compazine, 10 mg., I.M., every 6 hours as needed or Tigan 2 ml. (200 mg.) every 6 hours as needed.

(3) Amphetamine 5 mg., P.O., t.i.d., is sometimes helpful.

b. Vitamins P.O. or I.M., to supply 200 mg. each of thiamine, nicotinic acid, and vitamin C, 40 mg. riboflavin, 5 mg. folic acid, and Vitamin B_6.

c. Psychotherapy: hypnosis and psychoanalysis as indicated

6. Antepartum Fetal Evaluation

David H. Fields, M.D.

DEFINITION

1. Tests performed upon the fetus before the onset of labor may be biochemical, physical, or physiologic.
2. They may be used to evaluate: fetal well-being, fetal maturity, and fetal abnormalities.

TESTS OF FETAL WELL-BEING

General Principles

These tests indirectly assess placental function, since antepartum fetal jeopardy is usually secondary to placental insufficiency. There are four basic categories of tests:

1. Biochemical measurement of substances produced by healthy placentas (estriol, human placental lactogen)
2. Functional evaluation of fetal oxygen reserve (nonstress and stress testing of fetal heart response)
3. Evaluation of serial fetal growth (serial ultrasonography)
4. Direct observation of fetus and amniotic fluid to detect signs of distress such as meconium (amnioscopy, fetoscopy)

BIOCHEMICAL TESTS OF FETAL WELL-BEING

Estriol Measurement

Estriol is an estrogen produced by the placenta from fetal adrenal precursors and excreted by the mother in her urine. It may be measured either in a 24-hour maternal urine specimen or in maternal plasma.

1. Indications

a. *Suspicion of Placental Insufficiency* Although estriol measurement is most useful for detection of chronic, slowly progressive placental decompensation, if measured often enough, it may reveal more acute changes.

b. *Common Indications for Suspicions of Placental Dysfunction*

(1) Maternal hypertensive disease, including preeclampsia

(2) Postdate pregnancy

(3) Maternal diabetes

(4) Chronic maternal illness of any sort, especially renal, endocrine, and collagen vascular

(5) Suspicion of intrauterine growth retardation regardless of cause

(6) Previous stillbirth

2. Timing

Beginning at 30-weeks gestation, from once weekly to once daily depending on stage of pregnancy and specific indication (see specific diseases)

3. Interpretation

A SINGLE ESTRIOL LEVEL HAS LITTLE VALUE. Interpretation is based on trends.

a. Normal values vary from lab to lab with stage of pregnancy, so each lab must have its own table of acceptable ranges.

b. Rising or steadily high estriol levels indicate no fetal jeopardy on the basis of placental insufficiency.

c. Drops of 30- to 50 per cent or greater (from baseline values) indicate significant decrease in placental function and probable fetal danger.

d. Steadily low values are worrisome but require corroboration by other tests.

4. Pitfalls

a. *Low Estriols without Fetal Distress.* Since estriol production depends on fetal adrenal and maternal hepatic and renal function as well as a healthy placenta, a defect in any of these organs may affect estriol production and fetal distress.

(1) *Both Urine and Plasma Estriols*

(a) Maternal steroid ingestion (decreased fetal precursors)

(b) Fetal anencephaly (decreased fetal precursors because of associated adrenal hypoplasia)

(c) Fetal adrenal insufficiency

(d) Placental sulfatase deficiency (an inherited enzyme deficiency which does not affect fetal welfare but selectively blocks placental production of estriol sulfate—always associated with a male fetus—levels in the fetal death range)

(e) Lab error

(2) *Urine Estriol Only*

(a) Maternal Drug Administration. Ampicillin, aspirin, hydrochlorathiazide, mandelamine

(b) Maternal Renal Dysfunction. Decreased creatinine clearance

(c) Maternal Liver Disease. Decreased conjugation of estriol for urinary excretion

(d) Incomplete 24-hour urine collection

b. Falsely High Estriols

(1) Congenital adrenal hyperplasia (increased fetal precursors).

(2) Multiple gestation (increased placental bulk).

(3) Severe Rh hemolytic disease (increased placental bulk).

5. Management of a Low or Dropping Estriol Value

a. Repeat estriol determination immediately.

b. Check presence of immediate fetal jeopardy via nonstress or stress testing.

c. Crosscheck using assay of another hormone, e.g., human placental lactogen (HPL).

Human Placental Lactogen (HPL)

HPL is a substance produced solely by the placenta and secreted into maternal serum. As such, it has been suggested as an alternative to estriol measurement.

1. Indication

Same as estriol, although it is considered especially useful in pregnancy complicated by severe maternal hypertension or renal disease, when estriol levels may be falsely low. It is also considered especially unreliable in pregnancy complicated by diabetes or Rh disease because levels are high secondary to increased placental mass.

2. Timing

Same as estriol

3. Interpretation

Same method as for estriol, although 4 μg. per ml. after 30-weeks gestation seems to be a good dividing line between fetuses in distress and those who are well.

4. Pitfalls

a. Falsely high levels: maternal diabetes, Rh disease (large placental mass)

b. Low serum levels with healthy fetuses are not rare.

FUNCTIONAL TESTS OF FETAL WELL-BEING

Contraction Stress Test (CST) or Oxytocin Stress Test (OCT)

This test is based on the fact that a fetus suffering the effects of borderline placental insufficiency will show evidence of hypoxia via FHR monitoring during minimal stress. It requires the production of a certain rate of uterine contractions (3 per 10 min.), and electronic monitoring of the FHR to determine fetal status. Its major advantage over hormone studies is that it offers immediate evaluation of fetal condition.

1. General Indications

a. Suspicion of Utero-Placental Insufficiency (UPI). The CST offers an immediate method for evaluating fetal status with projected UPI which may be interpreted on the spot.

2. Specific Indications

a. Decreased Fetal Movement. To rule out hypoxia as the etiology of decreased fetal activity

b. Low estriol or HPL, while awaiting corroboration

c. Postdates pregnancy: usually after 41-weeks amenorrhea

d. Preeclampsia, hypertension

e. Diabetes

f. Other "high risk" pregnancy (hyperthyroidism, cardiovascular disease, collagen vascular disease, hemoglobinopathy)

g. Previous stillbirth

3. Timing

May be begun as early as 30 to 32 weeks gestation, and repeated at 5 to 7 day intervals, although there is usually no point in doing the test if delivery is not contemplated in the event of a positive finding. This is usually after 30 to 32 weeks gestation.

4. Procedure for Contraction Stress Test

a. Perform pelvic examination for status of cervix and membranes.

b. Begin I.V. infusion of D_5W (keep vein open).

c. External cardiotachometer and tocodynamometer affixed to patient. Baseline recording of fetal heart and uterine activity recorded for 20 minutes.

d. After recording the baseline for 20 minutes, if spontaneous uterine contractions are occurring less frequently than every 3 minutes and fetal heart recording shows no late deceleration, I.V. oxytocin infusion is begun via pump at the rate of 0.5 mu./minute (5 units oxytocin in 1,000 ml./D_5W at 0.1 ml./minute).

e. Vital signs (blood pressure, heart rate) of mother measured every 15 minutes during test.

f. Rate of infusion is doubled every 20 minutes until either (1) contractions lasting from 40 to 60 seconds are established at the rate of every 3 minutes or (2) repetitive late decelerations (at least 3) occur.

g. Oxytocin infusion is stopped when (1) patient has had adequate contractions at the rate of every 3 minutes for 10 minutes or (2) patient has had repetitive late decelerations.

h. The patient is monitored for 30 to 60 minutes after discontinuation of oxytocin for fetal heart changes and residual uterine activity.

i. Pelvic examination is repeated.

5. Interpretation

a. *Negative Test.* There are no late (Type II) decelerations in the FHR while the mother is having three contractions per 10 minutes. A negative test is very good evidence of a fetus not in distress at that moment who will tolerate continued intrauterine existence for one week. IT DOES NOT PREDICT THE OUTCOME OF LABOR, which involves much greater stress.

b. *Positive Test.* The FHR exhibits repetitive late decelerations while being stressed by NO MORE THAN three contractions per 10 minutes. Presumably, the fetus who shows this response with less stress is in greater jeopardy. A positive CST has been associated with a significant incidence of intrauterine death within one week, and even 72 hours. There is, however, the likelihood of a 25-per-cent false-positive rate.

c. *Suspicious Test.* If the FHR shows late decelerations after some but not all contractions, at a contraction rate of not more than three per 10 minutes, the meaning is unclear and the test should be repeated in 24 hours.

d. *Hyperstimulation* If uterine contractions occur too frequently, (more than four per 10 minutes) or last too long (greater than 90 seconds), one cannot interpret the significance of late deceleration. Under these circumstances the test should be repeated within 24 hours. If on repeat, there are no late decelerations, the test is negative.

e. *Unsatisfactory* The test cannot be interpreted if:

(1) There is a poor quality FHR recording, so that late deceleration cannot be determined.

(2) There are fewer than three contractions per 10 minutes, (unless the test is positive), so that the fetus has not been stressed enough to call the test negative. Repeat in 24 hours.

f. *Additional Interpretive Refinements*

(1) FHR variability greater than five beats per minute reflects a healthy fetus and rarely is associated with a positive test.

(2) Other Decelerations. Early (Type I) and variable (Type III) decelerations should not be interpreted as a positive test or as indicative of fetal jeopardy. Repeated variable decelerations, however, may reflect oligohydramnios or cord compression.

(3) Acceleration. Speeding of the FHR with contractions is generally considered to be favorable sign.

g. *Contraindications.* Because the CST requires the production of uterine contractions, any condition under which this might be dangerous should preclude the use of this test. Common contraindications include:

(1) Placenta Previa. Risk of hemorrhage

(2) Previous Classical Cesarean Section. Risk of uterine rupture

(3) Multiple Gestation. Risk of premature labor

(4) Premature Rupture of Membranes. Risk of premature labor

Non-Stress Testing

It is possible to evaluate fetal condition in utero by observation of fetal activity and corresponding FHR patterns. While there is less experience with this test than with the CST, it is currently felt that this is especially useful in conditions which contraindicate a CST. The NST, in time, may become the preferred first line functional test of fetal well-being with further evaluation via the CST when necessary.

1. Indications. Same as for CST, especially in pregnancies which contraindicate the CST

2. Timing. Same as for CST, but may be done more frequently because of its simplicity

3. Procedure

a. Begin with electronic FHR monitoring and uterine contraction monitoring.

b. Instruct the mother to depress the tocodynamometer each time the fetus moves.

c. Observe for five fetal movements in a 15 to 20 minute period, especially checking the reaction of the FHR. Various experiments have been tried to stimulate the quiet fetus who does not move sufficiently, but the meaning of these is unclear.

d. Terminate test upon five fetal movements or 40 minutes.

4. Interpretation

a. *Reactive NST.* Indicates a healthy fetus.

(1) Good baseline variability and rate.

(2) Five fetal movements within 15 to 20 minutes, each accompanied by acceleration of the FHR by at least 15 beats per minute.

b. *Nonreactive NST.* Fetal status is uncertain, perform CST.

(1) Baseline is abnormal or variability is lacking.

(2) Fetus will not move sufficiently.

(3) FHR does not change with fetal movement.

Ultrasonography (USG)

By using high energy ultrasonic pulses, it is possible to "draw" a scale picture of the fetus in utero. After approximately 15 years of widespread clinical experience, this is thought to be safe for the fetus. There are currently four uses for USG in antepartum evaluation of the fetus.

1. Gestational dating of pregnancy
2. Determination of fetal growing patterns and detection of growth retardation
3. Localization of intrauterine contents, (especially placenta), either for amniocentesis or to rule out abnormal presentation
4. Detection of multiple fetuses

Of these, #2 (determination of fetal growth pattern) may be used to assess intrauterine fetal well-being.

1. Advantages

a. Noninvasive

b. No x-irradiation

2. Basic Principles

a. Within the variation of normal curves for a specific population, the well-nourished fetus may be expected to grow at a certain rate.

b. This growth rate is assessable via combined measurement of the biparietal and transthoracic* diameters of the fetus at various states of pregnancy.

c. The fetus who shows a growth pattern that is slower than normal, or slows from his own previously established pattern *may* be suffering from nutritional deprivation.

d. Because placental reserve in early and midpregnancy so outweighs fetal needs, even severely compromised uteroplacental function usually does not result in early growth retardation.

e. Therefore, the key to serial sonography for fetal growth patterns is establishing a curve in the middle of pregnancy (16 to 26 weeks gestation) with which to compare growth in the third trimester.

3. Indications Suspicion that intrauterine fetal growth retardation is likely to occur, most likely in pregnancies complicated by:

a. Diabetes

b. Hypertension

c. Chronic disease

4. Contraindications. None

5. Method. At least two sonograms should be done 3 weeks apart demonstrating inadequate growth for the fetus, adjusted for gestational age and size. Three sonograms over a longer period may be more reliable. The earlier the first ultrasonogram (USG) is performed the better (see Basic Principles), as it will more likely correlate with fetal age.

6. Interpretation

a. If the first sonogram can be adequately correlated with gestational age (as opposed to size) as is the case in the early and mid-second trimester, the fetus can most likely be placed in a certain growth range. A second USG several weeks later should demonstrate adequate growth for a fetus of the specific size and age. If it does not, the fetus may be presumed to be growing too slowly.

b. If the first sonogram is later, or is inappropriate for dates, the fetus may be a different age than suspected, or already nutritionally deprived. In this case, a second USG (2 to 3 weeks later) will serve to define the growth pattern. Since growth retardation usually becomes progressively worse in cases in which the fetus is actually being starved, a third USG should show a growth rate decreased from that defined by the first two.

*Newer methods are constantly being introduced and will soon include measurement of total uterine volume and total fetal volume.

DIRECT OBSERVATION: AMNIOSCOPY/FETOSCOPY

These techniques are used primarily to detect meconium-stained amniotic fluid or fetal anomalies and are usually performed through a somewhat dilated cervix. Using either directly lighted scopes or fiberoptic equipment, there use is limited to later pregnancy when the cervix dilated.

1. Advantages

a. Easy to use
b. Immediate results

2. Indications. Suspicion of meconium in all high risk pregnancies

3. Contraindications

a. Ruptured membranes
b. Closed cervix

4. Risks. Unintentional rupture of membranes

5. Interpretation. Green amniotic fluid signals the likelihood of fetal distress and demands further investigation.

TESTS OF FETAL MATURITY

These are designed to predict the fetus' ability to survive in the outside world. They fall into two groups: tests on amniotic fluid, designed to assess functional maturity, and USG, which attempts to date the pregnancy accurately and enable the physician to statistically predict maturity based on age.

TESTS ON AMNIOTIC FLUID
LECITHIN/SPHINGOMYELIN RATIO, (L/S RATIO)

The most commonly accepted test of fetal maturity is determination of the L/S ratio of amniotic fluid. Since the major cause of morbidity and mortality in premature infants is respiratory distress syndrome (RDS), the most reasonable measure of fetal "survivability" should be lung function.

Basic Principles

As the fetal lungs begin to mature, Type II pneumocytes within the alveoli produce increasing amounts of surfactant, a substance which prevents atelectasis after birth. This is secreted into the amniotic fluid and results in more lecithin and less sphingomyelin, or a greater L/S ratio. The greater the L/S ratio, the more surfactant the lungs are producing.

Indications

Either planned or likely early delivery for any reason. Most commonly for:

1. Maternal diabetes
2. Preeclampsia
3. Premature rupture of membranes
4. Repeat Cesarean section
5. Rh-sensitized pregnancy

Contraindications

The only contraindication to amniocentesis is a relative one, the anterior placenta. Its importance varies conversely with the need to know about fetal maturity.

Interpretation

1. An L/S ratio of greater than 2 indicates a fetus with mature lungs. The incidence of RDS is very small (less than 2 per cent) and fatal RDS virtually nil (0.1 per cent) and is largely limited to fetuses who suffer intrapartum hypoxic distress.

2. An L/S ratio of 1.5 indicates a significant number (Hellman quotes Harvey, Ligett as 40 per cent) of fetuses will develop RDS, although only a small number (4 per cent) will die.

3. An L/S ratio of less than 1.5: Most fetuses will develop RDS and a significant number (15 per cent) will die.

Pitfalls

1. Infants of diabetic mothers seem to develop RDS more often than other infants in the face of an L/S ratio of 2 or

even higher. Some people have suggested 2.5 or even 3 as an L/S ratio for these fetuses.

2. Meconium staining lowers the L/S ratio at any level.

3. Contamination with maternal blood (serum) lowers the L/S ratio, if it is above 1.3.

4. Contamination of amniotic fluid with maternal urine (bladder tap) lowers the L/S ratio at any level.

FOAM TEST

This is a test to functionally assess surfactant activity, which the physician may easily do himself.

Principles

If the amniotic fluid contains enough surfactant, it will form a stable ring of bubbles upon shaking in a test tube. By diluting its concentration and repeating the test several times, one can measure surfactant activity.

Method

1. To each of five test tubes, add 1.0, 0.75, 0.50, 0.25 and 0.20 ml. of amniotic fluid, respectively. Then dilute the volume of the last four tubes to 1 ml. using normal saline.

2. Add 1 ml. of freshly prepared 95-per-cent ethanol to each tube.

3. Shake well, then rest in a stand. Do not move before reading.

4. Observe each tube for a stable ring of bubbles around the periphery.

Interpretation

1. Negative. No complete ring of bubbles in any tube; this usually correlates with L/S ratio of less than 1.5.

2. Intermediate. A complete ring of bubbles in one or two tubes—usually correlates with an L/S ratio of 1.5 to 2.

3. Positive. Complete ring of bubbles in three tubes, usually correlates with an L/S ratio of greater than 2.0. *N.B.* A positive test is a very good predictor of a fetus who will not develop RDS. A negative or intermediate test is less reliable and should be checked by L/S ratio measurement.

Pitfalls

1. False-negative results may occur from any of the following:

a. Dirty glassware

b. Old alcohol

c. Failure to shake sufficiently

d. Wrong diameter test tubes (8 to 14 mm. is acceptable)

2. False-positive tests may occur in the presence of meconium, vaginal secretions, or enough blood to result in a 3-per-cent hematocrit.

NILE BLUE SULFATE TEST

Principle

As the fetus matures, he sheds more and more "matrix" cells from the sebaceous glands into the amniotic fluid. The test is an attempt to stain and quantify the number of these cells and correlate with fetal maturity.

Method

1. Obtain amniotic fluid in standard fashion.

2. Stain amniotic fluid (0.1 ml.) with Nile blue stain (0.1 ml.)

3. Warm for 60 seconds.

4. Count number of orange-staining cells under high-power microscope field.

Interpretation

1. Greater than 30 per cent of cells stained orange indicate fetal maturity.

2. More than 10 per cent but fewer than 30 per cent of cells staining orange is indeterminate.

3. Fewer than 10 per cent of cells taking the orange stain indicates an immature fetus.

AMNIOTIC FLUID—CREATININE

Principle

As the fetus' kidney matures, its ability to excrete creatinine into the amniotic fluid increases and the concentration of creatinine in the amniotic fluid increases.

Method

1. Obtain amniotic fluid.
2. Laboratory determination of creatinine concentration

Interpretation

Levels greater than 2 mg. per 100 ml. have been associated with a mature fetus.

Pitfalls

Amniotic fluid creatinine varies directly with maturity of fetal kidney, muscle mass of fetus, and maternal serum creatinine levels. Falsely high levels may occur with high maternal creatinine or with a macrosomic fetus.

AMNIOTIC FLUID BILIRUBIN DETERMINATION

Principle

In the second half of pregnancy, amniotic fluid bilirubin tends to decrease, reaching zero at term.

Method

1. Obtain amniotic fluid.
2. Protect from light since bilirubin may be broken down from exposure to light.
3. Laboratory determination of bilirubin levels by spectrometry

Interpretation

Levels of zero usually indicate a mature fetus, otherwise prediction is very unreliable.

Pitfalls

a. Varies with maternal bilirubin

b. Increased in fetal hemolytic disease

ULTRASONOGRAPHY (USG)

Principle

This is an attempt to gauge fetal age by accurately measuring fetal size. If the fetus is indeed the age its size suggests, this method can be very helpful.

Gestational Dating

1. Early Pregnancy. Pregnancy may be dated using ultrasonographic measurement of the intrauterine contents. A gestational sac or ring becomes "visible" at 5 weeks gestation and is measurable until it fills the uterine cavity at 12 weeks gestation. By measurement of the sac during this period, the most accurate dating of pregnancy available is obtained.

2. Later Intrauterine Pregnancy

a. From the time the gestational sac echo merges with the uterine wall at 12 weeks, until the fetal skull becomes visible at 14, fetal age is undeterminable by USG. From 14 weeks to birth, the fetal age roughly correlates with the size of the fetal skull measured through the biparietal diameter.

b. There is a progressively widening variation in "normal" fetal sizes approaching term, due to genetic and environmental factors.

c. Therefore, the earlier in pregnancy the biparietal diameter measurement is obtained, the more likely it is to correlate with gestational age, uninfluenced by other factors. Optimal time for this measurement is probably from 16 to 24 weeks.

d. If the ultrasonography is after 30 weeks pregnancy, but is within 2 weeks of gestational age as measured by the last menstrual period, it may be presumed to certify gestational age.

Pitfalls

1. When using this test, the physician cannot accept the age predicted by USG, but should use the age suggested by menstrual history if it is confirmed (e.g., if a woman is 35 weeks by dates and her USG predicts a fetus of 36 weeks size, she presumably is 35 weeks pregnant, not 36 weeks).

2. In the third trimester, ultrasonographic gestational dating may be presumed to have a built-in error factor of plus-or-minus 2 weeks due to hereditary and environmental factors.

7. Conduct of Normal Labor

David H. Fields, M.D.

DEFINITION

Periodic contractions with progressive effacement and dilatation of the cervix

BASIC PRINCIPLES

Labor is an acute event terminating the chronic process of pregnancy. Its object is the delivery of a healthy baby to a healthy mother (and father). Today, labor has become a social event, as well, to be shared by the family unit. The aim of the obstetrician is to integrate all of the above factors to benefit all participants.

PREPARATION FOR LABOR

1. The patient and her husband should be advised to participate in a childbirth preparation course. She may not desire "prepared childbirth," but the physical exercises and psychological preparation from the course will ease her way, regardless of her needs during labor.

2. She should be advised to notify her physician early in the course of labor, so that careful observation of labor and preparation for delivery may be initiated with time to spare. *It is preferable to have a patient arrive in false labor rather than to have her arrive in the delivery room "fully dilated and pushing."*

3. She should be instructed in differentiating labor from Braxton Hicks contractions via the time-honored criteria:

a. Regular contractions at

b. Progressively shorter intervals which are

c. Painful in the fundus

d. Not alleviated by walking around

e. A useful guide is six contractions in 1 hour, of 45 seconds duration each.

ARRIVAL IN THE DELIVERY ROOM

1. A rapid but appropriate history should include the following information:

a. Expected date of confinement—last menstrual period

b. Time of onset of labor

c. Frequency of contractions

d. Presence or absence of amniotic fluid leakage

e. Presence of abnormal bleeding

f. Past obstetrical history, especially size, presentation, and mode of delivery of previous children

g. Past medical history which may affect labor and delivery, especially diabetes, heart disease, epilepsy, respiratory disease, allergic history

2. A rapid but appropriate physical examination should include the following:

a. Vital signs

b. Abdominal examination to determine fetal lie and fetal heart rate

c. Sterile vaginal exam (not performed if there is a suspicion by history or observation of placenta previa) to assess:

(1) Cervical dilatation and effacement

(2) State of membranes—if necessary, via use of nitrazine paper

(3) Fetal presenting part

(4) Pelvic architecture

d. Routine examination of heart,

lungs, extremities, neurologic condition

3. Routine orders for conduct of normal vertex labor are increasingly being questioned as inappropriate to the status of childbirth as a natural event, rather than a medical one. Each of those presented below is recommended for what we consider good reasons.

a. Modified nil per os (lollipops or similar hard candy)—because of decreased gastric motility and possible cesarean section. Since the danger of aspiration is due to gastric acidity, this may be obviated by administration of 30 ml. of antacid every 2 to 4 hrs.

b. Bedrest. If necessary, should be in left lateral recumbent position, especially for the patient who has received analgesia. For the unmedicated patient, sitting is preferable to lying supine to avoid the hypotension associated with uterine compression of the vena cava.

c. The partial perineal preparation should be used merely to remove the hair from the likely area of episiotomy, if anticipated.

d. A mild cleansing or Fleet's enema may be used to empty the rectum to prevent fecal soilage of the delivery area as the fetus descends in the second stage of labor. Contraindications to enema are:

(1) Ruptured membranes with unengaged fetal head

(2) Imminent delivery

e. Bladder function—spontaneous voiding should be encouraged; catheterization should be employed if necessary, but should not be routine.

f. Hematocrit should be determined, if not already known, on every patient on admission. If her hematocrit is less than 30, two units of crossmatched packed red blood cells should be available.

g. Urine for sugar, acetone, and protein, on admission, to check for diabetes, starvation ketosis, and preeclampsia.

h. Maternal vital signs should be recorded every hour.

i. Fetal heart rate and uterine contractions should be monitored continuously and electronically, if possible. If this is not possible, the fetal heart rate should be checked and recorded immediately at the end of a contraction, at least every 15 minutes in the first stage, and every 5 minutes during the second stage of labor. (For details of fetal monitoring, see Chap. 9.)

j. Intravenous glucose administered during labor helps to ward off starvation ketosis, provides a ready route for administration of medication if necessary, and need not interfere or inconvenience the patient if the catheter is placed in the forearm. Appropriate dosage is 5-per-cent glucose in water at the rate of 80 to 125 ml. per hour.

k. Analgesia/anesthesia administered as necessary. See Chap. 10.

(1) Subsequent vaginal examinations:

(a) To assess progress of labor, usually at 1- to 2-hour intervals;

(b) Immediately upon rupture of membranes to rule out cord prolapse and assess cervical dilatation;

(c) Upon notation of any FHR abnormality, to rule out cord prolapse and assess cervical dilatation.

CRITERIA FOR FOLLOWING LABOR WITHOUT INTERVENTION

1. Progressive cervical dilatation at least 1 to 2 cm/hr. after effacement.
2. Progressive descent of the fetal head and delivery within 1 hour after full cervical dilatation.
3. No ominous FHR changes, either by auscultation or electronic monitoring.
4. No excessive vaginal bleeding.
5. If any of the above criteria are not met, the obstetrician will need to either stimulate or interrupt labor, or provide additional support for the fetus (see Chap. 9).

8. Induction of Labor

David H. Fields, M.D.

DEFINITION

The artificial production of labor to terminate a pregnancy. This differs from *augmentation* of labor, which is increasing or strengthening contractions which have begun spontaneously.

There are two basic types of induction:

1. Third-trimester induction, the purpose of which is usually delivery of a live infant; and
2. Second-trimester induction, which is usually for purposes of abortion.

THIRD-TRIMESTER INDUCTION

Basic Principles

1. Should be performed when the physician wants to terminate pregnancy and there is no contraindication to labor.
2. Is best controlled using a quick-acting agent with a very short half-life, whose effects can be turned on and off quickly, i.e., intravenous oxytocin via continuous infusion.
3. Must be continuously monitored by a physician in attendance.

Indications

1. Maternal Jeopardy. Severe preeclampsia/eclampsia, severe cardiovascular disease, placental abruption, premature rupture of membranes, intrauterine fetal death with coagulation abnormalities, maternal malignancy

2. Fetal Jeopardy. Hemolytic Rh disease, placental abruption, fetal distress as determined by tests of fetal well-being, regardless of etiology. Although a positive oxytocin-challenge test makes a successful induction less likely, it does not make it impossible. Under these conditions, the induction should proceed carefully with cesarean section prepared for in advance and readily available if conservative management of fetal distress is unsuccessful.

3. High-Risk Pregnancy, Easily and Safely Delivered. If continued pregnancy poses a significant but not immediate risk to either mother or fetus (diabetes, premature rupture of membranes, mild preeclampsia, postdate pregnancy) and if the fetus is mature (L/S ratio >2, positive foam test, biparietal diameter >37 weeks) and if the cervix is easily inducible (soft, midposition to anterior, somewhat effaced) induction of labor should probably be undertaken.

4. Elective induction of labor for the convenience of either the patient or the obstetrician has become a very controversial area. If the fetus is unquestionably mature and the cervix ripe (see above) and if the labor is carefully conducted and monitored, elective induction should be as safe as spontaneous labor. However, the risks should be discussed with the patient in advance.

Contraindications

Since a carefully conducted induced labor should mimic an ideal labor, the contraindications to induction should be identical to the contraindications to labor and vaginal delivery:

1. Known or suspected cephalopelvic disproportion
2. Placenta previa

3. Abnormal fetal presentation or lie
4. Previous cesarean section
5. Previous vaginal reconstructive surgery
6. Grand multiparity—medically, this condition demands a very careful and gentle induction. Medicolegally, if uterine rupture were to occur, the physician would probably be defenseless.

Agents for Induction of Labor

1. Chemical

a. While many means have been tried to induce and augment labor, only one pharmacologic agent is clinically useful today: oxytocin.

b. Although it may be administered nasally, intramuscularly, or via buccal tablets, continuous intravenous infusion is the best method. Using a pump to guarantee continuous infusion, the physician can control the dosage with great precision.

c. In the near future, prostaglandins of the E and F2 α classes will probably be available for similar use.

d. Prostaglandins of the E and F2α classes are currently under investigation for third-trimester induction of labor. They may be administered orally, nasally, intravenously, vaginally, or intramuscularly. Due to the high incidence of disturbing side effects (nausea, vomiting, diarrhea, fever, flushing, and sweating), they offer no advantage over oxytocin.

e. Tocosamine, Spartocin, and ergot alkaloids have no place in the management of labor as their effects are unpredictable and frequently dangerous to the fetus and mother.

2. Physical: Amniotomy

a. Initially used as a method of induction by itself, artificial rupture of the membranes has become an adjunct to oxytocin-induced labor. Traditionally performed at the beginning of an induction, this practice often results in long labors with ruptured membranes, which are then complicated by amnionitis.

b. It makes more sense to postpone amniotomy until after good contractions have been established and some cervical change produced.

Techniques for Induction of Labor

1. All methods

a. All preparations as for natural spontaneous labor (see Conduct of Normal Labor, Chap. 8)

b. External fetal heart rate and uterine-contraction monitoring should precede induction to document fetal condition and absence of labor.

2. Intravenous Oxytocin (Pitocin, Syntocinon)

a. Prepare infusion by adding 10 units oxytocin to 1,000 ml. of 5-per-cent glucose in water or a balanced salt solution. Each milliliter will then contain 10 milliunits of oxytocin.

b. Begin infusion at 1 to 2 milliunits/minute (0.1 to 0.2 ml. per minute or 6 to 12 ml. per hour).

c. Observe 20 to 30 minutes. If adequate contractions are not produced, double the infusion rate and observe another 20 to 30 minutes.

d. Continue to double the infusion rate every 20 to 30 minutes, until contractions occur at least every 4 minutes; then increase in smaller increments until clinically acceptable contractions (2 to 3 minutes frequency, 40 to 60 seconds duration, fundus firm at peak of contraction) are obtained.

e. If adequate contractions cannot be obtained with 30 to 40 milliunits of oxytocin per minute, it is unlikely the induction will succeed.

3. Buccal Oxytocin (Pitocin)

a. Each tablet contains 200 units of oxytocin.

b. Place 1 tablet in buccal pouch; repeat in 30 minutes on the other side. If adequate labor is obtained, continue to place 1 tablet in alternating buccal pouches half-hourly.

c. If labor is not adequate after 1 hour, place 2 tablets in the pouch (first side); and repeat in 30 minutes (second side). If labor is satisfactory, continue at this dosage.

d. If labor is not adequate after 2nd hour, increase the dosage to 3 tablets and repeat in 30 minutes. If this does not succeed, buccal oxytocin will not suffice.

e. The above regime may be continued until delivery or until 15 tablets (3,000 units) have been used in one 24-hour period.

4. Intranasal Oxytocin (Syntocinon). No longer used for labor, but as an aid in breastfeeding to promote milk let-down.

5. Amniotomy

a. Standard prep for sterile vaginal examination.

b. Check fetal heart rate, preferably with continuous monitoring.

c. Feel amnion through dilated cervix and locate fetal head.

d. Rupture membranes as anteriorly as possible with Amnihook or similar device.

e. Allow fluid to escape while maintaining or guiding fetal head against the cervix using fundal pressure and intravaginal hand.

f. DO NOT REMOVE INTRAVAGINAL HAND UNTIL FETAL HEAD IS FIRMLY APPLIED TO CERVIX AND OVERT CORD PROLAPSE HAS BEEN RULED OUT.

g. Recheck fetal heart rate.

How to Judge the Quality of Induced Labor

1. If the monitor shows no evidence of fetal distress (late decelerations, fetal tachycardia or bradycardia) the labor is not too strong. Obviously if there is evidence of fetal distress, the labor, no matter how poor, is too vigorous.

2. If the cervix is showing the effects of labor (progressive effacement and dilatation), the labor is not too weak.

3. If the cervix is not dilating and contractions seem to be of good quality and frequency, two steps should be taken:

a. Rule out cephalopelvic disproportion, usually by x-ray pelvimetry.

b. Institute internal uterine contraction monitoring to measure the actual strength of contractions.

Risks of Induction

1. Fetal Prematurity. Traditionally, the most common complication of induced labor. If induction is for medical reasons, the risk of prematurity should be weighed against that of continued pregnancy. Before elective induction, fetal maturity should be documented by ultrasonography or L/S ratio.

2. Uterine Hypertonus. Early in induction, oxytocin may result in elevated resting uterine tone, rather than rhythmic contractions. This may be seen on the monitor as so-called "pit contractions" lasting upwards of several minutes. Unless there is an associated fetal bradycardia, the physician may observe, and it will pass as contractions become regular.

3. Fetal Distress. Usually secondary to too much oxytocin too quickly. The remedy is to turn off oxytocin infusion and begin other conservative measures for fetal distress (see Chap. 9, Fetal Distress). If there is no response in 5 minutes, delivery should be considered.

4. Water Retention/Hyponatremia. In dosages greater than 40 milliunits per minute, oxytocin can cause a significant antidiuretic effect. This blocks free water clearance, or the excretion of water without salt, and can result in significant hyponatremia. It may be avoided by administering oxytocin in a salt solution (Ringer's lactate or half-normal saline).

5. Ruptured Uterus. A rare complication secondary to excessive doses of oxytocin, usually when an I.V. has been left to run "wide open" by mistake.

6. Postpartum Hemorrhage. After a long oxytocin-stimulated labor, there is a tendency toward postpartum atony. This may be avoided by continuing the oxytocin for at least 1 hour after the delivery of the placenta.

SECOND-TRIMESTER INDUCTION

Basic Principles

1. Usually done between 16 and 24 weeks gestation, there is rarely expectation of delivering a live child.
2. All considerations are for avoiding maternal morbidity and mortality.
3. The cervix is tremendously resistant to dilatation in the second trimester.

Indications

1. Elective abortion (16 to 20 weeks gestation)
2. Maternal jeopardy (16 to 24 weeks), usually severe cardiovascular or renal disease or malignancy
3. Abnormal fetus documented by amniocentesis (16 to 24 weeks)

Contraindications

1. *To All Methods*

Previous uterine surgery predisposing to uterine rupture.

2. *To Saline Infusion*

Severe cardiac or renal disease, coagulopathy

Agents

1. Hypertonic saline, intra-amniotic installation
2. Hyperosmolar urea, intra-amniotic installation
3. Prostaglandins (F2α, E), intra-amniotic installation, extra-amniotic installation, vaginal suppositories, intravenous infusion, oral ingestion
4. Intravenous oxytocin, usually used in combination with one of above agents

Intra-amniotic Hypertonic Saline: 20-per-cent NaCl

1. Methods

a. Prepare patient as for labor (N.P.O., S.S.E., bladder evacuation).

b. Begin sedation prior to installation, usually a narcotic/tranquilizer combination (meperidine/promazine; morphine/diazepam).

c. Prepare and drape abdomen.

d. Infiltrate site of injection (usually 1 in. from midline and midway between symphysis pubis and top of fundus) with local anesthetic.

e. Perform amniocentesis using 14 or 16 gauge needle, and insert polyethylene tubing through needle into amnion. Remove needle.

f. Remove 100 to 300 ml of amniotic fluid (as much as possible up to 300 ml.) and replace with an equal volume +50 ml of 20-per-cent saline.

g. Begin infusion of high-dose oxytocin (50 to 100 milliunits/min.) intravenously within several hours.

h. Continue oxytocin infusion until at least 1 hour after delivery.

i. Delivery usually occurs within 48 hours. Installation of intra-amniotic saline may be repeated once after 2 days if there has been little effect.

j. If after 2 installations, delivery cannot be effected, hysterotomy should be performed.

2. Risks

a. Hyperosmolar crisis (precipitated by hypertonic saline infusion)

b. Congestive heart failure (saline loading)

c. Disseminated intravascular coagulation (saline loading and placental necrosis)

d. Water intoxication (high-dose oxytocin without electrolyte solution)

e. Postpartum hemorrhage

f. Septic shock (prolonged labor)

g. Incomplete abortion (Approximately 20 to 50 per cent of patients will require curettage for complete removal of the placenta).

Intra-amniotic Hypertonic Urea: 30- to 40-per-cent Urea in 5-per-cent Glucose

1. Method

a. Prepare patient as for labor (N.P.O., S.S.E., bladder evacuation).

b. Begin sedation prior to installation, usually a narcotic/tranquilizer combination (Meperidine/promazine; morphine/diazepam).

c. Prepare and drape abdomen.

d. Infiltrate site of injection (usually 1 in. from midline and midway between symphysis pubis and top of fundus) with local anesthetic.

e. Perform amniocentesis using 14 or 16 gauge needle, and insert polyethylene tubing through needle into amnion. Remove needle.

f. Remove 100 to 300 ml. of amniotic fluid.

g. Replace with an equal volume of 30- to 40-per-cent urea in D_5W.

h. Begin infusiuon of high-dose oxytocin (300 to 400 mu/min.) intravenously.

i. Continue oxytocin until 1 hour after delivery.

2. Risks

a. Water intoxication (high-dose oxytocin)

b. Postpartum hemorrhage

c. Septic shock (prolonged labor)

d. Incomplete abortion

Unlike hypertonic saline, hypertonic urea crosses membranes easily. Therefore the risk of hyperosmolar crisis and congestive heart failure is much less. Disseminated intravascular coagulation is also much less likely than with saline.

Prostaglandins

1. Intra-amniotic Installation

a. Prepare patient as for labor (N.P.O., S.S.E., bladder evacuation).

b. Begin sedation prior to installation, usually a narcotic/tranquilizer combination (meperidine/promazine; morphine/diazepam).

c. Prepare and drape abdomen.

d. Infiltrate site of injection (usually 1 in. from midline and midway between symphysis pubis and top of fundus) with local anesthetic.

e. Perform amniocentesis using 14 or 16 gauge needle and insert polyethylene tubing through needle and insert polyethylene tubing through needle into amnion. Remove needle.

f. Inject a test-dose of 5 mg. (1 ml.) of prostaglandin $F_2\alpha$ (PGF2 α—Prostin F2 alpha) slowly. Observe for reactions such as chest pain, vomiting, or bronchospasm.

g. After 5 minutes, inject an additional 35 mg. (7 ml.). Tape the catheter in place. Await labor.

h. If abortion is not imminent within 24 hours, a second dose of PGF2 α may be injected in the same fashion after verifying the catheter placement.

i. If labor and delivery are not imminent 24 hours after the second injection, or if the membranes rupture, oxytocin infusion is added until 1 hour after delivery.

2. Risks

a. Water intoxication (if oxytocin must be added)

b. Incomplete abortion (slightly higher than for hyperosmolar saline)

c. Nausea, vomiting, diarrhea, flushing, tachycardia, chest pain, and bronchospasm (all side effects of prostaglandins)

d. Sepsis (prolonged labor)

e. Postpartum hemorrhage

3. Other Routes for Prostaglandin Administration

Currently, these other methods of prostaglandin administration are experimental. In the near future they may be available.

a. *Extraovular.* Prostaglandin F2α may be injected via pump through a balloon catheter inside the cervix, or placed there in a gel. This may be useful when amniotic fluid is scant, such as from 13 to 15 weeks gestation.

b. *Vaginal Suppository.* PGE2 is currently under investigation as a vaginal suppository. Its side effects are basically those of prostaglandins.

c. *Intravenous and Oral Prostaglandins.* At present, seem to be characterized by a higher rate of side effects than the intra-amniotic or extraovular routes of administration.

9. Intrapartum Fetal Monitoring

David H. Fields, M.D.

BASIC PRINCIPLES

1. The most stressful and dangerous part of pregnancy for the fetus is labor and delivery.

2. Fetal damage during labor is due to interruption of the fetal oxygen supply. This is usually (but not always) a progressive series of hypoxic events.

3. The fetal heart is more sensitive to oxygen deprivation than the fetal brain, so the fetal heart rate (FHR) changes secondary to hypoxia and asphyxia precede brain damage and death and can be used as an early warning system.

4. Continuous electronic FHR monitoring is a sensitive *screening* method for detecting these changes. Determination of fetal *pH* is an accurate method for evaluating the extent of oxygen deprivation and overall fetal condition.

5. These two methods, in combination allow the doctor to detect fetal distress and correct it or terminate labor before permanent fetal damage occurs.

6. The gadgetry of fetal monitoring IS NOT a substitute for clinical judgment. It IS a tool to sharpen clinical judgment.

CONDUCT OF FETAL MONITORING DURING LABOR

External Electronic Monitoring (EEM)

1. All Labors

a. Begin monitoring of all labors with external fetal heart and uterine contraction sensors.

b. If adequate facilities are not available to monitor all labors, special consideration should be given to the following conditions, with initiation of electronic monitoring.

(1) Preeclampsia/eclampsia/chronic hypertension

(2) Diabetes mellitus

(3) Postdates labor

(4) Prematurity

(5) Suspected intrauterine growth retardation

(6) Oxytocin-induced or stimulated labor

(7) Prolonged labor

(8) Prolonged rupture of membranes

(9) Maternal cardiac or pulmonary disease likely to predispose to hypoxemia

2. Clear Recording Reassuring Patterns

a. Continue EEM as long as the recording is clear and only reassuring patterns (see Tab. 9-1) are noted. This is acceptable because a normal FHR recording is very good evidence of a fetus

Tab. 9-1. **Reassuring FHR Patterns**

a) Baseline FHR between 120 and 160 beats per minute (BPM). 100 and 120 BPM and 160 and 180 BPM, although not usual, are acceptable ranges if no other abnormal conditions are present.
b) Good short term baseline variability (5 to 15 BPM)
c) No change in FHR baseline with contractions
d) Accelerations of FHR with contractions or with fetal movement
e) Mild to moderate Type I decelerations

not in distress. IT IS ALSO NONINVASIVE.

3. Unclear Recordings

a. Unclear FHR recording

(1) The Doppler or phonosensor may not be in good apposition to the mother's skin. REAPPLY THE SONOLUCENT JELLY.

(2) The fetus may have descended in the birth canal during the course of labor

(a) RESEARCH MATERNAL ABDOMEN FOR AREA OF BEST RECORDING.

(b) ADJUST THE DEPTH FOCUS OF YOUR SENSOR IF YOUR EQUIPMENT HAS THIS FEATURE. Optimal depth is usually 8 to 12 cm.

(3) If it is impossible to obtain a clear recording of the FHR externally, SWITCH TO INTERNAL FHR MONITORING.

b. Unclear uterine contraction recording

(1) The tocodynamometer may be too tightly or loosely applied to the mother's abdomen. CHECK BY MANUAL PRESSURE ON THE TOCODYNAMOMETER TO MIMIC A UTERINE CONTRACTION (UC).

(2) Shifts in maternal position tend to change the pressure against the tocodynamometer. TRY SHIFTING MATERNAL POSITION.

(3) If an adequate recording cannot be obtained, and there are periodic FHR changes which must be correlated with contractions, SWITCH TO INTERNAL UC MONITORING.

4. Ominous Patterns *(See Tab. 9-2)*. If an ominous pattern is present on EEM, this must be investigated further. The first step in this process is to rule out an artefact by switching to internal electronic monitoring (IEM). In addition to being more reliable, IEM also gives more precise information regarding beat-to-beat variability.

Tab. 9-2. **Nonreassuring FHR Patterns**

a) Tachycardia (more than 180 beats per minute)
b) Bradycardia (less than 100 beats per minute)
c) Decreased beat-to-beat variability (less than 5 beats per minute, unless this is the only abnormality or the mother has received sedation or analgesia)
d) Severe early (Type I) deceleration (FHR drops to less than 60 beats per minute)
e) Late (Type II) deceleration of any magnitude
f) Variable (Type III) deceleration of any magnitude

Internal Electronic Monitoring (IEM)

1. When to Initiate

IEM should be used whenever an unclear recording or an ominous FHR pattern is obtained using EEM. Some physicians routinely use internal FHR monitoring when the fetal membranes are ruptured.

2. Clear Recording/Reassuring Patterns

If IEM is instituted and a clear recording and reassuring patterns are noted, continue until delivery. Like EEM, a normal FHR recording is very good evidence of a fetus not in distress.

3. Unclear Recording

a. Unclear FHR Recording

(1) Most monitors are keyed to respond to the R spike of the fetal EKG. If the electrode wires are reversed on the ground plate of the mother's legs, this may be read as a Q by the machine and not recorded properly. TRY REVERSING THE ATTACHMENT OF THE ELECTRODE WIRES TO THE GROUND PLATE. This is the simplest adjustment to make and should be tried first.

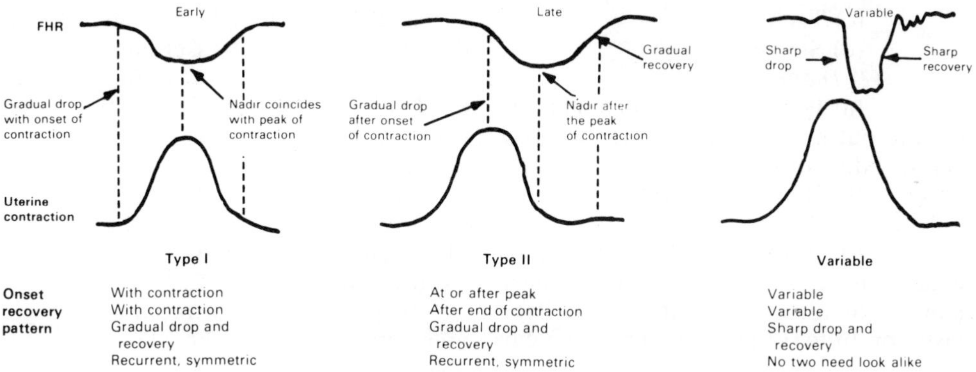

Fig. 9-1. Pattern of Contractions.

(2) Another common cause of an unclear FHR record using IEM is poor application of the electrode. CHECK THE APPLICATION OF THE ELECTRODE BY VAGINAL EXAM AND REAPPLY IF NECESSARY.

(3) If the recording is intermittently unclear and cannot be improved by the above measures, it may represent transient fetal arrhythmia. CHECK WITH A FETAL EKG STRIP.

b. Unclear UC Recording

(1) The problem easiest to remedy is a plug in the catheter. FLUSH THE SYSTEM WITH NORMAL SALINE AND RECALIBRATE.

(2) If the above does not work, the catheter may be out of position. ATTEMPT TO REPOSITION THE CATHETER.

4. Ominous Patterns. If IEM confirms the presence of an ominous pattern, a fetal scalp *p*H should be obtained and appropriate steps (see specific patterns below) taken immediately to correct the cause of the abnormal pattern (while awaiting *p*H results.)

a. *Tachycardia*

(1) *Causes*

(a) Fetal Hypoxia/acidosis

(b) Maternal or fetal fever (amnionitis)

(c) Fetal arrhythmia (especially paroxysmal atrial tachycardia, PAT)

(d) Maternal medication such as scopolamine and atropine

(e) Prematurity

(2) *Diagnostic Steps*

(a) Perform pelvic examination to rule out cord prolapse and evaluate cervical dilation.

(b) Obtain fetal *p*H.

(c) Take maternal temperature.

(d) Obtain fetal EKG to rule out PAT.

(e) Consider medications given.

b. *Bradycardia*

(1) *Causes*

(a) Hypoxia

(b) Arrhythmia (congenital heart block)

(c) Mistaken measurement of maternal heart rate

(2) *Diagnostic Steps*

(a) Perform pelvic examination to rule out cord prolapse and evaluate cervical dilatation.

(b) Obtain fetal *p*H.

(c) Obtain fetal EKG.

c. *Decreased Beat-to-Beat Variability (BBV)*

(1) *Causes*

(a) Asphyxia/acidosis

(b) Sedation and anticholinergic agents

(c) Tachycardia

(d) Sleeping baby

(2) *Diagnosis*

(a) Perform pelvic examination to rule out cord prolapse and evaluate cervical dilatation.

(b) Obtain fetal *p*H.

(c) Review medications.

(d) If after the above three procedures have been performed, no cause can be found, and the decreased BBV lasts for 10 to 30 minutes, the fetus can be presumed to be sleeping.

d. *Late Deceleration*

(1) *Causes:* Hypoxia

(2) *Diagnosis*

(a) Perform pelvic examination to rule out cord involvement and assess cervical dilatation.

(b) Obtain fetal *p*H, pO_2.

(c) Obtain maternal blood pressure.

e. *Variable Deceleration*

(1) *Causes.* Cord occlusion

(2) *Diagnosis*

(a) Perform pelvic examination to rule out cord prolapse.

(b) Shift maternal position to see if pressure is relieved.

(c) Test fetal *p*H to determine severity of fetal compromise.

THERAPY FOR ABNORMAL PATTERNS

While Awaiting *p*H Results

Once fetal compromise is suspected or diagnosed, begin conservative therapeutic measures pending return of *p*H results. These therapeutic measures are based on strengthening the following links in the maternal-to-fetal oxygen chain.

1. To increase maternal pO_2.

a. Nasal O_2 at 4 to 6 L. per min.

2. To increase maternal cardiac output.

a. Place mother in left lateral position relieving great vessel compression.

b. If regional anesthesia has been used, elevate legs and fluid load with Ringer's lactate solution.

c. Rule out shock.

3. To increase uterine blood flow.

a. Decrease intensity and frequency of uterine contractions by stopping oxytocin stimulation, if any.

b. In the near future, B-adrenergic uterolytic agents may be generally available to stop or slow spontaneous labors.

4. To increase placental function—NO MEASURES AVAILABLE.

5. To relieve obstruction of umbilical cord.

a. Change maternal position, usually to left lateral, then right lateral or Trendelenberg.

6. To increase fetal cardiac output—NO MEASURES AVAILABLE.

After Obtaining *p*H Results

1. If *p*H is more than 7.25, continue conservative therapeutic measures and repeat *p*H only if ominous patterns persist.

2. If *p*H is between 7.20 and 7.25, continue conservative measures and repeat *p*H in 20 to 30 minutes.

3. If *p*H is less than 7.20, repeat immediately and if confirmed, perform immediate delivery unless abnormal fetal heart rate patterns have reverted to normal. In this case, repeat *p*H in 15 minutes.

If *p*H Monitoring Is Not Available

If *p*H monitoring is not available, the abnormal FHR may be watched unless there are late decelerations, severe variable decelerations, or severe bradycardia or tachycardia. If any of these are present, the conservative therapeutic measures above should be applied for 15 to 30 minutes. If the fetal heart rate patterns have not reverted to normal by this time, immediate delivery should be performed, by forceps if safe, or by cesarean section.

GLOSSARY OF FETAL MONITORING

Fetal Distress. Danger to the welfare of a fetus, usually on the basis of hypoxia, acidosis, or asphyxia

Biochemical Terms

Hypoxia—pO_2 below normal (for fetus less than 20 torr)

Acidosis—*p*H below normal (for fetus less than 7.20 to 7.25)

Asphyxia—Combined hypoxia and acidosis

Electronic Fetal Heart Rate Monitoring

Instantaneous fetal heart rate—The number of beats which the heart would make in 1 minute calculated from the interval between any two consecutive beats (e.g., two beats are 1 second apart → 1FHR of 60 BPM; two beats are ½ second apart → 1 FHR of 120 BPM)

Baseline fetal heart rate—The rate between contractions of an unstressed fetus

Acceleration—Transient increase of fetal heart rate

Deceleration—Transient slowing of fetal heart rate

(Early) Type I deceleration (dip)—Repetitive, gradual decrease and recovery of fetal heart rate which inversely patterns associated UC.

Type II deceleration—Repetitive, gradual drop and recovery of fetal heart rate which begins after UC, peaks near end of UC, and recovers after UC.

Type III deceleration—Variable, sharp drop and recovery of fetal heart rate which may occur in any temporal relation to fetal heart rate and may or may not recur.

Combined—A late extension (functional Type II) may be superimposed over either Types I or III if they are complicated by hypoxia.

Bradycardia—Persistent slowing of fetal heart rate to less than 100 OR baseline of less than 100

Tachycardia—Persistent increase of fetal heart rate to more than 180 OR baseline of more than 180

Variability

Short-term—BBV of instantaneous fetal heart rate

Long-Term—Undulations of baseline over several minutes

10. Anesthesia and Analgesia

David H. Fields, M.D.

DEFINITIONS

1. Analgesia. Pain relief without loss of sensation

2. Anesthesia. Loss of all sensation

3. General Anesthesia. Anesthesia by induction of loss of consciousness, usually via a combination of injectable and inhalation agents

4. Conduction Anesthesia. Anesthesia created over an area of the body by anesthetizing a major nerve trunk, also known as regional anesthesia

5. Local Anesthesia. Anesthesia in a given area by injection in that area.

BASIC PRINCIPLES

1. Obstetrical anesthesia and analgesia are complicated by the attempt to provide the mother relief without affecting the fetus, treating "two patients at one time." This attempt is never wholly successful.

2. While anesthesia usually is needed for a given period of time, for a specific operative procedure, analgesic requirements during labor frequently seem open-ended.

3. The choice of analgesic agent or anesthetic method should be made taking into consideration such factors as its:

a. Duration of action

b. Likelihood of causing fetal depression

c. Effect on mother's cardiorespiratory status (especially in women whose labors are complicated by hypertension, hemorrhage or fetal distress)

d. Effect on labor

4. The need for analgesia during labor may be significantly decreased or eliminated by antepartum prepared-childbirth classes.

ANALGESIA

The basic purpose of analgesia during labor is to prevent undue maternal suffering. This is usually accomplished using a narcotic analgesic, with or without a tranquilizing agent.

NARCOTIC ANALGESICS: (e.g., Meperidine, Morphine)

Basic Principles

1. All agents in this class have essentially the same effect: pain relief and central nervous system depression (especially respiratory).

2. Their effects are roughly proportional to dosage.

3. They all cross the placenta to cause fetal neurologic depression.

Advantages

1. Their effects are short-lived. When given intravenously, or intramuscularly in reasonable doses, (meperidine 50 to 100 mg., morphine 5 to 10 mg.), their effects peak in one-half to 1 hour intramuscularly, and within minutes intravenously, and are gone in 3 to 6 hours.

2. They are easily and completely reversible. Virtually instantaneous and complete reversal of narcotic depression is obtained with naloxone (Narcan), a pure narcotic antagonist.

3. They may be administered by any physician.

Disadvantages

1. Fetal respiratory depression at birth may be severe. Narcotic analgesics are a major cause of low Apgar scores.
2. Fetal heart-rate patterns as seen on electronic monitoring lose variability.
3. Complete pain relief is not obtained without loss of consciousness.
4. They create reflex nausea and vomiting of short duration.

Administration

1. Given either intravenously (quicker onset, shorter duration) or intramuscularly, doses of 50 to 100 mg. of meperidine (5 to 10 mg. of morphine) may be used either alone or with a tranquilizer (e.g., promethazine) as needed.
2. One should attempt to use as little as possible, but enough to do the job. A good end-point is no discomfort between contractions, combined with easily tolerable contractions.
3. Avoid giving a dose within 1 to 2 hours of delivery, if possible, to avoid neonatal depression. Since the fetal liver is not fully functional at birth, narcotic effects tend to persist in the neonate once he is separated from the mother's metabolic system.
4. Avoid administration too early in labor. Heavy doses of analgesia before 3 or 4 cm. cervical dilatation may slow or even stop early labor.

NARCOTIC ANTAGONISTS

1. Until recently, all narcotic antagonists (e.g., nalorphine, levallorphan) also had an agonist effect, severely limiting their usage and effectiveness.
2. Today naloxone (Narcan), a pure antagonist with no depressive effect of its own, offers a safe effective method for reversing narcotic depression, both in the mother and the neonate.
3. NALOXONE DOES NOT REVERSE DEPRESSION CAUSED BY ANY OTHER MEDICATIONS OR SITUATIONS. IT IS ONLY EFFECTIVE FOR COUNTERACTING NARCOTICS.
4. Dosage is as follows:
   a. Adult: one ampule containing 0.4 mg.
   b. Neonatal: one ampule containing 0.02 mg.
5. These drugs should be administered in the following manner:
   a. Intravenous: onset of action in less than 1 minute
   b. Intramuscular: onset within 2 to 3 minutes
   c. In cases of severe neonatal depression suspected to be secondary to narcotics, naloxone should be administered via the umbilical vein, if it is readily available; otherwise it should be given intramuscularly.
   d. If severe neonatal respiratory depression is anticipated because of heavy maternal narcosis, the physician may give the mother an intravenous dose (0.4 mg.) several minutes before delivery.

TRANQUILIZERS

1. The most commonly used agents are phenothiazine derivatives (such as promethazine in dosages of approximately 25 mg.).
2. They are usually used in combination with a narcotic.
3. They offer the advantages of nausea relief and reduction of maternal anxiety.
4. They offer the disadvantage of not being reversible.
5. Agents of the benzodiazepine group (e.g., Valium, Librium) generally have long-lasting (several days) depressive effect on the fetus.
6. Scopolamine is sometimes used in doses of 0.3 to 0.4 mg. either I.V. or I.M., in combination with a narcotic or tranquilizer. However, this has become less common because of the fetal tachycardia which results.

ANESTHESIA

AGENTS FOR REGIONAL OR LOCAL ANESTHESIA

1. For most regional and local anesthesia in obstetrics, the injectable agents are largely interchangeable.

2. All agents listed below are indicated for all types of regional and local anesthesia except spinal, with the exception of procaine and tetracaine, which may be used for spinal anesthesia.

3. All should be used without epinephrine for two reasons:

a. Epinephrine may slow labor.

b. If oxytocin becomes necessary, it may cause severe hypertension when used in the presence of a vasopressor.

4. The side effects and risks of all the agents are essentially the same, with the exception of prilocaine, which in addition to its other effects, may precipitate an acute attack of methemoglobinemia or exacerbate a preexistent case.

5. The agents, with their average duration in hours, are listed below:

DURATION OF ACTION OF ANESTHETICS

chlorprocaine	(Nesacaine) ½–1 hr.
procaine	(Novocain) ½–2 hrs.
piperocaine	(Metycaine) 1–1½ hrs.
lidocaine	(Xylocaine) 1½–2½ hrs.
mepivacaine	(Carbocaine) 1½–2½ hrs.
prilocaine	(Citanest) 1½–3 hrs.
tetracaine	(Pontocaine) 1½–6 hrs.

ANESTHESIA FOR LABOR

Paracervical Block

1. Indication. Relief from the pain of uterine contraction and cervical dilatation. Additional anesthesia is necessary for delivery.

2. Method

a. Prep the vagina with povidone iodine (Betadine).

b. Determine cervical dilatation.

c. Use a needle director (e.g., Iowa trumpet which allows no more than 0.5 to 1 cm. of the needle to project beyond it).

d. Place the guide in the lateral vaginal fornix somewhere between the 3 and 4 o'clock position (or 8 to 9 o'clock). If injections are made at 3 and 9 o'clock positions, this is called a paracervical block. If they are at 4 and 8 o'clock, it is termed an uterosacral block. They are functionally the same.

e. Aspirate to be sure there is no blood.

f. Inject 10 ml. of anesthetic solution.

g. Repeat on the other side.

h. Observe the fetus with continuous fetal heart rate monitoring.

i. Since this anesthesia typically lasts 1 to 2 hours, it may have to be repeated.

3. Risks

a. Maternal toxicity with rapid absorption of repeated doses of large amounts of anesthetic agent are a real risk.

b. Fetal bradycardia has been described shortly after injection in up to 25 per cent of paracervical blocks. This is most likely secondary to high fetal levels of anesthetic.

c. If a large paracervical vein is lacerated, a considerable hematoma may result.

d. Inadvertent injection of the drug directly into the fetus is a real and very dangerous risk.

e. Allergic reaction may occur to any of the "caine" drugs.

4. Contraindications. The following conditions should prevent one from performing a paracervical block.

a. Fetal distress

b. Full cervical dilatation

c. Allergies to the "caine" drugs

Continuous Lumbar Epidural Anesthesia

See the following section on Anesthesia for Delivery.

ANESTHESIA FOR DELIVERY

Local Infiltration

1. Indications

a. Episiotomy

b. Cesarean section is rarely done using local anesthesia.

2. Method

a. After sterilely prepping and draping the perineum, infiltrate each side of the area requiring anesthesia with 10 to 20 ml. of local anesthesic.

b. Avoid injection directly into a blood vessel. This can be done by attempting to aspirate through the needle before every injection. If blood is obtained, reposition the needle and try again.

3. Advantages

a. There is essentially no risk of anesthetic mortality.

b. Performed in the delivery room, there is essentially no effect on the fetus if recommended dosages are used.

c. It is easily and quickly administered by any physician.

4. Risks. The complications of local anesthesia are rare and usually minor:

a. Allergic reaction to "caine" drugs

b. Local hematoma

c. Systemic toxicity, if too much is used, rarely

5. Contraindications. The only contraindications to local anesthesia are:

a. Allergy to the "caine" drugs

b. Local infection

Pudendal Block

1. Indications Relief of perineal pain during birth or episiotomy

2. Method

a. Holding a needle guard (e.g., Iowa trumpet) between two fingers of one hand, it is guided intravaginally to the lower edge of the ischial spine on one side.

b. A long 20- to 22-gauge needle which protrudes from the end of the guard by no more than 0.5 cm. is then passed through the vaginal mucosa and to the sacrospinous ligament.

c. Three to 4 ml. of anesthetic is injected after first attempting to aspirate blood (see local anesthesia).

d. The needle is then advanced past the ligament and another 3 to 4 ml. injected after attempted aspiration.

e. The needle is then withdrawn, a second puncture made slightly higher up the ischial spine, and another 3 to 4 ml. injected.

f. The procedure is then repeated on the other side.

3. Advantages

a. By blocking the pudendal nerve with its branches of the second through fourth sacral nerves, the perineum can be effectively anesthetized for delivery.

b. If recommended anesthetic dosages are not exceeded, and intravascular injection does not occur, maternal and fetal drug effects are essentially none.

c. It may be easily administered by any physician.

4. Risks

a. See Risks of Local Infiltration (facing column).

b. If the pudendal artery or vein is lacerated, a sizable hematoma may occur. This is usually prevented by the pressure applied by the descending fetal head. However, if the block is performed after delivery, for repair of the perineum, this safety precaution is absent.

Caudal Anesthesia

1. Indication

a. Relief of perineal pain during delivery or episiotomy, when lumbar epidural anesthesia cannot be performed.

b. If a greater volume of more dilute anesthetic solution is given, the level of anesthesia rises and relief from the pain of labor may be obtained.

2. Method

a. Prep and drape the sacrum and coccygeal area with the patient in the left lateral Sims' position.

b. After making a skin wheal over the sacral hiatus, the needle, (17 to 18 gauge), is passed through the skin at a

90° angle until it has entered the sacral hiatus. The sacrococcygeal membrane will be felt as it is pierced.

c. A syringe is now used to aspirate and inject a small amount of air. No blood or spinal fluid should be obtained on aspiration. No resistance should be encountered on injecting the air. If there is resistance, the needle may be either in maternal soft tissue, or in the fetus. Remove it.

d. Once entry to the caudal space has been verified, depress the needle almost parallel to the skin and advance it approximately 1 in. into the canal.

e. Now thread approximately 2 to 3 in. of a plastic catheter (19 to 20 gauge) through the needle into the caudal space. If resistance is met, try angulating the needle somewhat. *Never pull back on, or attempt to withdraw the catheter through the needle*. The bevel of the needle may cut the catheter leaving a piece inside the canal.

f. Once the catheter is placed, withdraw the needle, tape the catheter down, and inject a test dose of approximately 5 ml. of anesthetic agent.

g. If no evidience of spinal anesthesia, such as lower extremity paralysis, occurs in 5 min., an additional 20 to 25 ml. of anesthetic is injected.

h. The catheter is left attached to a syringe and may be left in place for additional anesthesia as required.

i. Maternal blood pressure and fetal heart rate are closely monitored.

3. Risks. Being a form of epidural anesthesia, caudal block carries all the risks of such including hypotension, drug toxicity from large volumes of anesthetic, and impaired labor. See Lumbar Epidural Anesthesia for a discussion of these.

4. Contraindications

a. Local infection
b. Pilonidal cyst
c. Neurologic disease
d. Maternal hypotension
e. Maternal hypertension
f. Fetal distress

Continuous Lumbar Epidural Anesthesia

1. Indications

a. Complete relief of the pain of both labor and delivery, whether vaginal or transabdominal, may be obtained using epidural anesthesia.

b. If used for labor and vaginal delivery, the anesthesia should extend from T10 to S4. For Cesarean section dermatomes up to T8 and possibly T6 need to be anesthetized.

c. Because of the risks and complexity of the method it is usually not used for short labors.

2. Method. Epidural anesthesia is usually performed by an anesthesiologist, especially in major centers.

a. Fluid load the patient with at least 500 ml. and up to 1,000 ml. of Ringer's lactate before performing the puncture. Keep a running I.V. throughout.

b. Measure the patient's blood pressure before performing the puncture. If it is not normal, stop.

c. Prep and drape the woman lying on her left side with her legs flexed and back straight. Her shoulders should be aligned perpendicularly to the table, to prevent spinal rotation.

d. Anesthetize the skin and underlying tissues of any one of the lumbar interspaces.

e. Introduce a Tuohy needle (16 gauge) with stylet into the center of anesthetized space until the ligamentum flavum is punctured. This will be accompanied by a sudden loss of resistance.

f. Attach a syringe and first aspirate. If neither blood nor spinal fluid is obtained, inject 2 to 3 ml. of air. It should enter without resistance.

g. Insert a plastic catheter (18 to 20 gauge) through the needle and advance it either up or down the canal. As stated in the section on caudal anesthesia, never withdraw the catheter through the needle inside the canal.

h. After again aspirating and checking position of the catheter, remove the needle and tape the catheter in place.

i. Inject a test dose of 2 to 5 ml. of anesthetic and wait 2 to 3 mintues.

j. If no evidence of spinal anesthesia occurs, (rapid anesthesia, lower extremity paralysis) inject an additional 10 to 25 ml. of anesthetic solution.

k. Turn the patient to her back and begin to check her blood pressure every 1 to 2 minutes for at least 20 minutes.

l. Institute continuous fetal heart rate monitoring as soon as the anesthetic is injected.

m. Administer additional anesthetic agent as required.

3. Risks

a. *Hypotension.* Maternal hypotension occurs much less frequently than with spinal anesthesia, but it is not rare. Because vascular pooling in the lower half of the body secondary to sympathetic blockade results in decreased venous return, cardiac output falls, resulting in hypotension. It is both more common and more dangerous in women who are hypovolemic, usually from hemorrhage or preeclampsia.

The best treatment is avoiding the problem by preloading with saline. If it occurs, it is usually corrected by rapid infusion of 500 to 1,000 ml. of Ringer's lactate or normal saline combined with elevation of the mother's legs or shifting her to the left lateral position. Vasopressors are rarely necessary but should always be available.

b. *Fetal Distress.* Fetal heart rate changes suggestive of distress occur commonly after epidural anesthesia. They may be due to maternal hypotension resulting in decreased uteroplacental blood flow or to the high fetal levels of anesthetic agent which may result from the large amounts necessary for continuous epidural anesthesia during labor.

c. *Interference with Labor.* If administered before active labor and cervical dilatation of 3 to 4 cm. have occurred, epidural anesthesia may considerably slow labor, perhaps by interference with Ferguson's reflex. It may also interfere with "pushing" in the second stage by eliminating sensations of rectal pressure and uterine contractions.

Early dysfunction can be overcome with oxytocin infusion. An attendant telling the patient when a contraction is beginning and enthusiastically urging her to "push" is usually sufficient to compensate for the lack of rectal pressure. If it is not, forceps rotation may be required.

d. *Postpartum bladder distention* frequently results if there is no catheter, because the patient is not aware of the urge to urinate.

e. *Risk of Spinal Blockade.* If the injection of anesthetic is inadvertently intraspinal, since such large volumes are used, total spinal blockade with cardiac and respiratory arrest may occur.

4. Contraindications

a. Maternal hemorrhage, either present or anticipated

b. Maternal hypertensive disease, especially preeclampsia

c. Fetal distress

d. Need for immediate anesthesia

e. Local infection

f. Neurologic disease

Spinal Anesthesia

1. Indications

a. Introduction of an anesthetic directly into the spinal canal may be performed for either vaginal or abdominal delivery.

b. Because it is a single injection technique, it is not indicated for labor itself.

c. Epidural anesthesia is preferable if it can be achieved, since the incidence of side effects is lower.

2. Method

a. Fluid load the patient with Ringer's lactate or normal saline. Keep a running I.V. in place.

b. Measure the patient's blood pressure. If it is not normal, stop.

c. With the patient sitting over the edge of a bed or table, her whole spine flexed (and held by an assistant), prep the area around the L3–L4 interspace.

d. Anesthetize the skin and underlying tissues.

e. Perform a "spinal tap" with a small gauge spinal needle and stylet.

f. Obtain a free flow of spinal fluid from the needle.

g. Inject a small amount of an appropriate anesthetic agent. For vaginal delivery 1.0 to 1.5 ml. will suffice, while 2.0 to 2.5 ml. may be needed to obtain a high enough level for cesarean section.

h. Remove the needle, apply pressure to the puncture site for a moment and turn the mother to the supine position with her head elevated slightly.

i. Measure maternal blood pressure every minute for 10 to 15 minutes after placement of the anesthetic.

j. Adjust the level of anesthesia as it develops, by tilting the patient up or down.

3. Risks

a. *Postspinal Headache.* Continued leakage of fluid from the puncture site may occur for several days and result in headaches which are very resistant to treatment. It is best to avoid this as much as possible by using a very small needle (25 or 26 gauge) for the puncture. Many also keep the woman flat for 12 hours after spinal anesthesia.

Once headaches have begun to occur, treatment by abdominal binders or placement of "spinal patches" yields variable degrees of success.

b. *Hypotension.* This tends to be more common, more severe, and more sudden than with epidural anesthesia.

c. *Fetal Distress.* See *Risks of Epidural Anesthesia.*

d. *Interference with Labor.* See *Risks of Epidural Anesthesia.*

e. *Bladder Dysfunction.* See *Risks of Epidural Anesthesia.*

f. *Arachnoiditis/Meningitis.* With the advent of sterile technique, disposable equipment, and single-dose containers of anesthetic, these have become rare complications.

4. Contraindications. The reasons to avoid spinal anesthesia are the same as those for not performing epidural blocks.

General Anesthesia

1. Indication

a. *Vaginal Delivery.* While general anesthesia used to be commonly used for vaginal delivery, it is now much less resorted to. The wide availability of prepared childbirth classes supplemented by local and regional anesthesia for operative vaginal deliveries has reduced the need for general anesthesia tremendously. It is now routinely used if:

(1) Anesthesia is needed on a moment's notice, e.g., repair of a cervical laceration or operative delivery for fetal distress.

(2) Intrauterine manipulation is attempted, e.g., delivery of a second twin, or difficult manual removal of a placenta.

(3) Postpartum curettage is necessary.

(4) Delivery of a malformed or stillborn child is anticipated.

b. *Cesarean Section.* General anesthesia is acceptable anesthesia for any Cesarean section, unless the mother has eaten very recently. It is the anesthesia of choice for abdominal delivery under the following circumstances:

(1) Any emergency delivery, where anesthesia is needed quickly, e.g., cord prolapse, fetal distress.

(2) Any condition is present which contraindicates regional anesthesia, e.g., fetal distress, maternal hypotension or hypertension.

2. Risks

a. Aspiration of gastric contents is the most common cause of obstetric anesthetic death. Since gastric emptying is so delayed in pregnancy, and especially during labor, there is a grave risk of aspirating acidic stomach contents during the reflex vomiting which may occur during anesthesia induction and reversal.

(1) *The following steps may be taken to reduce the risk:*

(a) Enforce at least an 8-hour, and preferably longer, fast before general anesthesia, if possible.

(b) Administer 30 ml. of an antacid before anesthesia. Even if she has fasted, never assume the patient has an empty stomach. Only a few ml. of highly acid fluid can be dangerous.

(c) Perform endotracheal intubation as soon as possible after induction of anesthesia.

(d) Extubate her when the patient is awake enough to cough and keep her head down and to the side.

(2) *If aspiration of gastric contents does occur, the following maneuvers should be taken:*

(a) Immediate removal of all particulate matter in the pharynx followed by examination of the vocal cords for other material. Bronchial lavage is no longer practiced.

(b) Immediate administration of large doses of corticosteroids, e.g., 1 g. of hydrocortisone I.V. followed by 250 mg. I.V. q.6h. Although the efficacy of this regime is unproven, there is a general feeling that it may help. If it is to be of any use, it must be given early in the course.

(c) Antibiotic coverage with a broad spectrum agent, e.g., ampicillin 1 g. I.V. every 6 hrs. or an appropriate dose of cephalosporin.

(d) Immediate chest radiograph, for baseline evaluation.

(e) Immediate blood gas measurement.

(f) Oxygen by mask, cannula or reintubation if necessary in concentrations sufficient to maintain pO_2 above 60 torr.

(g) Close observation of the patient for 24 hours, even if her condition does not seem to require it.

3. General Anesthetic Agents

a. *Inhalation Anesthetics*

(1) NITROUS OXIDE

(a) By itself, nitrous oxide cannot provide anesthesia. Used in a 40- to 50-per-cent mixture with oxygen for analgesia, it does not provide surgical anesthesia or relaxation until concentrations reach 80 to 85 per cent. At this level, maternal-fetal hypoxia is inevitable.

(b) However, in 60 to 70 per cent mixtures with oxygen it may be used very effectively for "balanced anesthesia" (see below) in combination with other agents.

(2) CYCLOPROPANE. This agent is being used less frequently because of major risks of cardiac arrhythmia, severe fetal depression, uterine atony, and serious explosion which accompany its use.

(3) ETHER. Illegal to even keep in many states, ether is no longer, to my knowledge, used in obstetrics in this country.

(4) HALOTHANE (FLUOTHANE), METHOXYFLURANE (PENTHRANE), AND ENFLURANE (ETHRANE)

(a) These are all halogenated agents used for general anesthesia.

(b) All are potent myometrial relaxants and may be used for intrauterine manipulation, although halothane and enflurane seem more effective. They also cause increased intrapartum and postpartum blood loss.

(c) All cause severe respiratory depression in both mother and fetus and are usually not used for delivery.

(d) Halothane may be hepatoxic.

(e) Methoxyflurane may be nephrotoxic.

b. *Intravenous Agents.* The ultrashort-acting barbiturates, such as thiopental when given intravenously, induce virtually instantaneous loss of consciousness without unpleasant sensations. Unfortunately, they do not provide adequate muscle relaxation or anesthesia for surgery, and would rapidly cross the placenta to cause severe fetal depression if used to maintain unconsciousness.

c. *Balanced Anesthesia*

(1) For cesarean section, the use of a short-acting barbiturate, a muscle relaxant, and a combination of nitrous oxide/oxygen with narcotic analgesia has evolved.

(2) It is used as follows:

(a) When everyone is ready to begin surgery, the patient is "put to sleep" with a dose of short-acting barbiturate, e.g., thiopental, after a small dose of d-tubocurarine to prevent fasciculation.

(b) She is then paralyzed with succinylcholine and intubated.

(c) Anesthesia is maintained with a nitrous oxide (70 per cent)/oxygen (30 per cent) mixture until the baby is born.

(d) After birth of the baby, anesthesia is continued with nitrous oxide/oxygen supplemented with intravenous narcotic analgesics.

(3) It offers the advantages of:

(a) Rapid, pleasant induction

(b) Minimal fetal depression

(c) Easy, safe reversal

11. Immediate Care of the Newborn

David H. Fields, M.D.

BASIC PRINCIPLES

1. The most immediately important aspect of making the transition from intrauterine to extrauterine life is the ability to breathe. If a newborn is breathing well, most likely he is not seriously ill. If he is not breathing adequately, he will need resuscitation.

2. Next in importance of consideration to the obstetrician, is the rapidity with which the newborn infant loses heat to his environment. He must be kept warm.

3. Apgar scoring at 1 minute gives a good indication of the need for resuscitation. At 5 minutes, it prognosticates subsequent perinatal course.

MANAGEMENT

1. Upon delivery of the infant's head, the obstetrician may choose to suction the nose and pharynx. If the delivery is complicated by the presence of thick meconium in the amniotic fluid, this should be done before the infant breathes. If there is no meconium, it may be postponed until the delivery of the infant is completed.

2. Following completion of the delivery, the infant is held, head down, and suctioned if it has not already been done.

3. Next, the cord is clamped. There has been considerable controversy in the past regarding delayed or immediate clamping of the cord. In most cases of otherwise normal babies it makes no particular difference. If there is reason to suspect fetal anemia, delaying the clamping and holding the infant below the level of the perineum will infuse him with extra volume and extra red cell mass. On the other hand, if the infant is premature, extra volume may overload him. One should not intentionally "transfuse" the premature infant.

4. After clamping the cord, the infant is placed in slight Trendelenberg position in a warmer, to prevent heat loss to the environment. Radiant heating devices have been found to be best for this.

5. At this time the 1-minute Apgar scoring is done. See Tab. 11-1.

6. Immediate further care is based on Apgar score.

a. If the score is 8 or above, no resuscitation is needed and routine care is instituted.

b. If the score is 4 to 7, the infant is considered moderately depressed and probably needs some stimulation, but not active resuscitation.

c. If the score is below 4, the infant

***Tab. 11-1.* Apgar Scoring.**

Sign	*0*	*1*	*2*
Heart rate	absent	below 100	over 100
Respiratory effort	absent	slow; weak cry	good
Muscle tone	flaccid	some flexion of extremities	well flexed active motion
Reflex irritability	none	grimace	vigorous cry
Color	blue	body pink; extremities blue	completely pink

is seriously depressed and active immediate resuscitation should be started.

CARE OF THE NEWBORN

Care of the Moderately Depressed Infant

1. Mild mechanical stimulation may "wake up" the infant. Tapping his soles, rubbing his back, or "puffing" him with air from a suction bulb are acceptable methods. Sphincter dilatation, thoracic compression, and vigorous slapping of the back may do more harm than good.

2. Simultaneously bathing the infant's face in a flow of oxygen without applying the mask to his face may be of help.

3. If neither of the above has sufficient effect and there is any question of narcotic suppression because of maternal medications, one ampule of naloxone (0.02 mg.) neonatal should be given I.M.

4. The above will almost always serve to "resuscitate" the moderately depressed infant, so routine care may resume.

Care of the Severely Depressed Infant

1. The severely depressed infant has a slow heart rate and poor respiration as well as being neurologically depressed. Usually these are on the basis of hypoxia, so immediate resuscitation after clearing the pharynx and nose should consist of administration of oxygen via face mask. This should be administered as short "puffs" in rapid sequence at a pressure of about 15 to 20 cm. of water.

2. If after 1 minute of this therapy, the infant's condition has not improved, endotracheal intubation with a search for a site of obstruction should be performed. Oxygen should then be administered in the same manner via the endotracheal tube.

3. While this is in progress, a second attendant should be placing an intravenous line, preferably in the umbilical vein. This line may then be used for administration of the following medications:

a. Naloxone 0.02 mg, I.V. if narcotic suppression is suspected

b. Sodium bicarbonate 3 to 4 mEq. initially; if resuscitation is not rapidly successful, further doses are guided by blood gas and *p*H measurements drawn from the umbilical artery line which should also be placed at this time.

4. Resuscitation may continue in this fashion as long as the infant is ventilated and has a cardiac output, as estimated by his heart rate.

5. In the event of cardiac arrest, artificial ventilation is continued at the rate of 30 to 40 "breaths" per minute. This is best done by light pressure with two fingers on the lower sternum. If there is a palpable femoral pulse in response to massage, effective circulation is being maintained. Intracardiac epinephrine may also be given in treating cardiac arrest.

6. If resuscitation is successful, the infant is transferred to a neonatal intensive care unit for further care.

Resumption of Routine Care

If the infant needed no resuscitation or only mild stimulation, routine care may be finished in the delivery room. This consists of:

1. Drying the infant

2. Applying a clamp and shortening the remaining umbilical cord

3. Applying silver nitrate 1-per-cent to the infant's eyes as prophylaxis for gonococcal ophthalmitis. Penicillin or tetracycline ointments may also be used.

4. Permanently identifying both fetus (foot print) and mother (fingerprint) on a single piece of paper before either leaves the delivery room

5. Conducting a rapid physical examination for congenital anomalies

12. Routine Postpartum Care

David H. Fields, M.D.

IMMEDIATE POSTPARTUM CARE

Definitions

1. Care rendered after the third stage of labor, but before the completion of the puerperium, is termed postpartum care.

2. The puerperal period begins directly after the delivery of the placenta and ends with the return of the reproductive tract to a normal nonpregnant condition, usually by 6 weeks postpartum.

3. Postpartum care may be divided into immediate postpartum care, subsequent in-hospital care, and late postpartum care, generally rendered at home.

Basic Principles

1. The most common early postpartum problem is hemorrhage, which most frequently becomes manifest during the first hour after delivery.

2. To focus awareness on the need for constant attendance with the mother during this period, it is sometimes called the "fourth stage of labor." It is usually managed in a "recovery room."

3. Like problems at other times during pregnancy, immediate postpartum problems are best dealt with before they occur.

Routine Immediate Postpartum Management

1. Account for all sponges and gauze pads before the patient leaves the delivery room. Always perform a final vaginal examination to insure the removal of any sponges.

2. Be certain the amount of blood draining from the vagina is normal before removal of the patient from the delivery table.

3. Check lochia, pulse, and blood pressure every 15 minutes for the first hour. If any begin to rise, further investigation is warranted.

4. Check firmness and height of the uterine fundus every 15 minutes for the first hour. If it begins to rise or soften, massage to enhance uterine contraction.

5. Many physicians routinely continue an infusion of oxytocin through the first hour, thereby avoiding the most common cause of postpartum hemorrhage, uterine atony. This may consist of 10 to 20 units of oxytocin per 1,000 ml. of D_5W or salt solution. It may be infused at the rate of 100 to 200 ml. per hour.

6. Ergot alkaloids (Ergotrate, Methergine) 0.2 mg. may be given I.M. immediately postpartum in place of the oxytocin, or in addition to it.

7. Many women desire to nurse their newborn child immediately after delivery. If the mother and child are both in good medical condition, there is no reason to discourage this. The physician might even encourage it, as the suckling will aid in contracting the uterus.

8. Even if all seems well, allow no food during the first hour. Sips of water may be taken.

9. If blood loss during labor was considered excessive, but vital signs are stable, measure hematocrit in the first hour.

10. Be alert for difficulty urinating. The patient can usually void using a bed pan or if allowed to the bathroom with assistance. If she cannot, however a full bladder may predispose to uterine atony.

If necessary, perform catheterization after 8 to 12 hours.

ROUTINE IN-HOSPITAL CARE AFTER THE FIRST HOUR POSTPARTUM

Basic Principles

1. As hospital stays have become shorter, more postpartum management must be conducted at home. Whereas women were previously routinely watched for several days to a week, most are now home within 3 to 4 days

2. The major problems in the first days after delivery are:

a. Postpartum bleeding and/or shock

b. Infection, especially of the uterus, episiotomy site, and bladder

c. Urinary difficulty

d. Poor return of bowel function

e. Breast problems, especially engorgement

f. Postpartum hypertension

g. Thombophlebitis

3. Care at this time is directed toward avoiding these problems, or detecting them early if they do occur.

Routine Postpartum Orders

1. Bedrest for several hours after delivery, then ambulation as soon as tolerated by the patient. Early ambulation is of singular importance in avoiding phlebitis.

2. Regular diet. The sooner a normal diet is resumed, the sooner normal bowel function begins.

3. Vital signs four times daily

4. Fundal palpation several times daily, with attention to quantity and quality of lochia

5. Void or catheterize every 6 to 8 hours, p.r.n. The use of catheterization can frequently be avoided if the patient is encouraged to use the bathroom rather than the bed pan; if necessary, however, it is preferable to a full bladder.

6. Perineal care, consisting of cleansing and drying several times daily

a. Frequent use of an ice pack in the first 24 hours, helps avoid swelling.

b. After the first 24 hours, witch hazel pads or a heat lamp may provide additional comfort.

7. Breast and abdominal binders, as needed for the patient's comfort

8. Hemoglobin and hematocrit determination on the second postpartum day

9. Analgesia with

a. A narcotic analgesic (codeine 30 to 60 mg. P.O. q.4h. p.r.n. or its equivalent)

b. A salicylate (aspirin gr. X P.O. q.4h. p.r.n.) or a nonsalicylate (acetaminophen gr. X P.O. q.4h. p.r.n.)

c. A combination of the above.

10. Sleeping medication (e.g., Seconal 100 mg. P.O. h.s. p.r.n. or Dalmane 30 mg. P.O. h.s. p.r.n.)

11. Cathartic (milk of magnesia 30 ml. P.O. h.s.) on the second night and if necessary, an evacuatory suppository (e.g., Dulcolax) or enema on the third day

12. Rh_0 D Immune Globulin (Rho GAM), 1 vial, should be administered to all unsensitized Rh_0 (D) negative or D^u negative mothers who deliver Rh positive infants, within 72 hours.

13. Agents to Suppress Lactation may be indicated for mothers not breastfeeding

a. *Deladumone OB 2 ml. I.M.* This combination of 180 mg. of testosterone enanthate and 8 mg. estradiol valerate, if given shortly before or directly after delivery, suppresses lactation in more than half of postpartum women, and decreases it in almost all. There is a risk of masculinization from the testosterone and possibly of an increased incidence of postpartum phlebitis and thromboembolism secondary to the estrogen.

b. *Diethylstilbestrol 5 mg. P.O. t.i.d. for 3 days.* This, like Deladumone, has been shown to be effective in suppressing lactation. It, however, has also been associated with an increased incidence of puerperal venous disease.

c. *Ice Packs, Support, and Compression.* While not as comfortable as hormonal suppressives, these simple mechanical measures will, when combined with mild analgesia, provide a safe method for dealing with engorgement. The patient usually tolerates them well if their safety is explained.

DAILY POSTPARTUM ROUNDS

Abnormalities in any of the following should be investigated:

1. Vital signs
2. Breasts
3. Uterine fundus
4. Lochia
5. Perineum
6. Bladder and bowel function
7. Extremities

Vital Signs

1. Pulse. Tachycardia in the sitting or standing position is frequently the first sign of excessive blood loss. It is also frequently secondary to fever.

2. Blood Pressure

a. Low blood pressure may reflect blood loss if the patient is experiencing dizziness or faintness, or if present with tachycardia. Otherwise, it is likely normal for a healthy young woman.

b. High blood pressure, if due to preeclampsia, may persist for several days or weeks postpartum, and should be treated as described under "Preeclampsia." If not secondary to preeclampsia, or another preexistent condition, it should receive appropriate workup and management.

3. Temperature

a. Febrile morbidity is defined as a temperature greater than 100.4 F (38°C) on any 2 of the first 10 postpartum days after the first 24 hours.[1]

b. Any fever should be investigated with an eye toward:

(1) Endometritis

(2) Urinary tract infection

(3) Infected episiotomy

(4) Thrombophlebitis of extremities or pelvis

(5) Breast pathology

(6) Upper respiratory infection or pneumonia if anesthesia was used during delivery

c. Appropriate workup should usually include examination of pelvic organs, lungs, breasts, extremities, as well as a complete blood count and clean-catch urinalysis, and special studies as indicated.

4. Breasts

a. Lactation and milk let-down generally occur within two or three days after delivery.

(1) Lactation is the result of the action of prolactin after the fall of progesterone levels effected by delivery of the placenta.

(2) Milk let-down occurs secondary to oxytocin's contractile effect on the myoepithelial cells of the breast.

(3) These are accompanied by tremendous breast engorgement and perhaps by mild fevers. Temperature, however, should not be elevated above 101°F, nor last more than several hours on the basis of breast engorgement.

5. Breastfeeding Mothers

a. Most medications are secreted in breast milk, and should be avoided as much as possible.

b. Nipple fissures secondary to overly aggressive suckling are both painful and dangerous because they provide a route for breast infection. If they occur, treatment should include:

---

1. Joint Committee on Maternal Welfare.

(1) Nursing with a breast shield

(2) Topical emolient and antibiotic creams

(3) Careful gentle cleansing and drying

c. If these are ineffective:

(1) Stop nursing from the affected side.

(2) Maintain lactation with breast pumping until the fissure is healed.

d. Good support for lactating breasts will make them much more comfortable.

6. Non-Breastfeeding Mothers

a. Hormonal suppression of lactation as described in immediate postpartum care, may be attempted. However, as noted, these are being used less frequently as more side-effects are described.

b. If hormonal suppression is not used, or is not successful, symptomatic relief can be achieved with:

(1) Tight support

(2) Frequent use of ice packs

(3) Analgesia

(4) Explanation to the mother that this is a self-limited problem which only lasts several days

7. Uterine Fundus

a. Directly after delivery, the fundus contracts to a level midway between the umbilicus and symphysis, then rises two or three finger-breadths above that. Over the next several days, it involutes at the rate of one or two finger-breadths per day, so that by the tenth postpartum day, it is a pelvic organ.

b. Apparent delay in involution should suggest possibly retained placenta, but is more likely due to incomplete emptying of the bladder, pushing the uterus upward.

c. Uterine tenderness after vaginal delivery suggests myoendometritis, and is usually accompanied by fever and abnormal lochia. (See section on Lochia).

d. Afterpains are the rhythmic contractions by which the uterus avoids atony. They are greater in multiparas and nursing mothers. Analgesia may be prescribed as needed.

8. Lochia

a. The vaginal discharge associated with involution of the uterus may persist and maintain a reddish color for several weeks after delivery, even until the first menstrual period.

b. The physician should be alert for lochia which is heavier and bloodier than normal, foul-smelling, or purulent. These suggest:

(1) Endometritis—usually associated with fever; lochia of streptococcal endometritis may be neither foul-smelling nor purulent.

(2) Retained secundines—usually associated with heavy bleeding and subinvolution of uterus.

(3) Retained vaginal sponge—odor is prominent.

c. Management of these consists of:

(1) Examination for foreign bodies and subinvolution

(2) Transcervical culture of the endometrial cavity

(3) Antibiotics after culture, if the patient is febrile. Ampicillin (500 mg. P.O. q.6h.) or a cephalosporin (same dose) is a good starting point in the not-too-ill patient while awaiting culture reports. If the patient is considered critically ill, treatment should be started with a combination of two or three parenteral antibiotics. This is usually an aminoglycoside (gentamicin 3 to 5 mg. per Kg. per day in 3 doses I.V. or kanamycin 500 mg. I.M. b.i.d.) in combination with a penicillin derivative (ampicillin 1 g. I.V. q.6h.) or clindamycin (1,200 to 2,400 mg. per day in 3 or 4 divided doses I.V.) or both. Inappropriate antibiotics may then be discontinued when culture reports return.

(4) Curettage as needed for retained secundines

9. Perineum

a. It is normal for the perineum to be swollen and sore for a day or so after delivery, especially if episiotomy was performed. After the first day, this is best managed with local heat or topical anesthetics.

b. If the episiotomy is hot or red or purulent, it may be presumed to be infected. Management in this case consists of:

(1) Culture of discharge, if any

(2) Local heat

(3) Antibiotics (ampicillin or cephalosporin 500 mg. P.O. q.6h., pending culture and sensitivity reports)

(4) Drainage of any collection of pus

c. If it is necessary to open an episiotomy because of infection, healing should be by secondary intention. Cosmetic or functional repair may be done at a later date.

10. Bladder

a. Bladder function may be impaired for up to several days after delivery secondary to

(1) Traumatic delivery

(2) Conduction anesthesia

(3) Immediate postpartum urinary retention with distention

b. A distended bladder may be detected as a suprapubic cystic mass or, indirectly, by its elevating the fundus to above the umbilicus. This should be checked several times daily in the first few days.

c. If the patient cannot void

(1) Catheterize every 6 to 8 hours

(2) If repeated catheterization is necessary or severe distention occurs, place an indwelling Foley catheter for 2 or 3 days.

d. If the patient has urinary incontinence in the first few days, catheterize for residual urine to rule out overflow incontinence.

11. Bowels

a. It is not unusual for the normal postpartum woman to go several days without a bowel movement, especially if she had enemas prior to delivery. This is not the medical emergency some patients think it is. It may be remedied with gentle laxatives (e.g., milk of magnesia, 30 ml. P.O. h.s.) for several days if necessary, or with enemas.

b. Soreness of the episiotomy site may inhibit bowel movements. This may be treated with stool softeners, glycerin suppositories, and local or systemic analgesia.

c. If there has been a fourth-degree laceration with repair, many physicians use parts or all of the following regime for bowel regulation:

(1) Low residue diet for one or two days

(2) Regular diet subsequently with stool softeners (e.g., Colace 100 mg. P.O. t.i.d. or Peri-colace, one capsule b.i.d., a mild cathartic).

(3) No rectal temperatures or enemas

(4) No mineral oil

(5) Systemic antibiotic (e.g., ampicillin 500 mg. P.O. q.6h. for several days)

d. Hemorrhoids regress several days after delivery. Symptomatic relief with seating cushions (doughnuts), topical analgesia (witch hazel, Anusol), and stool softeners usually suffices.

12. Extremities

a. The key to reducing postpartum phlebitis is early ambulation.

b. For patients who have varicose veins, (which tend to improve after delivery), support stockings are helpful.

REMAINDER OF THE PUERPERIUM

Discharge from the Hospital

This is usually between the second and fourth postpartum days and is permitted if the patient has no signs of infection, retained secundines, or urinary retention.

Patient Instructions

1. Sexual Activity

a. Most physicians recommend against sexual activity until the lochia has completely disappeared and many until after the postpartum check (traditionally at 6 weeks).

b. When the puerpeal woman resumes having sexual intercourse she should be warned of the following:

(1) Perineal tenderness secondary to an episiotomy is likely to persist for weeks.

(2) Vaginal dryness secondary to decreased estrogen levels is not uncommon and should not be a cause for concern. It will pass spontaneously within a few weeks. It can be overcome with patient foreplay and lubricating jellies if necessary.

(3) Prior to the first menstruation, conception is less likely than normal but quite possible. Contraception should be used from first coitus.

2. Mastitis

a. This may occur after the first postpartum week in a breastfeeding mother.

b. It is usually signaled by:

(1) Tender breasts, which are hot and engorged and may be locally reddened

(2) Fever and chills

(3) Possible breast abscess formation with fluctuance

c. It may be unilateral or bilateral.

d. Treatment consists of:

(1) Discontinuation of breastfeeding from both breasts since the infant is usually colonized and may infect the other breast in unilateral cases

(2) Antibiotics—since the most common organism is Staphylococcus aureus, either an appropriate semisynthetic penicillin, a cephalosporin, or erythromycin should be used.

(3) Drainage of abscess, if present, should be performed.

13. Forceps Delivery

David H. Fields, M.D.

BASIC PRINCIPLES

1. Obstetrical forceps are used to effect vaginal delivery which might otherwise occur after a longer period of time.
2. They should not be used in situations where a more effective second stage would not produce vaginal delivery (cephalopelvic disproportion).
3. Maximum force applied should not exceed 60 Kg. This is a crude number and has little meaning to the obstetrician. His experience must guide him.

DEFINITIONS

1. Low Forceps (Outlet Forceps). The fetal head is on the perineum and the sagittal suture is the midline (occiput anterior or posterior).

2. Midforceps. After engagement, until the head is on the perineum and in the direct occiput anterior or posterior position, the delivery will be midforceps. An artificial category of low midforceps, with the head on the perineum but in an oblique position, is used by some.

3. High Forceps. Use of blades prior to engagement of the fetal head. Although one never says "never" in medicine, this is about as close as one may get.

INDICATIONS

1. To shorten the second stage of labor for maternal benefit:
   a. Severe cardiac disease
   b. Cerebrovascular disease
   c. Severe preeclampsia
   d. Maternal exhaustion
2. To shorten the second stage of labor for fetal benefit:
   a. Fetal distress
   b. Premature placental separation during second-stage labor
   c. Correction of abnormal fetal position (e.g., persistent occiput posterior, asynclitism)
3. To deliver the aftercoming head in a breech delivery

APPLICATION OF FORCEPS DELIVERY

Prerequisites for Application of Forceps

1. Cervix fully dilated
2. Membrane ruptured
3. Fetal head engaged
4. Position of fetal head known
5. Adequacy of pelvis known

Additional Precautions

1. Bladder empty
2. Rectum empty
3. Pelvis well anesthetized

Application and Delivery

1. Always use a cephalic rather than a pelvic application, applying the blades appropriately to the fetal head.
2. If the left blade is always introduced first, crossing of the shanks will not be necessary.
3. Once the blades have been applied check position:
   a. Sagittal suture is midline between the blades and perpendicular to them.
   b. Fenestrations (if any) admit one finger on each side.

c. Posterior fontanelle is one finger's breadth above handle of blades.

4. If rotation is necessary, the handle of the blades should be swung in a wide arc so that rotation occurs around the midpoint of the blades, and the tips do not describe a wide arc. Rotation around the handles is a common cause of vaginal vault laceration.

5. Effect delivery by exerting traction in the axis of the pelvis. This may be accomplished by depressing the blades at their midpoint with one hand while exerting traction with the other.

6. Unless immediate delivery is necessary, pull rhythmically, mimicking uterine contractions and delivering gradually.

7. Perform an adequate episiotomy and deliver head slowly to avoid perineal lacerations and fetal brain damage.

8. Remove forceps either before or after delivery of the head. If before, there is less volume to be delivered through the vagina; if after, there is more control during the delivery.

Risks of Forceps Delivery

Maternal

1. Perineal, vaginal, rectal or bladder laceration

2. Cervical laceration or ruptured uterus (lower segment), especially if cervical dilatation is not complete or the fetal head has not descended enough.

3. Symphysis pubis separation, if outlet disproportion exists

Fetal

1. Bruises and cephalohematomas

2. Intracranial injury, especially tentorial tears and subdural hematomas

Specific Forceps Operations

1. Outlet Forceps

a. A low forceps delivery consisting of lifting the head over the perineum

b. Elliott forceps for unmolded heads; Simpson type forceps for molded heads

2. Rotations

a. From oblique or posterior positions to occiput anterior with the head well descended.

(1) May use Scanzoni (double application) or DeLee (key in lock) maneuver.

(2) Must have adequate pelvic room for rotation.

(3) May be better off with delivery as occiput posterior.

(4) Preferably, Tucker-McLean or other thin unfenestrated blades

b. From transverse arrest

(1) Usually done by Kielland's rotation.

(2) Tendency is increasingly to deliver by cesarean section.

3. Delivery of aftercoming head

a. Although the head is backwards, the blades are applied as if it were a vertex presentation.

b. Never hyperextend fetal body to avoid spinal cord injuries.

c. Use Piper long-handled forceps.

Trial and Failed Forceps

1. If under any circumstances, there is a question concerning the possibility of a successful forceps delivery and the criteria for the application of the blades have been met, forceps may be applied. This must be done with the knowledge that the trial may not be successful and with the judgment to stop and perform a cesarean section, if necessary, before damaging either mother or fetus.

2. *There are, unfortunately, no objective criteria for knowing when to stop.* CLINICAL JUDGMENT IS ESSENTIAL. Obviously, a failed forceps delivery indicates that delivery was not safely possible but was attempted. This should not occur too often.

14. Cesarean Section

David H. Fields, M.D.

DEFINITION

Delivery of the infant by incision of the uterine wall.

BASIC PRINCIPLES

1. Cesarean section is a surgical procedure requiring anesthesia and postoperative recovery and carrying all the risks of these. Maternal mortality is two per thousand deliveries or approximately 10 times higher than for vaginal delivery.

2. Cesarean section rates have increased tremendously over the last several years to rates of up to 25 per cent at some centers, and approximately 15 to 20 per cent in most areas.

3. This is

a. Because of the increasing safety of anesthesia and improved postoperative care (electrolyte and fluid management, antibiotics, early ambulation)

b. Because of the increasing indications for cesarean section, especially in the areas of fetal distress and abnormal presentations

TYPES OF INCISION

1. Transverse Lower Uterine Segment Incision (Intraperitoneal). This is the uterine incision of choice unless contraindicated (see classical incision). It usually involves less blood loss, carries a lower risk of rupture during subsequent pregnancy, and lowers the risk of postoperative bowel adhesions when compared with the classical incision. The major disadvantage is a risk of extension laterally, tearing the major uterine vessels.

2. Vertical Lower Uterine Segment Incision. Used much less commonly, this incision requires extensive dissection of the bladder from the uterus. It does offer the option of extension upwards, if necessary, but also carries the risk of tearing down into the vagina or bladder.

3. Classical Incision. Beginning above the lower uterine segment and coursing upward to the fundus, this incision is usually only indicated in cases of placenta previa, transverse fetal lie, or carcinoma of the cervix which may make lower segment surgery dangerous or difficult.

INDICATIONS FOR CESAREAN SECTION

A cesarean section is indicated when delivery is required and cannot be performed vaginally because it will take too long or because it will endanger the mother or the fetus.

1. Cephalopelvic Disproportion. This is the most common indication for cesarean section during labor. It is diagnosed either by pelvimetry or by trial of labor with careful monitoring (vertex presentation only).

2. Fetal Distress. Diagnosed by intrapartum fetal monitoring, this is an indication for cesarean section when conservative measures (see Chapter 9 on Fetal Monitoring) fail and vaginal delivery is not imminent. A true medical emergency, it is usually performed with general anesthesia for utmost speed.

3. Prolapsed Umbilical Cord. Another true emergency, this situation requires immediate delivery. This can be accomplished only by cesarean section unless full dilatation is present and the patient is multiparous.

4. Placenta Previa. If total, this is a mandatory indication for cesarean section. If marginal or partial, vaginal delivery may be attempted, but extreme watchfulness must be the rule and immediate cesarean section must be available, and should be prepared for in advance.

5. Placental Abruption. If attended by torrential hemorrhage, maternal shock or fetal distress, this should be treated by immediate cesarean section. Otherwise, labor may be induced as long as there is careful fetal and maternal monitoring and cesarean section is immediately available if necessary.

6. Abnormal Presentation

a. There is essentially no choice but cesarean section in cases of:

(1) Transverse lie or shoulder presentation

(2) Face presentation with posterior chin

(3) Footling breech or hyperextended breech

(4) Interlocking twins

b. In addition, cesarean section is increasingly used (although not mandatory) for the following situations related to abnormal presentation:

(1) Breech complicated by almost anything (prematurity, postmaturity, large fetus, mild pelvic abnormality, uterine dysfunction, maternal disease such as diabetes or preeclampsia, desire for sterilization)

(2) All face presentations

(3) Brow presentations

c. Finally, in some centers cesarean section is being used to deliver all breech presentations.

7. Preeclampsia/Eclampsia. If this necessitates delivery prematurely and induction is unsuccessful or will take too long, cesarean section is indicated. Usually induction is possible.

8. Diabetes. Like preeclampsia, diabetes frequently requires early fetal delivery. Currently, long inductions are out of favor, and cesarean section is becoming increasingly popular.

9. Erythoblastosis Fetalis. This is another disease frequently requiring early delivery, although it is becoming increasingly rare. If induction is not possible, ceasarean section should be performed.

10. Maternal Gynecologic Malignancy. Carcinoma of the cervix or ovary discovered in the third trimester should indicate cesarean section followed by appropriate therapy. For carcinoma of the cervix, a classical incision should be made to avoid cutting through tumor.

11. Previous Surgery. If the patient has had previous surgery invading the endometrial cavity through the uterine wall, elective cesarean section is usually performed. This includes previous cesarean section, transmural myomectomy, and correction of uterine abnormalities.

12. REPEAT CESAREAN SECTION. While most physicians routinely advocate repeat cesarean section even if the original indication was a nonrecurring one (cord prolapse, breech, etc.), some physicians will allow subsequent labor.

The following conditions should be met:

a. Initial postoperative course should have been without infection.

b. The mother should have had a successful delivery prior to the cesarean section.

c. Intensive fetal and maternal intrapartum surveillance should be conducted.

d. Cesarean section should be prepared for in advance and literally available "at a moment's notice."

e. Labor should be uneventful.

PREPARATION FOR CESAREAN SECTION

1. Nothing by mouth, preferably for at least 8 hours.
2. 30 ml. of antacid P.O. prior to surgery
3. Abdominoperineal prep
4. Preoperative CBC and urinalysis
5. Preoperative Foley catheterization
6. Type and crossmatch 2 units packed red blood cells, preoperatively
7. Running intravenous system, preferably through 18-gauge catheter
8. Preoperative medication with anticholinergic agent only, usually atropine sulfate, 0.4 mg.

ANESTHESIA

Almost always general, epidural or spinal. (See Chap. 10, Anesthesia/Analgesia.)

POSTOPERATIVE MANAGEMENT

1. Bedrest for 24 hours, followed by progressive ambulation
2. Vital signs every 15 minutes until stable, then every 4 hours.
3. Nothing by mouth for first 12 to 24 hours, then progressive increase in diet depending on patient's condition
4. Intravenous fluids providing 2,500 to 3,000 ml. of water, 70 to 140 mEq. of NaCl, and at least 100 g. of sugar per 24 hours. Continue until oral intake is adequate. Add 40 to 60 mEq. of potassium chloride on the second day.
5. Foley catheter discontinued within the first 24 hours after surgery, unless there has been bladder trauma
6. Hemoglobin and hematocrit measurement of the first evening and following morning of the surgery
7. Pain relief as required, usually with narcotics analgesics (e.g., 50 to 100 mg. Demerol q.4h. p.r.n.)
8. Sleeping medication as required

15. Complications of Labor

David H. Fields, M.D.

DYSFUNCTIONAL LABOR

Definitions

1. Normal labor is divided into three stages.

a. *Stage I.* From beginning of labor to full cervical dilatation

b. *Stage II.* From full dilatation to birth

c. *Stage III.* From delivery of the child to delivery of the placenta

2. Stage I labor is also divided into several phases:

a. *Prodromal or Latent Phase.* Contractions are mild, irregular and short (less than 45 seconds); usual duration several hours; some cervical effacement, little dilatation.

b. *Active Phase.* Contractions are strong, regular (usually every 2 to 3 minutes) and last longer (more than 45 seconds); complete effacement, dilatation up to 8 cm. at the rate of at least 1.2 cm. per hour in primiparas and 1.5 cm. per hour in multiparas.

c. *Deceleration Phase.* Contractions are somewhat shorter, perhaps weaker, and less often; completes dilatation.

3. Dysfunctional labor is an abnormality in any of the stages or phases of labor (usually either Stage I or Stage II). It is characterized by lack of appropriate progress, either in cervical dilatation or descent of the presenting part.

4. Hypotonic dysfunction is characterized by contractions of less than normal intensity.

5. Hypertonic dysfunction (much rarer) is characterized by strong, painful contractions which are uncoordinated.

Hypotonic Dysfunction

When due to contractions of less than normal intensity, prolongation of any stage or phase of labor is hypotonic dysfunction. The following categories have been created:

1. Prolonged Latent Phase

a. *Definition.* Duration of latent phase greater than 20 hours in a "primip" or greater than 14 hours in a "multip." Occurs very early in labor.

b. *Etiology*

(1) Excess sedation

(2) Patient not actually in labor

c. *Risks to Mother/Fetus.* These are essentially created by aggressive intervention. If the membranes are intact, prolonged latent phase is not associated with fetal or maternal risk, only discomfort.

d. *Management.* Most important is to determine that the patient is actually in labor. This can be done by:

(1) *Sedation* for the mother, either a barbiturate (Seconal or Nembutal 100 mg. I.M.) or a narcotic (Demerol 50 mg. I.M.). This will usually result in several hours of good rest after which the patient will awaken either out of labor or in active labor.

(2) *Oxytocin stimulation.* If the mother awakens from sedation and her condition is unchanged, she is most likely in labor. Augmentation with oxytocin infusion then becomes the treatment of choice.

2. Prolonged Active Phase

a. *Definition.* Dilatation of the cervix at less than 1.2 cm. per hour in a primipara and less than 1.5 cm per hour in a multipara, after the active phase of labor has begun.

b. *Etiology*

(1) Cephalopelvic disproportion (CPD)

(2) Fetal malposition

(3) Conduction anesthesia applied too early

(4) Overdistention of the uterus with twins or hydramnios

c. *Risks to Mother/Fetus*

(1) If membranes are ruptured, prolonged labor with risk of amnionitis, fetal distress

(2) Iatrogenic fetal distress with intervention

d. *Management*

(1) *Oxytocin* if CPD is ruled out. Oxytocin stimulation, with all precautions as for augmented induced labor, is indicated.

(2) *Amniotomy*, if membranes are intact

(3) *Cesarean section*. If oxytocin and amniotomy fail to effect dilation in an effaced cervix over 2 to 3 hours, or if fetal distress occurs, Cesarean section should be performed.

3. Prolonged Acceleration Phase

a. *Definition*. Failure of the cervix to reach full dilatation after approximately 8 cm.

b. *Etiology*

(1) CPD

(2) Uterine exhaustion

c. *Risks*. Same as for prolonged active phase

d. *Management*. Same as for prolonged active phase

4. Prolonged Second Stage

a. *Definition*. Second-stage labor lasting longer than 1 hour in multiparas or 2 hours in a primipara.

b. *Etiology*

(1) CPD

(2) Malposition, especially occiput posteriors

(3) Maternal exhaustion with poor expulsive efforts

(4) Conduction anesthesia with poor expulsion efforts

(5) Uterine exhaustion

c. *Risks*. Most of the risks of prolonged second stage are incurred when the physician makes heroic attempts to deliver the baby "from below."

(1) *Fetal Distress*. Damage from prolonged labor or augmentation

(2) *Maternal Injury*

(a) Uterine rupture—secondary to either oxytocin or untended second stage for many hours—this rarely occurs today.

(b) Lower uterine segment, vaginal bladder injury secondary to forceps deliveries

(c) Amnionitis secondary to prolonged labor

d. *Management*

(1) *Oxytocin*. If there is no CPD and the fetal vertex is beyond easy reach of forceps, oxytocin infusion done cautiously is the treatment of choice.

(2) *Forceps*. If there is no CPD and the vertex is at + 2 or + 3 station, forceps delivery may be chosen.

(3) *Cesarean Section*. In cases of oxytocin failure, high vertex, fetal distress, or CPD, transabdominal delivery is the method of choice.

Hypertonic Dysfunction

1. Definition. Uterine contractions which seem to cause pain out of proportion to their strength or effect.

2. Etiology. The uterine musculature contracts in a discoordinated fashion, with midsegment predominance. The result is painful contractions with poor or no cervical dilatation and a soft fundus.

3. Risks

a. Fetal distress from elevated uterine tonus

b. Fetal distress from mistaken attempts to correct this problem with oxytocin

4. Management. Sedation

ABNORMAL PRESENTATIONS

Breech Presentation

1. Definitions

a. *Frank Breech.* Buttocks presenting, flexed hips, extended knees.

b. *Full Breech.* Buttocks presenting, flexed hips, flexed knees.

c. *Footling Breech.* One or both feet presenting

2. Etiology

a. The fetus is assumed to choose the most comfortable position in utero. Therefore, most of the etiologic factors predisposing to a breech position create either less room in the pelvis or more room in the fundus, or a vertex which will not fit in the pelvis under any circumstances (hydrocephalus).

b. They are:

(1) Multiparity
(2) Prematurity
(3) Hydramnios
(4) Hydrocephalus
(5) Placenta previa
(6) Low uterine fibroids
(7) Uterine anomalies
(8) Twins

3. Incidence. Three to 4 per cent of all pregnancies present as breeches.

4. Diagnosis

a. If discovered before the onset of labor, optimum diagnosis is achieved by ultrasonography which involves no radiation.

b. If discovered in labor, the diagnosis is usually made or confirmed by cervical examination.

c. This should be complemented by a flat plate of the abdomen to definitively demonstrate a breech and to define curvature of the cervical spine.

d. If vaginal delivery is contemplated, the physician should also perform x-ray pelvimetry.

5. Risks

a. *Maternal.* There is no appreciable increase in risk for the mother.

b. *Fetal.* There is considerably increased risk for the fetus.

(1) Overall mortality in several series of breech deliveries has ranged up to 25 per cent.

(2) Even when corrected for prematurity and congenital anomalies, (increased twice in breeches), the mortality rate for breech deliveries is still at least two to five times that for vertex deliveries.

c. The major causes of fetal morbidity and mortality are:

(1) Traumatic delivery—especially to the brain, spinal cord, liver, spleen, and adrenal glands
(2) Cord prolapse
(3) Congenital anomalies
(4) Prematurity

6. Management

a. *Cesarean Section.* Increasingly, breech presentation has become an indication for abdominal delivery. Some physicians advocate cesarean section for all breech deliveries, since for all practical purposes, the morbidity and mortality which seems to be inherent in breech vaginal delivery can be essentially eliminated by cesarean section. This is an argument which cannot be refuted. It can only be weighed against the increased maternal morbidity and mortality attendant to cesarean section and possibly repeat cesarean section. Below is a generally accepted list of indications for abdominal delivery of a breech fetus, according to Pritchard and MacDonald:

(1) Fetus with estimated weight over 8 pounds

(2) Premature breech with estimated weight 1,000 to 2,500 g.

(3) Any contracture of the maternal pelvis

(4) Hyperextension of the fetal spine or head

(5) Breech not in labor or not engaged

(6) Footling breech

(7) Dysfunctional labor

(8) Previous perinatal death

(9) Concurrent desire for tubal sterilization

(10) Primiparous breech

b. *Vaginal Delivery.* If the fetus weighs between 2,500 g. and 4,000 g., is a frank breech who has an older sibling, has chosen a mother with a good pelvis, and the physician opts for vaginal delivery, there are several measures that should be taken:

(1) X-ray pelvimetry to verify an adequate pelvis

(2) Careful monitoring of labor with external fetal monitoring until rupture of membranes and internal monitoring after

(3) Maintenance of intact membranes as long as possible to effect a good dilating wedge

(4) Allow spontaneous delivery to the umbilicus, if possible.

(5) Perform a very generous mediolateral episiotomy, preferably under pudendal or caudal block.

(6) From this point the fetus may be grasped by the hips or legs but never around the abdomen, as this is how intra-abdominal organs are traumatized.

(7) After delivery of the arms, maintain flexion of the head by continuous supra-pubic pressure provided by an assistant.

(8) Deliver the head by raising the fetal body above the midline until the chin becomes visible. The Mauriceau maneuver may be used to aid flexion, but should not be used for traction, since it may result in serious injury to the fetus.

(9) Continue the delivery of the head by *slowly* easing out the rest of the fetal skull to avoid tentorial tears and intracranial injury.

(10) If the delivery of the head is not accomplished easily, one should use Piper forceps. These should be on the table, unwrapped and ready for use if needed.

c. ALWAYS TREAT A BREECH DELIVERY WITH THE RESPECT ACCORDED A CESAREAN SECTION. It should always be attended by

(1) Someone skilled in breech delivery

(2) A competent anesthesiologist, and

(3) Someone skilled in neonatal resuscitation

Face Presentation

1. Definition. Extreme extension of the fetal head so that facial organs present against the cervix

2. Etiology. Anything that prevents flexion of the head predisposes to face presentation. This includes:

a. Pelvic inlet contraction

b. Pendulous abdomen

c. Anencephaly

d. Multiple loops of cord around the neck

e. Fetal cervical ligament contracture

f. Low pelvic tumors

3. Risks

a. Usually all major risks are from traumatic intervention.

b. If the chin rotates posteriorly, vaginal delivery is impossible.

4. Management

a. Rule out contracted pelvis.

b. If no pelvic contracture exists and the chin is anterior, spontaneous vaginal delivery may be allowed.

c. If there is any pelvic contraction, if the chin rotates posteriorly, or if operative intervention is contemplated, perform cesarean section.

Brow Presentation

1. Definition. The fetal vertex is midway between full extension (face) and full flexion (occiput). The presenting part at the inlet is essentially the forehead.

2. Etiology. Usually pelvic contraction

3. Risks

a. Engagement cannot occur as long as the brow presentation persists.

b. Rupture of membranes with an unengaged head predisposes to cord prolapse.

4. Management

a. If the fetus can be monitored, labor may be observed to see if the brow spontaneously converts to an occiput or a face presentation.

b. If it converts to an occiput, vaginal delivery is anticipated.

c. If it converts to a face presentation, management is as described in the preceding section.

d. If conversion does not occur, or if fetal distress or dysfunctional labor occur, perform cesarean section.

Transverse Lie (Shoulder Presentation)

1. Definition. The fetus lies perpendicular to the long axis of the uterus. The presenting part may be either a shoulder or the back. A slight variation of this is the *oblique* lie, with the fetus not quite perpendicular.

2. Etiology

a. Contracted pelvis

b. Pendulous abdomen in a grand multipara

c. Placenta previa

d. Prematurity

e. Hydramnios

3. Risks. Vaginal delivery is impossible with a transverse lie; if attempted, maternal and fetal death are significant risks.

4. Management

a. X-ray flat plate of the abdomen to verify the diagnosis.

b. Cesarean section if the lie is transverse at the onset of labor.

Compound Presentation

1. Definition. A combination of an extremity (usually an arm) and either the vertex (usually) or the breech presenting together

2. Etiology. Prematurity is the most commonly identified.

3. Risks

a. Prolapsed cord from failure to occlude the inlet

b. If prolapsed cord does not occur, there is no inherent risk in a compound presentation since labor usually proceeds normally.

4. Management

a. Treat as normal labor until full dilatation.

b. If the prolapsed extremity is not withdrawn by full dilatation, it may be pushed upwards. It is sometimes more effective to pinch the hand or foot so that the fetus retracts it by itself.

Persistent Occiput Posterior (OP)

1. Definition. Vertex presentation which remains in the occiput posterior position after full dilatation. This occurs in about 5 per cent of vertex labors.

2. Etiology

a. Persistent OP with an unengaged vertex is usually due to inlet contraction.

b. OP with an engaged vertex is most likely due to midpelvic dystocia, usually with an anthropoid or android pelvis.

3. Risks

a. If engagement occurs and satisfactory descent follows, the only major risk of an OP delivery is the likelihood of an episiotomy extension because of the greater excursion of the vertex.

b. If descent is impaired or labor dysfunctional, the risk of performing an unintentionally high forceps delivery is also present. This is because in the OP position, unusual elongation of the fetal skull with formation of tremendous caput may occur. In extreme cases, fetal hair may protrude at the vagina with an unengaged head.

4. Management

a. *Spontaneous rotation* to occiput anterior (OA), or *spontaneous delivery* as an OP may occur, especially if labor is aided with oxytocin, and if there is no CPD.

b. *Manual rotation* to OA followed by spontaneous or forceps delivery may be attempted.

c. *Forceps delivery* as an OP or forceps rotation to OA may be performed if there is no CPD. Be sure of the station of the vertex before applying forceps.

d. If any of the above is not easily feasible, cesarean section becomes the preferred method of delivery.

Persistent Occiput Transverse

1. Definition. Arrest of the fetal vertex with the sagittal suture in the transverse position after full cervical dilatation

2. Etiology. Transverse arrest may be divided into two categories, with and without CPD.

a. When complicated by pelvic dystocia, transverse arrest is commonly associated with android or platypelloid pelves.

b. When occurring without CPD, transverse arrest is usually due to hypotonic labor and conduction anesthesia.

3. Risks. The major risk of transverse arrest is an attempted forceps delivery in the face of unsuspected CPD.

4. Management

a. Determine presence or absence of CPD.

b. If CPD is not apparent and labor is not of good quality, an attempt to rotate the head with oxytocin infusion is warranted. If this is not successful, the physician should recheck for the presence of CPD.

c. If the physician is still confident that there is no disproportion, and the head is at plus 2 station or lower, a cautious attempt at forceps delivery may be made.

d. If at any time there is a suspicion of CPD, or measure 2b. and 3c. fail, cesarean section should be performed.

HYDROCEPHALUS

Definition

Internal hydrocephalus is the collection of excess fluid within the ventricles of the brain, resulting in a very large head filled with fluid, and very little brain tissue.

Etiology

Usually due to a blockage in the cerebrospinal pathways at the level of the upper spinal cord, hydrocephalus is frequently associated with spina bifida.

Diagnosis

1. Suspect hydrocephalus when there is an unusually large fundal mass, or when widened fontanelles are felt through the dilated cervix.
2. If hydrocephalus is suspected antepartum, almost certain diagnosis may be made using ultrasonography.
3. If the diagnosis is suspected during labor, confirm it with an A-P film of the abdomen. In vertex presentations this should make the diagnosis. In breech presentations because of the magnification factor, even an A-P film may not be diagnostic of hydrocephalus.

Risks

1. CPD is almost invariable with clinically evident hydrocephalus.
2. If the condition is undiagnosed and labor is allowed to continue without drainage, or even worse, if labor is stimulated, uterine rupture is a real risk.
3. There are essentially no additional fetal risks to decompression since even in mild cases fetal mortality is well over 50 per cent.

Management

The key to management is drainage of the hydrocephalus using a large-bore (16 to 18 gauge) long needle. This may be accomplished:

1. Transcervically in vertices when the cervix is 3 to 4 cm. dilated
2. Transcervically in breeches when the body has been delivered
3. Transabdominally in vertices prior to induction
4. Transabdominally in breeches after the body has been delivered

ANENCEPHALY

Definition

Complete or partial absence of the brain and overlying skull, associated with adrenal and pituitary hypoplasia, is termed anencephaly.

Etiology

1. Probably inherited as a polygenic predisposition, anencephalus may be precipitated by an environmental agent. Currently suspected as an etiologic agent is an enzyme produced by the potato blight organism. About 70 per cent are female.

Diagnosis

1. The first case of anencephalus in a family is frequently diagnosed in the labor room as the infant moves convulsively during each vaginal exam. It may be confirmed by x-ray flat plate or ultrasonography.

2. Subsequent cases are detected by second-trimester amniocentesis for α fetoprotein levels which are elevated in this and other open neural tube defects.

Risks

1. The recurrence rate for future pregnancies is currently accepted to be between 4 and 5 per cent.

2. Prolonged gestation is the rule. This may be due to the hypoplastic or absent pituitary gland.

3. The presentation is usually breech, but this is actually a benefit since the breech is larger than the head. In vertex presentations, which are usually face, shoulder dystocia at the incompletely dilated cervix is not uncommon.

4. Hydramnios is a common complication. In fact, anencephalus is the most common cause of hydramnios.

5. The risk of a surviving child is very small. Most die within a few hours after birth.

Management

1. If anencephalus is diagnosed during the second trimester, the treatment is therapeutic abortion.

2. If it is diagnosed in the third trimester, pregnancy should be terminated by amniocentesis to remove excess amniotic fluid and subsequent oxytocin infusion to induce labor. This may be difficult.

HYDRAMNIOS

Definition

Collection of amniotic fluid in volumes of greater than 2,000 ml. is defined as hydramnios. Clinically significant hydramnios, however, usually involves volumes over 3,000 and 4,000 ml.

Etiology

Excess fluid is associated with a number of conditions and may result from various disturbances of amniotic fluid circulation:

1. Esophageal atresia of the fetus results in impaired swallowing with a very high incidence of hydramnios.

2. Anencephaly and spina bifida result in transudation of fluid across the meninges secondary to direct exposure of cerebrospinal membranes to amniotic fluid.

3. Twin gestation (monoamniotic) may represent greater placental mass and greater urine output into the amnion.

4. Diabetes and erythroblastosis fetalis are frequently associated with hydramnios. This may be related to a large placenta, but this is uncertain.

5. Pulmonary hypoplasia, by inhibiting fetal respiratory inbibing of amniotic fluid, may predispose to hydramnios.

Diagnosis

1. Suspect hydramnios when the uterus is larger than dates and the fetus is difficult to palpate. Fetal heart sounds may also be distant.

2. Document it by ultrasonography or flat-plate radiograph of the abdomen. At the same time, evaluate the fetus for abnormalities.

3. Be alert to the fact that "hydramnios" may be a large cyst.

Risks

The risks of hydramnios may not be generally recognized. Perinatal mortality may approach 50 per cent because of the following factors:

1. Fetal

a. Clinically evident hydramnios is associated with congenital anomalies in up to 20 per cent of cases. Most commonly these are:

(1) Anencephalus

(2) Esophageal atresia

(3) Pulmonary hypoplasia

b. Premature labor secondary to uterine distention is frequent. In acute-onset hydramnios, labor commonly occurs before 28 weeks gestation.

c. Prolapse of the umbilical cord with rupture of the membranes is not uncommon.

2. Maternal

a. Extreme uterine distention leads to an increased risk of placental abruption, dysfunctional labor, and postpartum hemorrhage due to uterine atony.

b. Because of uterine enlargement, dyspnea and venous-compression symptoms of the lower extremities may be severe.

c. There is also a risk of other maternal disease, most notably diabetes.

Management

1. Determine, if possible the presence of fetal abnormalities, by radiograph or ultrasonography.

2. Treat underlying maternal disease such as diabetes, if any.

3. If necessary, for maternal dyspnea or pain relief, perform amniocentesis with removal of several hundred ml. at a time. This may precipitate labor and is used only for maternal necessity, not to prolong pregnancy.

4. If labor begins and seems to be dysfunctional, amniocentesis with removal of several liters of fluid may help in more severe cases.

5. In less severe cases, transvaginal rupture of the membranes with gradual release of the fluid may be attempted. This is accompanied by the risk of cord prolapse.

6. Diuretics and salt restriction are generally ineffective.

PREMATURE LABOR

Definition

Onset of labor before the thirty-seventh week of gestation

Etiology

While a great percentage of premature labors occur for no known reason, the following conditions predispose to prematurity:

1. Multiple gestation
2. Hydramnios
3. Premature rupture of the membranes
4. Preeclampsia
5. Chronic maternal diseases, especially diabetes, heart disease with hypoxia, and urinary tract infection
6. Fetal congenital anomalies

Diagnosis

The diagnosis of premature labor is essentially the diagnosis of labor. Unfortunately, if treatment is likely to be successful it must be begun early, preferably before significant cervical dilatation has occurred.

Risks

Prematurity is the number-one cause of perinatal mortality, principally on the basis of respiratory distress syndrome.

Management

1. Early in threatened premature labor, bedrest in the lateral position will frequently be helpful.

2. Active attempts to stop labor are indicated if:

a. The membranes are intact.

b. The cervix is less than 4 cm. dilated.

c. There is no evidence of fetal anomaly.

d. There is no evidence of fetal distress.

3. Agents currently in general use for arresting premature labor are:

a. *Alcohol*

(1) Use a 10-per-cent solution of 95-per-cent ethanol in D_5W.

(2) Infuse 7.5 ml. per Kg. of maternal weight per hour for the first 2 hours as a loading dose.

(3) Continue at the rate of 1.5 ml. per Kg. for the next 10 hours.

(4) If labor resumes after the first course, it may be repeated, with the repeat loading dose being 10 per cent of the initial loading dose for every hour which the infusion has been stopped.

(5) Suppression of maternal vomiting with an agent such as hydroxyzine (50 to 75 mg. I.M. q.4h.), and protection against aspiration of vomitus with an antacid (30 ml. P.O. q.2h.) are also helpful.

(6) The major risk of alcohol infusion is fetal sedation. If cervical dilatation progresses to beyond 4 cm., the infusion should be stopped.

(7) In various studies, the success of alcohol averaged about 70 per cent, not statistically better than bedrest.

b. *B-adrenergic Agents*

(1) Still under experimental protocol B-2 adrenergic agents such as ritodrine and salbutamol seem to be very effective for stopping labor.

(2) Their usefulness may be limited by autonomic side effects such as tachycardia, nausea, vomiting, dyspnea.

c. *Prostaglandin Inhibitors.* Aspirin, indomethacin, and a host of recently available anti-inflammatory agents may postpone the onset of labor. They are not useful once labor has begun.

4. Whether labor is allowed to continue or whether an attempt is made to stop it, careful monitoring is indicated.

5. Sedation and analgesia should be kept to a minimum to reduce fetal risks.

6. Wide episiotomy is recommended to spare the fetal head. The use of elective forceps is an individual choice which may or may not decrease fetal trauma.

7. A neonatal specialist should be present at the delivery of severely premature infants (less than 32 weeks).

PREMATURE RUPTURE OF MEMBRANES

Not strictly a complication of labor, premature rupture of the membranes poses one question: Should the physician induce labor?

Active intervention after premature rupture of the membranes is a highly controversial issue, with opinion ranging from delivery of all infants within 24 hours, to extremely conservative watchful waiting. The management presented here might be considered middle-of-the-road.

Definition

Rupture of the membranes before onset of labor

Etiology

Unknown

Diagnosis

1. Identification of amniotic fluid leaking from the vagina is frequently possible by:

a. Testing *p*H (amniotic fluid is alkaline, whereas the normal vagina is acidic), using Nitrazine paper

b. Testing fluid for ferning by allowing it to dry on a slide

c. Staining it for fetal cells

2. Pitfalls in diagnosis include alkaline vaginal discharges and the loss of alkaline urine, especially with infection.

Risks

1. Prematurity, if delivery is accomplished, with attendant risk of respiratory distress syndrome

a. Whether prolonged rupture of the membranes protects against respiratory distress is undetermined.

2. Severe fetal and maternal infection if delivery is delayed.

Management

1. Determine fetal maturity, if possible.

a. Obtain ultrasonography for biparietal diameter and correlate with dates.

b. If there is a question about maturity, obtain amniotic fluid either vaginally at the introitus (without examination) or by sonographically directed amniocentesis (for L/S ratio).

2. If the pregnancy is beyond 36 weeks or the L/S ratio is mature, after 12 hours, perform a vaginal exam to verify membrane rupture and rule out cord prolapse, then induce labor.

a. As a general rule, delivery should be accomplished within approximately 24 hours of vaginal examination.

3. If the pregnancy is under 36 weeks gestation or the L/S ratio is immature, avoid vaginal examination and allow the pregnancy to continue.

4. If waiting is the choice, the following precautions must be taken:

a. Bedrest until fluid leakage stops

b. Vital signs, including oral temperatures, every 4 hours

c. White blood cell counts daily

d. External fetal monitoring to rule out symptomatic cord prolapse

e. Hospitalization for 2 to 3 days after leakage stops

5. Antibiotics before delivery are of questionable value in forestalling amnionitis or fetal infection. If, however, the mother becomes febrile, broad-spectrum antibiotic therapy should be started after obtaining cultures. Delivery at this point is indicated, preferably by induction of labor, but by cesarean section if necessary.

6. Birth after Prolonged Rupture of Membranes

a. Infants born after prolonged rupture should be cultured at birth, especially from the gastric fluid and ear. The decision to begin antibiotics at birth should depend on the pediatric service.

b. Cultures of the fetal side of the placenta, the inside of the uterus, and the amniotic fluid should be obtained. If the mother is afebrile and there is no suspicion of infection, antibiotics may be withheld.

7. Enhancement of Lung Function. It has been shown that treatment of the mother with corticosteroids (betamethasone, 12 mg.) at least 24 hours (but less than 7 days) before delivery will significantly reduce the incidence of RDS in infants between 28 and 32 weeks gestation. Its effectiveness before 28 weeks and after 32 weeks is under investigation.

a. Long-term effects of this treatment are unknown, at present, and it is still considered an experimental protocol for investigation.

PROLAPSE OF THE UMBILICAL CORD

Definitions

1. Occult Prolapse. The umbilical cord falls into the pelvis next to the presenting part but not beyond it and cannot be reached by the examining finger.

2. Forelying Cord. The cord is in front of the presenting part but the membranes are intact.

3. True Prolapsed Cord. The membranes are ruptured, and the umbilical cord is in front of the presenting part, usually compressed by it.

Etiology

All conditions which interfere with good engagement predispose to cord prolapse: prematurity, pelvic inlet contraction, hydramnios, and many others.

Diagnosis

1. Occult cord prolapse is detected by variable decelerations on fetal heart rate monitoring during labor.
2. Forelying cords and true prolapses are suspected by monitoring and can be confirmed by vaginal examination.

Management

1. Occult Prolapse. See "Variable Deceleration," Chap. 9, Fetal Monitoring.
2. Forelying Cord. Cesarean section
3. True Prolapse

a. If vaginal delivery can be anticipated within 5 minutes either spontaneously or by forceps it may be attempted.

b. If vaginal delivery is not imminent:

(1) Position patient in deep Trendelenberg or knee-chest position.

(2) Elevate presenting part out of the pelvis and hold it there until cesarean section is performed.

(3) Prepare for immediate cesarean section.

SHOULDER DYSTOCIA

Definition

Inability to deliver the shoulders after the delivery of the fetal head

Etiology

A large fetus, especially over 4,000 g., predisposes to dystocia. This is especially to be suspected in pregnancies complicated by diabetes.

Diagnosis

1. Suspect shoulder dystocia if the estimated fetal weight is 4,000 g. or more.
2. Final diagnosis is made as the shoulders resist delivery.

Risks

Perinatal mortality ranges as high as up to approximately 15 per cent.

1. Hypoxia. As the head is delivered, the umbilical cord is placed on traction and compressed in the birth canal. If delivery of the shoulders takes too long, hypoxia results.

2. Fetal Injury

a. Attempts to deliver the shoulders may result in spinal cord injury to the fetus.

b. Fracture of the clavicle is sometimes necessary for delivery.

Management

Optimal management consists of avoiding shoulder dystocia.

1. If a fetus over 4,000 g. is suspected, x-ray pelvimetry may be performed. If cephalopelvic disproportion is likely, cesarean section should be performed.
2. If shoulder dystocia is diagnosed after the head is delivered, management should be as follows:

a. Clear the infant's nose and mouth by aspiration.

b. Prevent impaction of the anterior shoulder under the symphysis by rotating the fetus to an oblique position.

c. Perform or extend the episiotomy to generous proportions.

d. With the fetus still oblique, attempt delivery by combined cephalic traction and fundal pressure.

e. If this does not succeed, sweep the posterior arm out and repeat.

f. If this does not succeed, rotate the opposite shoulder to the posterior oblique position, remove that arm, and repeat *d*.

g. As a last resort, fracture a clavicle by pressure with a finger from the supraclavicular fossa OUTWARD. This helps avoid pleural puncture by the fractured clavicle.

TWINS

Definitions

1. Monozygotic (Identical) Twins. Cleavage of one zygote to form two embryos

2. Dizygotic (Fraternal) Twins. Separate fertilization of two ova

3. Monoamniotic Twins. Two fetuses within one amnion and one chorion. Always monozygotic.

4. Monochorionic, Diamniotic Twins. Two fetuses within one chorion, but two amnions. Always monozygotic.

5. Dichorionic, Diamniotic Twins. Each fetus with its own chorion and amnion. May be either monozygotic or dizygotic.

Etiology

1. Dizygotic twinning accounts for most cases, and is increased in frequency in women who

a. Are black

b. Are over 35 years old

c. Have a family history of twins

d. Have received clomiphene citrate (7-per-cent incidence) or menopausal gonadotropins (20- to 40-per-cent incidence)

2. Monozygotic twinning is invariable in incidence at approximately one per 250 pregnancies.

Diagnosis

1. Antepartum

a. Diagnosis requires an index of suspicion precipitated by a uterus larger than dates.

b. Detection of two fetal heartbeats whose rates differ by at least 10 heartbeats per minute strengthens suspicion.

c. Certain diagnosis may be made by ultrasonography or x-ray flat plate of the abdomen.

2. Intrapartum

a. A significant percentage of twins are not suspected until delivery of the first twin reveals an infant much smaller than expected.

b. Always explore the uterus after delivery of any infant, before draining the umbilical cord.

Risks

Twinning is associated with an increased risk of:

1. Premature labor
2. Intertwin transfusion syndrome
3. Congenital anomalies
4. Maternal anemia
5. Preeclampsia
6. Hyperemesis gravidarum
7. Labor complications, including:
   a. Hypotonic dysfunction
   b. Cord prolapse
   c. Premature placental separation
   d. Abnormal presentation
   e. Postpartum hemorrhage

Management

1. Antepartum. The aim of management is to prevent premature delivery and be alert for maternal complications. The only effective method to date for decreasing prematurity is strictly enforced bedrest, preferably from mid-second trimester until time of delivery.

2. Labor. Once labor has begun, the following steps should be taken:

a. If labor is premature, attempt to stop it (see section on premature labor).

b. If labor is to continue:

(1) Institute fetal monitoring of both fetuses.

(2) Start a running intravenous system.

(3) Type and crossmatch 2 units of packed red blood cells.

(4) Keep analgesia and anesthesia during labor to a minimum. Conduction anesthesia carries a greater risk of precipitating hypotension in women who are at risk for hypertension and hemorrhage.

(5) While the use of oxytocin in dysfunctional labor complicated by twin gestation is generally not advocated, many physicians will use it cautiously.

3. Delivery

a. *First Twin*

(1) If the first fetus is a vertex, deliver it as a normal single birth.

(2) DO NOT UNCLAMP THE CORD.

(3) Explore the uterus immediately to determine the status of the second twin, including the presence of another amniotic sac, presentation, and position.

(4) If the first twin is a breech, many physicians will treat it as a premature breech because of its likely smaller size. One has the option of cesarean section or breech delivery.

b. *Second Twin*

(1) If the presenting part of the second twin is directly over the pelvis, guide it into the pelvis, then rupture the membranes.

(2) Monitor the fetal heart carefully with a stethoscope or fetal monitor if it is available in the delivery room.

(3) As long as there is no bleeding from the uterus (placental separation), and the fetal heart remains good, a normal breech or vertex delivery may be conducted. Oxytocin may be used cautiously.

(4) If the presenting part of the second twin is not directly over the pelvis, the fetal parts must be identified.

(5) Then rupture the membranes, locate the feet, grasp them and perform a breech extraction. This is best done under general anesthesia.

(6) Double-clamp the cord of the second twin, for later identification.

c. *Placenta and After*

(1) Immediately after the delivery of the second twin, the placenta is delivered, frequently by manual removal.

(2) Explore the uterus and cervix for lacerations.

(3) Begin oxytocin infusion to insure contraction of the uterus, combined with uterine massage.

(4) After repair of the episiotomy, inspect the placentas and membranes for evidence of monozygosity.

Indications for Cesarean Section

1. Interlocking twins are an absolute indication for abdominal delivery. This diagnosis may be made when x-ray flat plate reveals the presenting twin to be a breech, while the second presents a vertex with its head below the head of the first.

2. Many physicians perform cesarean section when the first twin presents as breech, regardless of the presentation of the second.

3. Conjoined twins usually are delivered by cesarean section.

MULTIPLE GESTATION

Triplets or greater pose all the risks and problems of twin gestation, except more so. Antepartum management is essentially the same as for twins. If the fetuses are large enough at the time of delivery to be reasonably sure of survival, cesarean section is probably the best method for delivery.

AMNIOTIC FLUID EMBOLISM (AFE)

Definition

Infusion of amniotic-fluid particulate matter into the circulation through the uterine veins

Etiology

Requiring a simultaneous opening in the amnion and the uterine veins, AFE is most often associated with placental abruption.

Diagnosis

This relatively rare syndrome should

be suspected when a woman in labor develops severe dyspnea, cyanosis, and shock.

Risks

1. Death. Most physicians question the diagnosis of AFE if the patient SURVIVES. Pulmonary vascular obstruction and systemic vascular collapse are usually rapidly fatal.

2. Coagulation Defects. If death is not rapid, potent thromboplastins in the amniotic fluid initiate disseminated intravascular coagulation. This is usually manifested by severe bleeding from the genital tract and all puncture sites.

Management

Therapy is usually not successful but is directed at improving oxygenation, maintaining blood pressure and cardiac output, and combating coagulation defects. This is as much an emergency as cardiac or respiratory arrest. Resuscitation should involve the cardiac arrest team.

INVERSION OF THE UTERUS

Definition

The fundus of the uterus is prolapsed, inside out, through the cervix.

Etiology

This rare occurrence is almost always the result of traction placed upon a fundally implanted placenta directly after delivery.

Diagnosis

Manual exploration of the vagina and uterus after every delivery will identify this when it occurs.

Risks

Hemorrhage and shock secondary to blood loss are the major immediate risks.

Management

1. Immediate replacement of the fundus tremendously decreases morbidity by cutting down on blood loss. This is accomplished by:

   a. Starting two intravenous lines and beginning simultaneous infusion with a salt solution and whole blood

   b. Instituting deep anesthesia

   c. Replacing the fundus by applying simultaneous traction on the dilated cervix and upward pressure on the center of the fundus with a closed fist

   d. After replacement, insuring uterine contraction by oxytocic stimulation and bimanual compression and massage

2. If bimanual replacement is not possible because the cervix has constricted, immediate laparotomy should be performed.

16. Hemorrhage in Pregnancy

David H. Fields, M.D.

DEFINITIONS

1. Vaginal bleeding during pregnancy is usually classified by the time of its occurrence. For practical purposes, it may be divided into bleeding during:
   a. The first half of pregnancy
   b. The second half of pregnancy, including labor
   c. The postpartum period
2. The bleeding may vary in quantity from a few drops, presaging an impending problem, up to torrential hemorrhage.

ETIOLOGY

1. Bleeding in the First half of Pregnancy. This type of bleeding may be due to:

a. Threatened or incomplete abortion, especially before 16 weeks gestation

b. Ectopic pregnancy, especially in the first 8 to 10 weeks of pregnancy

c. Vaginal or cervical lesions, which may present at any time

d. Placenta previa, which is usually a complication of the second half of pregnancy, but may present as early as 16 weeks gestation

2. Bleeding in the Second Half of Pregnancy. The major causes of bleeding beyond the time of fetal viability are:

a. Abnormal placental implantations, e.g., placenta previa, vasa previa

b. Premature placental separation, varying from marginal sinus rupture to clinically severe abruption

c. Abnormally formed placentas, e.g., placenta membranacea and circumvallate placenta

d. Labor, accompanied by heavier than normal "bloody show" or rapid cervical dilatation

e. Vaginal or cervical lesions

3. Postpartum Hemorrhage

a. Uterine atony is by far the major cause of postpartum hemorrhage, accounting for 90 per cent of the early cases. Other causes include:

b. Uterine, cervical, and vaginal lacerations from traumatic delivery

c. Retained placental fragments

d. Coagulation abnormalities

MANAGEMENT

Specific management of bleeding in the second half of pregnancy and postpartum periods is discussed under individual headings in the rest of this chapter. For management of earlier bleeding, see other chapters throughout this book.

PLACENTA PREVIA

Definition

Implantation in such a fashion that part of all of the placenta overlies the internal os of the cervix.

1. Total Placenta Previa. The internal os is completely covered.

2. Partial Placenta Previa. The internal os is partially covered.

3. Marginal Placenta Previa. The placenta may be touched through the cervix, but does not extend beyond it.

It is important to realize that the relation of the cervix and the placenta may change as the cervix becomes effaced, or dilated.

Etiology

While there is no specific etiology, placenta previa seems to be more common in:

1. Multiparas of older age
2. Diseases complicated by large placentas such as diabetes and hemolytic Rh disease
3. Previous lower segment scarring as from cesarean section and perhaps curettage

Diagnosis

1. Ultrasonography (USG)

a. The key to diagnosis of placenta previa is ultrasonographic investigation of all painless, bright red bleeding before the onset of labor.

b. Other, older methods have been rendered obsolete by USG.

c. An added benefit of this is that fetal biparietal diameter and an estimation of fetal age can be obtained at the same time.

2. Double Set-up Examination. If bleeding is heavy enough to demand immediate delivery, or the patient is in labor, a sterile vaginal exam may be performed under double set-up conditions. This means that the patient is on the operating room table, prepped and draped, ready for immediate cesarean section if necessary, at the time of the examination.

Risks

1. Maternal

a. *Hemorrhage with shock* is the major risk for the mother.

b. The initial bleeding episode is almost always self-limited and not fatal. However, with repeated episodes of bleeding, the mother may be brought to the "edge of shock," and pushed over by the next.

2. Fetal

a. *Premature delivery*, forced by repeated bleeding episodes, accounts for most of the fetal mortality.

b. Since the blood loss is usually maternal rather than fetal, fetal shock if present is usually due to asphyxia secondary to maternal shock and decreased uteroplacental blood flow.

General Mangement

1. Once the diagnosis is made, the physician must decide whether to deliver the fetus immediately or allow continued pregnancy. The rationale for allowing pregnancy to continue is only to await fetal maturity. Either way, hospitalization is mandatory.
2. Continuation of pregnancy is preferable if all the following circumstances are met:
   a. Gestational age less than 37 weeks
   b. Bleeding stopped, or slow enough to not threaten mother
   c. No labor or abdominal pain
   d. No fetal distress as demonstrated by nonstress fetal monitoring
3. Immediate delivery is preferable if any of the following occur:
   a. Fetal maturity—gestational age 37 weeks or greater
   b. Labor
   c. Deteriorating maternal condition as evidenced by tachycardia, hypotension, or severe hemorrhage
   d. Fetal distress

Hospital Orders for Conservative Mangement

1. Bedrest until there has been no bleeding for 24 hours
2. Vital signs q.1h. until bleeding has stopped; then q.4h.
3. N.P.O. until bleeding has stopped for 24 hours
4. Running intravenous (D_5W or salt solution at 100 to 150 ml. per hour) as long as patient is N.P.O.
5. Hematocrit/hemoglobin on admission and as necessary
6. Type and crossmatch for 2 units of packed red blood cells.

7. Transfusion for H/H under 10/30 or as clinical condition warrants

8. If placental localization has not yet been performed, obtain ultrasonography.

Method of Delivery

1. Cesarean Section. This is almost always the method of choice after placenta previa is documented, either by USG or double set-up examination.

a. The uterine incision will depend on the location of the placenta. If it extends over the anterior wall of the uterus, a vertical incision above the placenta is necessary. Otherwise, a transverse low segment incision may be made.

b. If placental implantation is low enough that lower segment bleeding cannot be stopped after delivery, hysterectomy may be required.

2. Vaginal Delivery

a. If the diagnosis is made by double set-up examination and the placenta can be documented as partial or marginal, amniotomy may allow the fetal head to descend and tamponade the bleeding.

b. If this does not occur, or if maternal shock or fetal distress occurs, immediate cesarean section should be performed.

LOW LYING PLACENTA

Basic Principles

1. Diagnosed when placenta previa is suspected, this condition should be treated in almost the same manner as a partial or marginal placenta previa, but with expectations for successful vaginal delivery.

2. What this means is that the causes of bleeding and dangers to the mother and fetus are of the same origin, but not usually as severe.

Management

1. If the criteria for conservative management of placenta previa are met, observation is justified.

2. When there is labor, amniotomy generally suffices to control bleeding. Labor is conducted with careful maternal and fetal monitoring.

3. If amniotomy does not control the bleeding and maternal or fetal condition deteriorates, cesarean section is indicated.

MARGINAL SINUS RUPTURE

Definition

Minimal premature separation of the edge of the placenta

Etiology

Unknown; however, this is a mild form of marginal placental abruption.

Diagnosis

1. Clinically, this is indistinguishable from placenta previa, being characterized by painless antepartum bleeding, although it is, in fact, a mild form of placental abruption.

2. The diagnosis is one of presumption when ultrasonography reveals a normally placed placenta and subsequent vaginal examination reveals no lesions.

Risks

This may progress to more severe placental abruption, although there is no way to predict this. If it does not, risks are minimal and related to total maternal blood loss.

Management

1. As long as the bleeding remains, the patient should be maintained on bedrest. This may be at home once placenta previa has been ruled out if blood loss is minimal.

2. If the bleeding remains mild, one should pursue expectant management

awaiting spontaneous labor or attainment of fetal maturity.

3. When delivery is planned, either due to spontaneous labor or attainment of fetal maturity, amniotomy allows for better labor and a more accurate assessment of blood loss.

PLACENTAL ABRUPTION

Definition

1. Premature separation of an otherwise normally implanted placenta after the twentieth week of gestation is termed placental abruption.

2. The degree of separation may vary from minimal as in marginal sinus ruptures, to total.

3. Separations may be at the periphery of the placenta in which case they tend not to extend because the blood can escape; or, they may be central and progressive with bleeding causing further dissection of the placenta from its bed, causing further bleeding and so on.

Etiology

While no single cause for placental abruption is known, several maternal conditions seem to predispose to its occurrence.

1. Hypertension is the most commonly found predisposing factor, being found in almost 50 per cent of cases.

2. Multiparity

3. History of previous placental abruption

4. Other less common predispositions include: hydramnios, trauma, and delivery of a first twin.

Diagnosis

1. Suspect placental abruption whenever there is antepartum vaginal bleeding in combination with abdominal pain.

2. Physical findings such as uterine tenderness, and a tetanically contracted uterus strengthen the diagnosis.

3. When placental abruption is severe, signs of maternal and fetal distress occur.

Risks (Maternal)

1. Shock secondary to blood loss is the major risk for the mother with placental abruption.

2. Defibrination with secondary coagulopathy may occur. This is most likely due to disseminated intravascular coagulation precipitated by release of placental thromboplastins; however, with central abruption, the formation of a large retroplacental clot may result in hypofibrinogenemia.

3. Renal shutdown has classically been described with severe placental abruption. This is almost certainly secondary to hypovolemic shock.

4. The classically described Couvelaire uterus, secondary to extravasation of blood through the myometrium to below the uterine serosa, may not result in functional impairment.

Management

Once the diagnosis of placental abruption has been established, the need for delivery is apparent, unless the fetus is very immature or the symptomatology so mild that only a marginal separation is suspected.

The following plan of treatment optimizes fetal salvage and minimizes maternal morbidity.

1. Evaluation

a. Vital signs every 30 minutes

b. Frequent palpation of the uterus for signs of rigidity or increase in the height of the fundus

c. Frequent evaluation of the amount of uterine bleeding

d. Continuous fetal heart rate and uterine contraction monitoring

e. Hemoglobin/hematocrit on admission

f. Platelet estimation or count

g. Urinalysis

h. Coagulation workup consisting of fibrinogen levels, prothrombin time, partial thromboplastin time, thrombin time and fibrin split product measurement. If a plain tube of blood is taken and observed for clot formation, coagulatory status can be roughly gauged in a matter of minutes. If a good clot is formed within several minutes, fibrinogen levels are almost certainly higher than 100 mg. per 100 ml. If not, all the above tests will most likely be abnormal.

i. Type and crossmatch for 4 units of packed cells with fresh frozen plasma if needed for coagulopathy. If fresh frozen plasma is not available, fresh whole blood should be used.

2. Therapy

a. Begin fluid replacement with intravenous Ringer's lactate or normal saline solution AND blood as necessary. It is far better to stay ahead rather than get behind on blood replacement.

b. Begin induction of labor by amniotomy and oxytocin infusion if ALL of the following conditions are met:

(1) There is no evidence of maternal shock.

(2) The fetal heart rate on continuous electronic monitoring shows no evidence of fetal distress. After amniotomy, internal monitoring is preferred.

(3) The uterus is not tetanic, but is capable of rhythmic contraction.

(4) Continuous vaginal blood loss is not alarmingly heavy.

(5) Coagulation studies are not severely abnormal.

c. Because of uterine irritability, after cervical effacement occurs, labor can usually be expected to progress rapidly.

d. Indications for cesarean section are a worsening in maternal or fetal condition as evidenced by any of the parameters directly above. Whereas it used to be a "rule" to perform abdominal delivery after 6 to 8 hours of labor, this is not necessary as long as maternal and fetal condition can be adequately monitored.

e. If gross evidence of disseminated intravascular coagulation develops, such as bleeding from puncture sites, fibrinogen 4 g. I.V., cryoprecipitate or several units of fresh frozen plasma may be used for immediate correction. Platelet counts should be done, and platelet transfusions given if the counts are low in the presence of active bleeding.

f. If there is laboratory evidence of coagulopathy, but no evidence of active maternal hemorrhage, delivery itself will usually result in correction of these within one or two days.

g. If the fetus is dead on arrival at the hospital, the management should be as in section (b) above, without fetal monitoring. Cesarean section may still be necessary if maternal condition necessitates immediate delivery.

CIRCUMVALLATE PLACENTA

Definition

1. A placenta in which a thickened ring consisting of a double fold of amnion and chorion surrounds the fetal portion of the placenta, is termed a circumvallate placenta.

2. When this ring is at the placental edge rather than on the fetal surface, the placenta is called circummarginate.

Etiology

Unknown

Risks

Painless antepartum hemorrhage may occur with this rare condition.

Management

1. Distinguish from placenta previa via sonography.

2. Conduct labor and/or cesarean section as described under marginal separation of the placenta.

PLACENTA MEMBRANACEA

Definition

When the chorion laeve fails to degenerate, chorionic villi develop all around the ovisac. This results in a very thin layer of functioning placenta all around the uterine cavity.

Etiology

Unknown

Risks

Since there is placenta in contact with the entire lower uterine segment (including over the os), placenta membranacea may behave as a total placenta previa, with increasing bleeding during the second half of pregnancy.

Management

As for placenta previa

VASA PREVIA

Definition

Abnormal implantation of the fetal vessels into the placenta, in such a fashion that some traverse the amnion overlying the cervical os.

Etiology

Unknown

Risks

Rupture of a vessel, especially at the time of rupture of the membranes, may result in fetal exsanguination.

Diagnosis

If amniotomy is accompanied by the onset of excess vaginal bleeding, test the blood for the presence of fetal cells. The Kleihauer-Betke acid elution test (Apt test) is suitable for this.

Management

1. Vaginal delivery may be performed if it can be accomplished in less time than it takes to arrange a cesarean section.

2. Prepare for a shocky baby at birth. The blood loss from vasa previa has been fetal.

VAGINAL AND CERVICAL LESIONS

A multitude of vaginal and cervical lesions may cause bleeding during pregnancy. The list is essentially the same as for vaginal and cervical lesions which may cause nonpregnant bleeding, and the diagnosis and workup are essentially the same: speculum exam followed by microbiologic, cytologic, and histologic studies as necessary.

POSTPARTUM HEMORRHAGE

Early Postpartum Hemorrhage

1. Definition. Blood loss greater than 500 ml. in the first 24 hours after delivery.

2. Etiology

a. Approximately 90 per cent of early postpartum hemorrhage is due to uterine atony after delivery. Common conditions predisposing are: general anesthesia, overdistended uterus (twins, hydramnios), prolonged labor, oxytocin-stimulated labor, multiparity, precipitate labor.

b. Cervical or vaginal lacerations which are unrecognized at delivery may continue to ooze blood.

c. Retained placental tissue may prevent uterine contraction and result in hemorrhage, somewhat after delivery.

d. Coagulation abnormalities rarely cause postpartum hemorrhage in and of themselves. They may, however, exacerbate other bleeding.

Uterine Atony

1. Diagnosis

a. Uterine atony is diagnosed by feeling the fundus. Since it is so common, if the fundus is softer or higher than it should be, postpartum atony is presumed.

b. If the uterus is well contracted, another cause for the bleeding must be sought. Inspection of the cervix and vagina will detect lacerations if present.

c. Bleeding may occur in the presence of a well-contracted uterus from uterine rupture or laceration secondary to trauma of labor or delivery. This is diagnosed by manual exploration of the uterus after suspect deliveries. Many physicians advocate routine exploration of the uterus after every delivery.

d. Sometimes, in the face of a well-contracted uterus, blood will ooze from the cervix. Especially if it had not been effaced well before dilatation (as in multiparas), the cervix may bleed within the canal from torn vessels. This may be diagnosed by excluding uterine rupture.

2. Management

a. Atony is best treated by a combination of immediate bimanual uterine massage and oxytocin stimulation, using either oxytocin (20 units per 100 ml. Ringer's lactate at 200 to 300 ml. per hour) or an ergot alkaloid (Methergine or Ergotrate 0.2 mg. I.V. or I.M.) or both.

b. Lacerations of the genital tract obviously require suturing. Good exposure is critical for this. If an assistant is not present, get help.

c. Uterine rupture requires laparotomy with either repair of the laceration or hysterectomy.

d. If examination reveals retained placenta, remove it manually. If this is not possible, resort to curettage.

e. Adequate fluid replacement and transfusion when necessary are central to proper therapy.

Late Postpartum Hemorrhage

1. Definition. Blood loss greater than 500 ml. after the first postpartum day but within the first month

2. Etiology

a. Retained placental tissue or fetal membranes is the most common cause of late postpartum hemorrhage.

b. Subinvolution of the placental site is a second major reason for abnormal bleeding and may be due to endomyometritis.

3. Diagnosis. The diagnosis of late postpartum bleeding is best made by a therapeutic trial. See directly below.

4. Management

a. Begin by attempting therapy with oxytocin infusion (20 units in 500 to 1,000 ml. D_5W).

b. If this results in a decrease in the bleeding, continue with an ergot alkaloid (Ergotrate, Methergine 0.2 mg P.O., or I.M. q.4h. × 6 doses). This is frequently combined with systemic antibiotic administration (ampicillin or tetracycline is a good initial choice) on the theory that local infection of the placental site predisposes to late hemorrhage.

c. If the above regime does not control the bleeding, or if the bleeding recurs, curettage is indicated.

PHILOSOPHY OF BLOOD REPLACEMENT

Basic Principles

1. Blood replacement therapy may be used for three general purposes:
   a. Replacement of red cell mass
   b. Replacement of volume
   c. Replacement of clotting factors
2. Since all three are rarely necessary simultaneously, the art has changed its name to "Blood Component Replacement Therapy."
3. The implication of this is that one does not replace "blood" any longer, except in unusual circumstances, but rather one replaces what is needed with the appropriate blood component.
4. Blood should not be used as a tonic. Even with the use of packed cells

and screening for hepatitis B, there is a significant risk of hepatitis C with each transfusion.

Definition of Blood Components

1. Packed Red Blood Cells. One unit of "packed cells" is 250 ml. It contains the red cell mass of one unit (500 ml.) of blood with a hematocrit of 50 per cent.

2. Plasma. The liquid portion of blood, before it clots, is plasma. If frozen before it has a chance to stagnate, it contains all the fibrinogen and clotting factors of blood. One unit of fresh frozen plasma (250 ml.) contains approximately 2 g. of fibrinogen.

3. Platelets. Platelets are centrifuged off and stored as a separate component for specific use in cases of severe thrombocytopenia.

4. Fibrinogen. Pooled from the plasma of many donors, fibrinogen may be used specifically for correction of defibrination syndromes in obstetrics. However, because it is pooled, its use carries an unacceptably high risk of hepatitis. The use of cryoprecipitate is preferable if it is available, or of fresh frozen plasma if there is associated hypovolemia.

Correction of Loss in Specific Situations

1. Chronic Blood Loss. If transfusion is necessary, chronic blood loss is best corrected with packed red blood cells. Because in chronic situations intravascular volume is slowly replaced, volume-supplying blood components are not necessary.

2. Acute Blood Loss. In this situation both red-cell mass and volume need replacement. This can be accomplished with packed red blood cells and either crystalloid solutions (normal saline, Ringer's lactate) or fresh frozen plasma. The reasons for avoiding whole blood, if possible, are twofold:

a. To reduce the risk of hepatitis

b. To enable the whole blood to be fractionated for components (e.g., platelets, cryoprecipitate)

If blood loss is greater than 6 units, coagulation factors need replacement as well and frozen plasma or FRESH whole blood are necessary instead of crystalloids.

3. Coagulopathies. In obstetrics these can usually be corrected by delivery of the fetus. However, if necessary,

a. Platelets may be transfused separately.

b. Cryoprecipitate, frozen plasma, or fibrinogen are available for hypofibrinogenemia.

c. Frozen plasma is therapy of choice for other coagulation factor deficits, except factor VIII.

17. Sepsis and Septic Shock

Hugh R. K. Barber, M.D.

DEFINITION

1. Septic shock is defined as that condition seen in a patient with an apparent infection, a temperature either elevated or depressed above or below normal, a thready pulse of 110 or over, hypotension (usually systolic 80 mm. Hg or below), and a decrease in urinary output below 20 ml. per hour.

2. Shock is defined as a state in which capillary perfusion is inadequate to sustain life. Vital cells are starving for lack of oxygen and other nutrients and metabolic products are not being removed from tissues because capillary flow is too slow or does not exist at all.

3. Shock is an emergency situation no matter whether it is due to a severe injury with blood loss, a severe infection, heart failure, or other causes. The situation must be dealt with immediately or cellular injury and death will soon progress to organ failure and death of the patient.

BASIC PRINCIPLES

1. Bacteremic shock is one of the emergencies of medicine. It carries a mortality rate of 80 per cent, which is higher when *Proteus* or *Cl. welchii* is the infecting organism.

2. The gram-negative organisms most frequently seen in this group are: *E. coli* (most common), *Proteus mirabilis*, *Pseudomonas aerogenes*, and *Aerobacter aerogenes*.

3. Among the most frequent gram-positive bacteria cultured are enterococcus, anaerobic streptococci, *Bacteroides*, *B. welchii* and *Clostridium perfringens*. *B. welchii* and *Clostridium* secrete exotoxins. Infections due to *Bacteroides* are now being reported frequently.

4. Shock is noted especially in conjunction with infected abortion, premature rupture of the membranes (chorioamnionitis), pyelonephritis, especially in pregnancy, and diffuse peritonitis. It may be associated with gynecological cancer or following extensive radical surgery. Sepsis and septic shock may follow chemotherapy for pelvic malignancy or trophoblastic disease.

5. Although the entire mechanism has not been completely elucidated, most physicians accept the theory that the basic physiopathology is generalized intravascular clotting initiated by the release of endotoxin (lipopolysaccharide) by the above named gram-negative bacteria.

6. Currently, two main mechanisms have been involved to explain the findings in endotoxic shock: selective vasospasm and disseminated intravascular coagulation (DIC). The pathophysiology can be attributed to both these mechanisms as well as to reduce myocardial response to sympathetic stimuli.

7. *Clostridium perfringens* (*B. welchii* and *Clostridium*) secrete exotoxins. These are probably the most serious of all infections. The exotoxins become irreversibly bound to tissue soon after they are liberated from the infecting organism.

8. Since toxin is fixed to tissue, specific antitoxins are therefore of questionable value. The exotoxin contains the

enzyme lecithinase (which causes necrosis of tissue as well as rapid lysis of red and white blood cells) as well as collagenase (a proteolytic enzyme that causes necrosis of muscle tissue).

9. There is lack of oxygen to vital organs, owing to compensatory generalized vasoconstriction which gives rise to impaired tissue perfusion.

The clinical syndrome is characterized by:

a. A change in the sensorium

b. A sudden drop in blood pressure below 70 systolic

c. A weak thready pulse

d. Respiratory disturbance (respiratory alkalosis)

e. Electrolyte deficits and urine suppression

10. The usual laboratory findings are a rise in the hematocrit, SGOT, SGPT, LDH, catecholamines, BUN, blood amylase, and blood sugar.

11. Metabolic acidosis occurs later.

DIFFERENTIATION OF SEPTIC ABORTION AND SEPTIC SHOCK

1. There is some confusion between these two terms. Septic abortion is defined as one associated with an elevation of temperature to 100.4°F (38°C) or more of two days duration, not necessarily consecutive, or a single elevation of 102°F (38.9°C) or more caused by uterine infection. Only about 1 to 5 per cent of septic abortions develop septic shock. All cases of septic abortion are potential candidates for this dreaded complication. Only by exercising constant vigilance and instituting prophylactic measures can one prevent this.

2. Septic shock can occur at any time but the infected abortion with a 12-plus-week size uterus that is tender with a closed cervix and a puslike discharge exuding from the cavity is an especially likely candidate.

Diagnosis

1. Delay in diagnosis and delay in early institution of therapy are the most important factors in the production of mortality in septic shock. Although the diagnosis and management will be considered separately, the urgency of the time factor makes it necessary that these two overlap. The emergency nature of this condition is not too dissimilar to the diabetic presenting with hypoglycemic shock.

2. At the time that the initial blood is drawn for laboratory evaluation, the treatment is started.

3. Hyperventilation and respiratory alkalosis are helpful aids in making an early diagnosis of gram-negative bacteremia.

4. One of the earliest signs of impending shock is mental confusion and inappropriate behavior. When these occur in a patient with infection and fever, it usually indicates that the next step, hypotension, is about to occur. The importance of this triad in early diagnosis cannot be overemphasized: hyperventilation, mental confusion, and fever. Awareness of this may permit the diagnosis of shock at its very inception.

5. It must be stressed that the adrenergic effect is not prominent at this stage. The patient is warm, skin is dry, cardiac output and tissue perfusion is adequate.

6. It is only as the case progresses that the classic signs and symptoms of severe septic shock supervene and here the adrenergic component takes over (vasoconstriction).

7. Signs of advancing septic shock are as follows:

a. Hypotension associated with fever or a subnormal temperature

b. Chills

c. Tachypnea and respiratory distress

d. Tachycardia (110 to 180 beats per min. with narrow pulse pressure)

e. Progressive oliguria (usually less than 20 ml. hr.). The urinary output is one of the best clinical indicators of tissue perfusion!

f. Cold, moist skin

g. Drop in temperature of extremities with peripheral cyanosis

h. Mental obtundity, primarily marked anxiety and inappropriate behavior

i. Unexplained ileus

j. Unexplained petechia with occasional bleeding

k. Jaundice

8. Laboratory findings that help confirm the diagnosis are as follows:

a. Drop in blood *p*H

b. Drop in serum bicarbonate

c. Blood gas determination indicates drop in pO_2 and rise in pCO_2

d. Rise in blood urea nitrogen and phosphate

e. Drop in serum sodium, potassium, and calcium levels

f. Positive toxicology studies

g. Positive cultures—from any site—organisms that usually cause bacteremic shock (only about 25 to 30 per cent have positive blood cultures)

h. Rising hematocrit

i. Drop in platelet count, serum fibrinogen, or prothrombin

j. Elevation of SGOT, SGPT, LDH, and serum amylase

9. There is probably no specific laboratory test that absolutely confirms the diagnosis, but several positive tests lend credence to the supposition.

10. As usual, the clinical manifestations are paramount. The laboratory results merely reinforce the physician's clinical judgment.

OMINOUS SIGNS

Signs Usually Indicating a Lethal Outcome

Any of these should be disturbing, but the patient has a good chance of recovery. With two or three in combination, the prognosis must be guarded since these are usually lethal.

1. Coma
2. Increasing oliguria or anuria that does not respond to therapy, combined with a significant rise in BUN
3. Respiratory difficulty with a pCO_2 of 55 mm. Hg or more
4. Marked drop in fibrinogen or platelets
5. Severe sepsis that does not respond to antibiotics
6. Jaundice (hemolysis)
7. Marked acidosis with blood *p*H of 7.29 or less and a bicarbonate of less than 9.9 mEq./L.
8. Impaired liver function with jaundice
9. Cardiac failure or marked arrhythmia
10. Old age and/or debilitation from cancer, etc.
11. Any combination of the above suggests a grave prognosis.
12. Disseminated intramuscular coagulopathy is discussed elsewhere.

Treatment

Time is the keystone of therapy in treating septic shock. An outline of treatment for the first 12 hours is given as follows:

1. Careful monitoring is essential.
2. The clinical measurements most useful are pulse rate, blood pressure, pulse pressure (reflecting stroke volume), central venous pressure (or pulmonary wedge pressure or pulmonary artery pressure), blood volume estimation (early shock only), and hourly urinary output. These factors also designate the type and volume of fluid replacement.
3. Thorough and complete history and physical examination, including pelvic and speculum examination.
4. I.V. fluids to augment fluid and electrolyte intake, but especially to keep

a vein open in case of emergency. Use an 18-gauge needle.

5. Keep a catheter in the bladder so that hourly output of urine can be monitored. Record hourly intake and output.

6. Order gram-stained smears and cultures of blood, urine, cervix, draining wounds, and secretions from areas in which drains are inserted.

7. Get baseline complete blood count, hematocrit, and platelet count.

8. Order baseline serum electrolytes (sodium, potassium, chloride, carbon dioxide, calcium, phosphates) and *p*H.

9. Serum fibrinogen, prothrombin, and clotting time

10. Blood urea nitrogen and toxicological studies when indicated

11. Routine examination and culture of urine, plus bilirubin and toxicological studies when indicated

12. Radiograph of chest and abdomen for pathology, foreign bodies, or gas under the diaphragm

13. Baseline blood gas studies

14. Check the following hourly:
   a. Blood pressure
   b. Pulse
   c. Respiratory rate
   d. Rectal temperature
   e. Urinary output
   f. Urinary specific gravity
   g. Any inappropriate mental aberrations

15. After the initial orders are instituted additional procedures are indicated:

a. Where a removable septic focus is present, surgery is the keynote of treatment.

b. Where the septic nidus cannot be removed, therapy is medical by necessity.

c. Treatment is tailored to the needs of the patient.

d. An adequate airway should be ensured.

e. Fluid and blood replacement should be guided by central venous pressure, urinary output, and blood volume estimation.

f. Blood, plasma, or 5-per-cent dextrose in saline should be given as indicated.

g. Low-molecular-weight dextran provides volume replacement and reduces sludging in the microcirculation.

h. Metabolic acidosis is common, becoming progressive if not corrected; 0.45 per cent saline with one or two ampules of sodium bicarbonate added is useful in this case.

i. Lactate should not be used to correct acidosis in these patients because conversion to carbon dioxide requires aerobic metabolism. Sodium bicarbonate, however, acts rapidly and provides good buffering action.

Antibiotic Therapy

1. Garamycin (gentamycin sulfate) 1.5 to 3 mg. Kg/day I.M. in divided doses, or Coly-Mycin (colistin) 120 to 300 mg. I.M. in 2 to 4 divided doses o.d. plus kanamycin 1 g. I.M. initially, followed by 0.5 g. q.12h., or Keflin 2 g. initially and then 1 g. I.M. initially, followed by 0.5 g. q.12h. In some instances all three may be required.

2. If these drugs fail to control the infection, chloramphenicol is given as an I.V. bolus, 1 g. every 8 hours. Penicillin or ampicillin should also be given as crystalline penicillin G in dosage of 10 million units every 4 hours in intravenous fluids. As an alternative to penicillin, ampicillin 500 mg., or cephalothin, 2 g. every 4 hours I.V. may be used. Nephrotoxic drugs should be avoided in the presence of oliguria.

Corticosteroids (If Indicated)

1. Solu-Medro (methylprednisolone) 240 mg. I.V. as a bolus and then q.4 to 6 h. or

2. Hydrocortisone 1 to 2 g. I.V. as an initial bolus and then 1 g. I.V. q.4 to 6 h.

Vasomotor Drugs (If Indicated)

1. In the warm-hypotensive phase, a vasopressor rather than a vasodilator is indicated.

a. The most potent vasopressor, metaraminol (aramine) is given only in the least amount that will keep the systolic pressure just high enough to ensure adequate urinary output, and for as short a time as possible.

b. Aramine (metaraminol) is best administered in 500 ml. 5-per-cent glucose to which 100 to 200 mg., of the drug is added.

c. In critical cases where vasoconstrictors failed, Isuprel (isoproterenol) in doses of 5 ml. (5 mg.) in 500 ml., of glucose may be administered.

Currently the best catecholamine to begin treatment of shock is dopamine. Dopamine is essentially three drugs in one, depending on the dosage used and the patient's response. Very small dosages (2–5 μg./kg./min.) produce a specific dilation of gut and kidney vessels to increase blood flow to essential viscera. Moderate doses (5–30 μg./kg./min.) have, in addition, an inotropic effect (increased heart forces) that increases cardiac output. Very high doses (more than 30 μg./kg./min.) cause vasoconstriction that is just as powerful as that of norepinephrine or epinephrine. In other words, very high doses of dopamine have the same pressor effects as norepinephrine.

2. In the cold-hypotensive phase, however, there is generalized vasoconstriction and usually hypovolemia.

a. Volume replacement plus vasodilator drugs in small doses is the treatment of choice at this phase.

b. Chlorpromazine (Thorazine) in a dose of 5 to 10 mg. I.V. every half hour, as needed, up to four times, is one of the best vasodilators in septic shock.

3. When the central venous, wedge, or pulmonary artery pressure is elevated and the pulse rate is in the normal range, isoproterenol (Isuprel) may be used for its inotropic and vasodilator (beta-receptor) effects. Because of its tendency to produce cardiac arrhythmia, proterenol should not be used when pulse rate is above 120 beats per minute.

4. Digitalization should be carried out when the central venous pressure is above 12 cm. of water and tachycardia is present. Cedilanid (lanatoside C) should be given in 2 or 3 divided doses I.V. until 1.6 mg. to 3.5 mg. is given to produce digitalization.

5. With evidence of intravascular clotting, heparin sodium may be administered by I.V. bolus q.4 h., the initial dose being 10,000 units; subsequent doses usually 5,000 units. The total daily dose of 25,000 to 35,000 units may be divided into four doses q.6 h.

Treatment for Specific Infections

1. Welchii Infections

a. Same regimen as for gram-negative bacterial infections plus penicillin 50 million units I.V. in 24 hours or ampicillin 8 g. I.V. in 24 hours

b. Although controversial for the protection it provides, some give polyvalent gas gangrene antitoxin, 60,000 to 100,000 I.U. I.V., with doses repeated every 2 to 4 hours depending upon the clinical situation.

c. Early D and C to be followed by hysterectomy at once if there is more than minimal uterine involvement or if there is spread outside of the uterus

d. In the absence of severe kidney involvement with oliguria or anuria, dialysis is indicated.

e. Hyperbaric oxygen, if available, might be efficacious.

2. Gram-Positive Cocci Infections

a. Same regimen as listed under gram-negative

b. Use of vasoconstrictors early (see previous dosage)

c. More liberal use of plasma and fluids

Clinical Evaluation

Although electronic gadgets and sophisticated laboratory procedures are helpful, the patient can be managed successfully without them. A clinical evaluation is summarized as follows:

1. Peripheral Resistance

Examine the patient—if cold and clammy, the peripheral resistance is increased.

2. Blood Volume

Observe the central venous pressure. Circulating blood volume is more important than the findings of the peripheral blood volume.

3. Cardiac Output

A narrowed pulse pressure correlates with a decreased cardiac output. A fast thready pulse indicates that there is incomplete filling of the heart with a diminished output.

4. Visceral Organ Blood Flow

Measure the output of urine. The urine output is proportional to renal blood flow. Since the kidney is the target-sensitive organ and the renovascular bed is particularly sensitive as far as response to endotoxin is concerned, it is obvious that if the kidney is responding, as evidenced by an adequate urinary output, the other organs are being adequately perfused.

Surgical Treatment

1. In the presence of chorioamnionitis, if vaginal delivery is not accomplished within 12 hours, abdominal delivery should be seriously considered. For the patient with severe infection or endotoxic shock, Cesarean hysterectomy should be performed, together with ligation of the inferior vena cava and ovarian veins as indicated.
2. In an occasional patient with persistent anuria, dialysis may be required. Consultation with a nephrologist is indicated.
3. An infected abortion should be removed with adequate supportive measures, within 12 hours.
4. Usually, dilatation of the cervix and evacuation of the uterus with ring forceps followed by digital and sharp curettage are adequate to remove the septic focus.
5. Suction curettage is probably more effective than sharp curettage up to the fourteenth week of pregnancy.
6. When the disease has advanced to the stage of microabscess formation in the myometrium, hysterectomy is the only logical surgical treatment. Hysterectomy should be considered in the following situations:
   a. The patient continues in shock after curettage and adequate supportive measures.
   b. The uterus is over 14 weeks size.
   c. The uterus is perforated.
   d. The patient is oliguric.
   e. Intrauterine Clostridium welchii infection is diagnosed.
   f. The technique should be tailored to the problem.
   g. In the presence of clostridial infection, minimum of devitalized tissue should be left behind.

Thrombotic Complications

1. Septic pelvic thrombophlebitis involving both ovarian and hypogastric vessels is not uncommon in patients with long-standing septic abortion, postpartum endometritis, chorioamnionitis, pelvic inflammatory disease, and peritonitis.
2. Septic pulmonary embolization may occur.
3. Sepsis complicated by embolization is the basic problem. Therefore, ligation of the inferior vena cava and ovarian veins is the treatment of choice.
4. Vena caval plication is not adequate because the infected thrombi are small.
5. Heparinization is indicated as outlined earlier.

SHOCK LUNG SYNDROME

Basic Principles

1. The syndrome is often referred to as acute respiratory distress syndrome.

congestive atelectasis, shock lung, respirator lung, and postperfusion lung.

2. The term *acute respiratory distress syndrome* is attractive because it does not attribute the pathologic changes of the lung to one mechanism.

3. Shock lung is not a new disease, but it is being seen more frequently as progressively more sophisticated means of combatting profound hypotension and other perfusion problems save more severely ill patients.

4. Pulmonary complications are one of the leading causes of death in hemorrhagic or endotoxic shock successfully treated for the initial insult.

Basic Mechanism

1. Complications Predisposing to Shock Lung

a. Hypotension
b. Sepsis
c. Rapid blood volume restoration

2. Four Phases

a. First is the initial phase of injury and usual resuscitation; respiratory alkalosis commonly occurs.

b. Second is that of circulatory stabilization. The patient is often lucid and oriented but may show early signs of respiratory difficulty, such as tachypnea.

c. Third is one of progressive pulmonary failure that responds poorly to an increase of oxygen to the alveoli.

d. Fourth is characterized by severe hypoxia, hypercarbia, acidosis, and cardiac arrest.

Pathology

1. Shock lung has been confused with such pathologic diagnoses as bronchopneumonia, patchy atelectasis, and agonal changes.

2. In the acute stage the lung grossly shows edema, congestion, hemorrhage, heaviness, and relative airlessness.

3. Microscopically, there is patchy atelectasis, intra-alveolar edema, interalveolar edema, congestion, and hemorrhage. There may or may not be microthrombi.

Treatment

1. Is outlined earlier for the treatment of septic shock. However, there are additional cautions to be used in these critically ill patients.

2. Initial fluid replacement is important. Early, one unit of plasma or plasmanate should be given for each L. of crystalloid solution.

3. All fluids infused or perfused in the patient with shock lung should be multiple-filtered to remove microemboli and to eliminate aggregation of colloids.

4. Serum salt-poor albumin (50 g. over a one-hour period) or low-molecular-weight dextran enhances the colloidal osmotic pressure of the pulmonary perfusate. This helps to prevent pulmonary edema.

5. Fluid therapy is monitored by urine output.

6. Central venous pressure (CVP) is not an infallible indicator of myocardial efficiency. Its use should be accompanied by frequent auscultation of the lungs to determine the presence of moist rales and of the heart to determine the presence of protodiastolic gallop sounds. CVP monitoring measures only the function of the right side of the heart.

7. Pulmonary artery pressure (PAP) and pulmonary wedge pressure (PWP) monitoring by means of a Swan-Ganz catheter gives an index of left ventricular competence.

8. In the critically ill, the auscultation of blood pressure by the cuff method is inaccurate and it is better to cannulize a peripheral artery and connect it to a strain-gauge transducer measuring device. It also affords easy access for sequential arterial blood gas determinations and other laboratory blood samples.

9. Fluid replacement is adequate when

either urine output returns to adequate levels (more than 40 ml./h.) or CVP or PWP rise rapidly.

10. If urine output is not reestablished by fluid loading, furosemide (80 mg.) is given.

11. In most patients, arterial blood pressure, CVP, PWP, urine output, and pulse rate will be restored to normal or near normal levels with the measures above. If, however, urine output does not return to adequate levels, indicating adequate perfusion, the patient should be rapidly digitalized.

12. Regulation of breathing with a machine that can maintain a positive-end expiratory pressure (PEEP) is perhaps the most important treatment that can be given to the patient when the shock lung syndrome develops.

a. The end expiratory pressure is first set at 8 cm. H_2O and gradually increased to 18 to 20 cm. H_2O, a level that maintains arterial pO_2 at the desired level of 60 to 90 mm. Hg on a minimum percentage of inspired oxygen.

b. A volume-cycled respirator is more useful in these patients than the traditional pressure-cycled ventilators.

18. Gestationally Induced Hypertension

David H. Fields, M.D.

DEFINITIONS[1]

1. Hypertension

a. Systolic blood pressure greater than 140 mm. Hg, or a rise greater than 30 mm. Hg

b. Diastolic blood pressure greater than 90 mm. Hg or a rise greater than 15 mm. Hg

2. Proteinuria. Greater than 0.3 g. excreted per 24 hours

3. Edema. Persistent edema of lower extremities after overnight bedrest, or edema of hands or face

4. Preeclampsia. This is the development of hypertension with proteinuria or edema or both after the twentieth week of gestation.

a. Mild preeclampsia: The occurrence of preeclampsia uncomplicated by neurologic symptoms, severe hypertension, or proteinuria.

b. Severe preeclampsia: Preeclampsia complicated by the occurrence of any of the following:

(1) Systolic blood pressure greater than 160 mm. Hg or diastolic blood pressure greater than 110 mm. Hg at bedrest

(2) Proteinuria of 5 g. or greater per 24 hours

(3) Oliguria (output less than 500 ml. per 24 hours)

(4) Cerebral or visual disturbances or hyperreflexia

(5) Right upper quadrant or epigastric pain

(6) Pulmonary edema or cyanosis

5. Eclampsia. When convulsions occur in a preeclamptic woman, the condition is upgraded to eclampsia.

6. Gestational Hypertension. The development of hypertension in the second half of pregnancy without either proteinuria or edema

7. Gestational Edema. The isolated accumulation of 5 pounds of edema fluid in one week

8. Chronic Hypertension. Hypertension existing before the twentieth week of pregnancy or persisting after the puerperal period

9. Superimposed Preeclampsia. Preeclampsia occurring in a woman who has pre-existing hypertension

PREECLAMPSIA

Basic Principles

1. Preeclampsia is still a disease whose etiology is unknown. However much of the underlying pathology is beginning to be understood. Central to the condition is generalized vasospasm. This results in many of the symptoms and signs of preeclampsia:

a. Hypertension secondary to increased arterial constriction

b. Edema, probably secondary to increased transudation of fluid out of the vascular system

c. Multiple organ symptomatology secondary to spasm in the vessels supplying them, with associated decreases in blood flow

c. Fetal malnutrition and distress secondary to decreased uterine and placental blood flow and functional placental insufficiency

1. Committee on Terminology of the American College of Obstetrics and Gynecology.

2. Although the cause of the vasospasm is unknown, it has been determined that preeclamptic women exhibit an increased sensitivity to infused angiotensin II.

a. This is the most potent vasopressor identified in the body. It is an end product of the reaction initiated by renin acting on renin substrate to produce angiotension I, a decapeptide, which is further cleaved by angiotensinase to angiotensin II, an octopeptide.

b. Angiotensin, renin, and aldosterone levels all increase during normal pregnancy, but sensitivity to them apparently decreases so that a drop in blood pressure occurs during much of normal gestation. In preeclamptic women, although these hormones are, in fact, present in lower concentration, vascular reactivity to them seems increased. As stated above, this is for unknown reasons.

3. Secondary to vasospasm, the preeclamptic woman has a decreased intravascular volume. The more severe the preeclampsia, the lower the circulating blood volume is likely to be. *Understanding this is of key importance to the management of preeclampsia.*

4. Preeclampsia threatens pregnancy in two ways:

a. At any time it may progress to eclampsia. Eclamptic convulsions carry a significant risk of death for both mother and fetus.

b. With progressively worse vasospasm and decreased uteroplacental blood flow, the fetus is in danger of intrauterine growth retardation and fetal distress.

5. All therapy for preeclampsia currently available is ameliorative. The only cure for the disease is termination of pregnancy.

6. Eclampsia is an immediate threat to the life of both mother and fetus and requires termination of the pregnancy as soon as possible.

7. All the changes of preeclampsia and eclampsia are reversible with termination of the pregnancy except for infarction in specific organs.

SPECIFIC ALTERATIONS IN PREECLAMPSIA AND ECLAMPSIA

Renal

These have been most extensively studied and are primarily related to two factors:

1. Decreased Glomerular Filtration Rate (GFR) proportional to the severity of the disease

a. Because of decreased renal blood flow secondary to decreased intravascular volume, GFR also decreases. In very severe preeclampsia, it may even fall to or below nonpregnant levels.

b. This lowered GFR results in a fall in clearance by the kidney of substances such as creatinine, urea nitrogen, and uric acid and accounts for increased serum levels of these substances found in preclampsia.

c. In very severe preeclampsia, renal blood flow and GFR are lowered to the point of creating oliguria. This requires aggressive therapy.

d. Renal blood flow may occasionally be lowered to the point of developing renal cortical necrosis. This is rare and is thought to be caused by renal artery spasm.

2. Glomerular Capillary Endotheliosis

a. The deposition of what may be a fibrin derivative within the endothelial cells of the glomerular capillaries is considered to be the pathognomonic lesion of preeclampsia. The origin of this substance is unknown.

b. Damage to the glomerular capillary endothelium is probably responsible for the proteinuria characteristic of the later stages of preeclampsia.

Uterus and Placenta

1. Uteroplacental blood flow is typi-

cally compromised in the more severe cases of preeclampsia. It has been posited in the past that uterine ischemia might well "fuel the fire" of preeclampsia by resulting in release of a toxin. This has not been demonstrated.

2. Decreased uteroplacental blood flow is apparently responsible for the detrimental effects of preeclampsia on the fetus, by decreasing nutritional and oxygen supply. This has been demonstrated.

3. The uterus seems to be more irritable in preeclamptic and eclamptic pregnancy, accounting for the ease with which induction is frequently performed. Whether this is related to decreased blood supply is unknown.

Liver

1. Hepatic blood flow is somewhat decreased in severe preeclampsia, as are tests of liver function such as BSP excretion. In addition, serum glutamic oxaloacetic transaminase (SGOT) may also be elevated.

2. Pathologic changes in the liver such as periportal necrosis and hemorrhage seem to be a result of eclampsia.

3. Edema of the liver, or subcapsular hemorrhage, resulting in stretching of Glisson's capsule and right upper quadrant pain are considered grave prognostic signs.

Brain

1. Cerebral edema as documented by fundiscopic examination may occur in severe preeclampsia. It is usually attended by blurred vision and unrelenting headache, and is a grave sign.

2. Cerebral lesions, including thrombosis and cerebrovascular hemorrhage, have been documented on postmortem examination of eclamptic women. Their occurrence may be either a result or a cause of eclamptic convulsions and death.

Cardiopulmonary Changes

1. With the exception of decreased cardiac output secondary to decreased circulating blood volume, all the cardiopulmonary alterations are related to eclampsia.

2. During a convulsion, lack of respiration results in carbon dioxide retention and respiratory acidosis, with subsequent compensatory hyperventilation.

3. Pulmonary edema and congestive heart failure are rarely seen except on postmortem examination, where they are common findings.

Hematologic Changes

1. Hemoconcentration results from the decrease in intravascular volume. A progressively rising hematocrit is a sign of worsening preeclampsia.

2. Coagulation abnormalities have been among the most extensively studied in recent years, partly on the premise that preeclampsia might be due to a chronic form of disseminated intravascular coagulation (DIC).

a. Thrombocytopenia may be found in a significant percentage of severely preeclamptic women, with or without other clotting abnormalities. It is generally taken as an indication for delivery. Hemorrhage on the basis of thrombocytopenia is not common and does not occur until the count falls below 20,000 per cubic millimeter.

b. Evidence of intravascular coagulation consisting of elevated fibrin degradation products, prolonged thrombin time, and less often elevated prothrombin and partial thromboplastin times and hypofibrinogenemia, have been identified in severe preeclampsia and eclampsia with varying frequency. Current feeling is that they are more likely to be results of the disease process rather than a cause for it.

c. Microangiopathic hemolysis may occur in severe preeclampsia and eclampsia. It is probably secondary to intravascular fibrin deposition.

Eyes

1. Visual changes are usually secondary to retinal edema and ischemia and are transient.
2. Rarely retinal detachment will occur. This usually spontaneously reattaches within a few weeks.

Fluid and Electrolyte Changes

1. Vasoconstriction, decreased intravascular volume, and decreased glomerular filtration rate, all of which have been discussed, are the major changes.
2. Although total-body sodium may be somewhat low, serum concentrations of sodium and other elecrolytes are unchanged.

Diagnosis

1. The key to diagnosis of preeclampsia is suspicion. Careful watching for early signs is indicated in cases of:
   a. First pregnancies
   b. Previously existing hypertension, renal disease, or vascular disease
   c. Diabetes
   d. Multiple gestation
2. Be alert for
   a. "Transient" increases of blood pressure, especially diastolic pressures approaching 90 mm. Hg
   b. Edema of the lower extremities which is present upon arising in the morning
   c. Rapid weight gain, greater than 2 pounds in any week
   d. All the later signs, such as proteinuria, visual disturbances, headaches, epigastric or right upper quadrant abdominal pain
3. Perform the roll-over test on all suspect nulliparas between 28 and 32 weeks gestation. This test is performed by measuring blood pressure in the lateral recumbent position, then repeating the measurement after rolling-over to the supine position. A rise of 20 mm. Hg or more in the diastolic pressure is an excellent predictor for the development of preeclampsia.

Management of Preeclampsia

The management of preeclampsia is directed to two objectives:

1. Prevention of maternal injury, especially convulsion.

2. Delivery of a healthy, if possible, mature infant.

3. Once the diagnosis of preeclampsia is made, subsequent care should usually be in the hospital in all but the very mildest cases. Orders on hospital admissions should be as follows for mild preeclampsia.

Maternal Management

1. Bed Rest. Rest in quiet surroundings preferably in a lateral recumbent position. This serves both to lower maternal blood pressure and to increase uterine blood flow. Bathroom privileges should be allowed.

2. Vital Signs. Especially blood pressure q.4h. except 4 A.M.

3. Diet. Should provide ample protein and at least 2,400 calories daily. Salt should not be restricted in uncomplicated cases of preeclampsia, nor should fluids.

4. Weight. On admission and daily thoughout

5. Intake. Fluid sufficient to maintain an *output* of at least 1,000 ml. per 24 hours.

6. Complete urinalysis. On admission, and urine for protein at least twice daily

7. CBC

8. Electrolytes, BUN, creatinine, uric acid, liver, enzymes, serum total proteins and albumin, glucose (SMA6–SMA12).

9. Baseline coagulation studies. Fibrinogen, fibrin degradation products, thrombin time, prothrombin time, and partial thromboplastin time

10. Mild sedation. Phenobarbital 30 to 60 mg. q.i.d., is traditional but of questionable efficacy.

11. Diuretics. Once popular, these are not indicated in the treatment of preeclampsia. While they may lower blood pressure, they do not lessen the risk of convulsion and may even make fetal condition worse because of further decreases in uterine blood flow.

12. Eclamptic precautions. Airway, anticonvulsant, and tracheostomy set in the room

Management of Severe Preeclampsia

If the blood pressure is greater than 160/90 mm. Hg, or the mother has neurologic signs such as hyperreflexia or visual disturbance or epigastric pain, the following additions are made to the above orders.

1. Magnesium Sulfate

a. Administration: This may be given either I.V. or I.M. and is the cornerstone of management.

(1) I.V. solution is made with 10 g. $MgSO_4 \cdot 7H_2O$ in 1,000 ml. D_5W. This is infused at 1 g. (100 ml.) per hour after an initial loading dose with 4 g. (20 ml. of 20-per-cent solution).

(2) I.M. initial dosage of 10 g. (20 ml. of 50-per-cent solution) injected into buttocks (one-half on each side), followed by 5 g. (10 ml. of 50-per-cent solution) every 4 hours on alternating sides.

b. Magnesium sulfate therapy must be carefully monitored to avoid hypermagnesemia. It should only be continued as long as:

(1) A patellar knee jerk is obtainable

(2) Urine output is at least 25 to 30 ml. per hour

(3) Respiratory rate is greater than 8 per minute

c. Signs of magnesium toxicity of increasing severity which should be watched for are:

(1) Loss of patellar reflex

(2) Respiratory depression

(3) Complete paralysis

d. If necessary, the antidote for magnesium toxicity is calcium gluconate I.V., 10 ml. of a 10-per-cent solution.

e. Magnesium sulfate therapy should not be continued beyond 2 or 3 days, so that once it is begun, preparations for delivery should not be far behind.

2. Antihypertensive Therapy

a. Specific control of blood pressure in indicated if levels are such that the physician fears the risk of cerebral hemorrhage. Therapy is begun for systolic levels greater than 180 mm. Hg and diastolic levels above 110 mm. Hg.

b. Hydralazine (Apresoline) is the agent of choice as it not only lowers pressure by direct vasodilatation, but it also increases cardiac output. The preferred method of administration is I.V., 5 to 10 mg. every 20 minutes until desired control is achieved.

c. Diazoxide (Hyperstat) has been used. It has the advantages of long duration of action and no need for titration. A dose of 300 mg. by rapid I.V. push is given. Blood pressure usually drops within several minutes and remains lowered for several hours. It should be given with a dose of furosemide, 40 mg., because it causes salt retention and may precipitate circulatory overload. It also causes uterine muscle relaxation and may stop labor.

Fetal Studies

Preeclampsia threatens the fetus by progressively decreasing uteroplacental blood flow. If delay in delivery is anticipated because of prematurity, the following studies should be performed to ensure fetal well-being, while the mother's condition is being controlled.

1. Estriol determinations, either plasma

or urine, should be performed once or twice weekly to assess placental blood flow and function. They must be interpreted with the knowledge that decreased creatinine clearance will result in lowered urinary and increased plasma levels. They should be initiated upon diagnosis of preeclampsia, but not before 30 weeks gestation.

2. Human placental lactogen levels may be more useful than estriol in preeclampsia with renal impairment. The schedule and interpretation of testing is in the same fashion as for estriol (see Chap. 6, Antepartum Fetal Evaluation).

3. Contraction stress testing and nonstress testing may be initiated on a weekly basis beginning at approximately 32 to 33 weeks gestation.

4. Ultrasonography for determination of fetal size should be obtained as soon as the diagnosis is made and repeated in 2 to 3 weeks to assess fetal growth.

5. Amniocentesis for fetal maturity studies should be performed. It will most likely be rewarding after 36 weeks gestation, but possibly even at 34 weeks.

Termination of Pregnancy

1. Indications

a. Development of severe preeclampsia unresponsive to therapy as described above

b. Development of eclampsia, regardless of response to therapy

c. Fetal jeopardy as determined by which ever tests are being used, perferably a combination of stress or nonstress testing, a hormonal assay, and ultrasonography

d. Development of fetal maturity

e. Spontaneous labor may be awaited if preeclampsia remains mild and fetal distress does not supervene

2. Method

a. The preferred method is induction of labor via oxytocin infusion. This is usually quite successful because of uterine irritability, but special attention should be paid to the likelihood of uterine hypertonus. Continuous fetal heart rate monitoring should be performed during labor, with scalp *p*H determinations used as necessary.

b. If induction is not successful or if fetal distress in labor occurs, cesarean section should be performed.

3. Conduct of Labor

a. All precautions as for routine labor

b. Vital signs every 30 minutes

c. Check patellar reflexes hourly.

d. If magnesium sulfate has been begun, continue through labor.

e. Running I.V. throughout labor

f. Continuous fetal monitoring

g. Avoid conduction anesthesia, since epidural or spinal blockade may provoke precipitous drops in blood pressure in these already unstable patients. Shock will endanger both the mother and fetus.

h. Substitute instead analgesia during labor and local or pudendal block anesthesia for delivery.

i. Outlet forceps may be used to shorten the second stage.

4. Conduct of Cesarean Section

a. All normal preparations for Cesarean section as outlined in Chapter 14, Cesarean Section.

b. Avoid conduction anesthesia, as above. Balanced general anesthesia is the method of choice as it forestalls convulsions, causes little in the way of hypertension, and results in minimal fetal depression.

Postpartum Management

1. The risk of convulsion remains during the first 24 hours postpartum. Therefore, careful observation beyond normal postpartum care should be maintained for at least that long. After the first day, convulsions are extremely rare and may not be eclampsia.

2. If magnesium sulfate has been previously begun, continue for 24 hours postpartum. If not, mild sedation in the form of phenobarbital 30 mg. q.6h. may be used.

3. Avoid ergot alkaloids in the postpartum patient as these may precipitate a hypertensive episode.

4. Check for persistence of proteinuria daily until it subsides.

5. All other routines are as for normal postpartum management.

ECLAMPSIA

The occurrence of convulsions in a preeclamptic woman is a true emergency. It must be prevented if possible (see management of preeclampsia) or treated immediately. The foregoing precautions for preeclampsia are designed to avoid convulsions. If they fail and eclampsia occurs, the following steps should be taken.

Termination of the Convulsion

1. This may effectively be done using parenteral magnesium sulfate as described above (the loading dose of 4 g. I.V. is essential).

2. If this fails diazepam (Valium) 10 mg. I.V. or amobarbital 250 mg. I.V. should promptly arrest the convulsion.

Prevention of Further Convulsions

This is most effectively done by continuing magnesium sulfate therapy until delivery and 24 hours into the postpartum period.

Maternal Support Pending Delivery

1. Complete bedrest
2. Vital signs every 30 minutes
3. Nothing by mouth
4. I.V. fluids (D_5W) to keep vein open and maintain urinary output at a minimum of 30 ml. per hour
5. Foley catheter to monitor urine output
6. Continuous oxygen by nasal catheter at 5 L. per minute
7. Frequent observation to detect congestive heart failure or impending pulmonary edema. Therapy for these with digitalization as indicated.

Fetal Monitoring

Continuous monitoring should be instituted and continued until delivery.

Delivery

Termination of pregnancy should be begun by induction of labor as soon as maternal condition is stable. The previously arbitrary rule of waiting 12 to 24 hours after a convulsion should be disregarded, as the best way to avoid a second or third or fourth convulsion is to end the pregnancy.

Postpartum Management

Same as for severe preclampsia.

Prognosis

1. After delivery, the disease remits with no known permanent sequelae, unless there has been specific organ infarction or hemorrhage.

2. Subsequent pregnancies in women who have had preeclampsia or eclampsia are likely to be similarly affected in 15 to 20 per cent of cases.

3. Nonpregnancy hypertension does not appear to be any more common as a result of preeclampsia or eclampsia.

19. Chronic Hypertension in Pregnancy

David H. Fields, M.D.

DEFINITION

The presence of hypertension (blood pressure greater than 140/90) before the onset of pregnancy or occurring before the twentieth week in pregnancy not complicated by multiple gestation or molar disease is termed pre-existent or chronic hypertension.

BASIC PRINCIPLES

1. This is essentially hypertension unrelated to pregnancy which happens to be present. As such it occurs more often in women at increased risk for hypertension:

   a. Black females
   b. Gravidas over the age of 35
   c. Obese women
   d. Diabetics

2. Its cause may be any of the causes of hypertension. Most commonly this is essential hypertension, but it may also be

   a. Renal disease (either acute or chronic)
   b. Hormonal abnormality (e.g., hyperaldosteronism)
   c. Tumor (e.g., pheochromocytoma)
   d. Renovascular disease
   e. Collagen vasular disease (e.g., systemic lupus or periarteritis nodosa)
   f. Diabetic nephropathy

3. Since blood pressure tends to drop during the second trimester, a pregnant hypertensive woman first seen at this time may have a pressure within the normal range. Blood pressures at the upper end of normal during the second trimester should be suspect. They may be pushed out of the normal range by the expected third-trimester rise.

4. Hypertension may be grouped into mild and severe cases, and used to predict outcome:

   a. Mild hypertension—blood pressure remains below 160/100. There is no associated renal or cardiovascular disease.
   b. Severe hypertension—blood pressure is above 160/100. There may be associated renal, hypertensive cardiovascular or retinal disease.

5. The diagnostic workup for chronic hypertension during pregnancy should be the same as outside of pregnancy except for the radiographic studies.

   a. A particular search for pheochromocytoma should be made since this rare tumor carries a 50 per cent maternal mortality in pregnancy if not treated. The major symptoms are: headache, sweats, palpitations, nausea, vomiting, tachycardia, blurred vision, vertigo, and tremulousness.
   b. If the hypertension persists after pregnancy, x-ray studies, including a hypertensive IVP should be done at that time.

RISKS OF HYPERTENSION DURING PREGNANCY

1. Preeclampsia. There is an increased risk of preeclampsia superimposed on the woman with chronic hypertensive vascular disease. This may vary from 15 to 50 per cent depending on the study and criteria used. It is usually a very severe disease with poor prognosis.

2. Fetal Jeopardy and Growth Retardation. If maternal blood pressure remains below 160/100, there is no statistical increase in fetal loss over normal pregnancies.

3. Placental Abruption. Chronic hypertension is one of the only conditions that has been well documented as predisposing to premature separation of the placenta.

4. If pheochromocytoma is the cause of the hypertension, maternal mortality may approach 50 per cent.

5. Prognosis. Pregnancy does not worsen the course of hypertension after the end of gestation.

ANTEPARTUM MANAGEMENT

Diagnostic Studies

1. Upon diagnosis the following maternal studies should be obtained. If normal they should be repeated as the need arises.

a. Urinalysis

b. SMA-6 electrolytes, BUN, glucose

c. Serum creatinine and creatinine clearance

d. Fundiscopic exam

e. Oral glucose tolerance test

2. The following studies of fetal well-being should also be done:

a. *Ultrasonography.* Initially between 20 and 24 weeks gestation and then every 3 to 6 weeks, if there is any evidence of maternal hypertensive vascular disease

b. *Estriol or human placental lactogen* measurement beginning weekly at 30 to 32 weeks gestation and biweekly from 35 weeks

c. *Stress and Nonstress Testing.* Weekly from 32 to 34 weeks, depending on the severity of the disease

d. *Amniocentesis* for fetal maturity, when elective delivery is contemplated

3. Early termination of pregnancy may be necessary for preeclampsia, if it occurs, or fetal distress. Otherwise spontaneous labor is awaited.

Therapy

1. Biweekly visits until the 30th week and then weekly until delivery should be the rule.

2. Minimal salt restriction is unnecessary unless the mother has heart disease.

3. Antihypertensive Medication. Therapy is only indicated for pressures above 160/100. The risk of decreasing placental blood flow must be weighed against the benefits of lowered blood pressure. Pressures should be maintained at the upper limits of normal to minimize this risk. The following agents may be used:

a. *Hydralazine* (Apresoline) is the drug of choice because it is a direct vasodilator which simultaneously increases cardiac output and tends to maintain placental blood flow. It may be used orally in doses ranging from 10 to 50 mg. q.i.d.

b. *Methyldopa* (Aldomet) is also an excellent drug. Acting as a false transmitter, it lowers blood pressure without decreasing cardiac output. Starting in its lower range, the dosage may vary from 250 mg. P.O. t.i.d. to up to several g. per day.

c. *Diazoxide* (Hyperstat) may be indicated for control of acute severe hypertension unresponsive to hydralazine. Since it may cause salt and water retention, it should be followed by a dose of 40 mg. furosemide (Lasix). The dose of diazoxide is 300 mg. by rapid I.V. injection. It is followed within minutes by a maximal response, if any is going to occur. Blood pressure rarely falls below normal limits.

d. *Reserpine-containing compounds* are rarely used in pregnancy because of fetal side effects, such as nasal stuffiness and because other drugs are as, or more, effective.

e. *Diuretics* are *not* indicated for

the treatment of hypertension during pregnancy.

MANAGEMENT OF LABOR

Labor is conducted normally with the following exceptions:

1. Electronic fetal monitoring is mandatory.
2. Blood pressure should be checked frequently to detect intrapartum preeclampsia.
3. Avoid the use of spinal or epidural anesthesia.
4. Avoid ergot alkaloids in the third stage of labor.

POSTPARTUM MANAGEMENT

The postpartum orders are essentially unchanged from those of normal pregnancy, except for:

1. Frequent blood pressure checks
2. Avoiding the use of ergot alkaloids

20. Diabetes and Pregnancy

David H. Fields, M.D.

DEFINITION

1. Diabetes is an endocrine disorder characterized by inadequate insulin secretion to meet metabolic needs. This results in an inability to move sugar from the plasma into the cells. "Intracellular starvation," in the face of high blood sugar (with a switch to fatty acid metabolism and the formation of ketone bodies), results in the typical picture of hyperglycemic keto-acidosis of the "out of control" diabetic.

2. While the metabolic effects are most dramatic, in the long run, changes in the vascular system may be more significant. This is also true for complications of pregnancy in the severely diabetic woman.

BASIC PRINCIPLES

Effects of Pregnancy on Diabetes

1. Pregnancy is a diabetogenic state, mostly because of the anti-insulinic effects of huge amounts of human placental lactogen, estrogen, and progesterone produced by the placenta.

2. Women who are borderline or chemical diabetics before pregnancy may become overtly diabetic while pregnant. This condition reverts in the postpartum period and tends to recur with the next pregnancy.

3. Two to 4 per cent of otherwise normal women will develop chemical diabetes while pregnant (gestational diabetes, Class A diabetes) which reverts to normal after delivery. While up to 30 per cent of these women may later become diabetic, there is no evidence that pregnancy increases this tendency (only that it unmasks it).

4. Overt or insulin-dependent diabetics who become pregnant tend to become more severely diabetic with increases in insulin needs averaging between 50 and 100 per cent.

Effects of Diabetes on Pregnancy

1. *Increased perinatal mortality*. Prior to careful blood sugar control and antepartum fetal evaluation, perinatal mortality varied from 4 per cent in the mildest (Class A) diabetics to upwards of 50 per cent in the most severe cases. These figures are being revised sharply downwards as modern management begins to be widely used, into a Class A perinatal mortality approaching that of the population at large, and the rest at between 3 and 10 per cent. Major causes are:

   a. Sudden intrauterine death (etiology unknown)

   b. Prematurity

2. Increased risk of preeclampsia—up to four times

3. Increased risk of infection, especially of the urinary tract

4. Hydramnios

5. Increased incidence of postpartum hemorrhage

6. Fetal macrosomia

7. Fetal respiratory distress syndrome even with good L/S ratio

BASIC PRINCIPLES OF MANAGEMENT

1. Detect diabetes with a high index of suspicion and a liberal use of oral glucose tolerance testing.

2. Control maternal diabetes through diet and insulin, aiming for normal fasting blood sugar levels and 2-hour post-

prandial sugar in the 140 to 150 mg. per 100 ml. range.

3. ORAL HYPOGLYCEMIC AGENTS ARE CONTRAINDICATED IN PREGNANCY.

4. Be alert for maternal complications such as preeclampsia and infection.

5. Monitor fetal condition by various antepartum tests of well-being (estriol, oxytocin stress testing and nonstress testing, ultrasonography). Human placental lactogen measurement is not as useful in diabetes because of abnormal placental mass.

6. Terminate pregnancy when there is evidence of fetal jeopardy or of fetal maturity, whichever comes first. An L/S ratio of 2 generally suggests fetal maturity. In pregnancy complicated by diabetes, there is an increased likelihood of respiratory distress syndrome and some people suggest 2.5 or even 3 as a more likely safe L/S ratio.

DETECTION OF DIABETES

1. Basic Parameters. The cornerstone for the detection of diabetes is blood sugar measurement. If the patient has an elevated fasting blood sugar (more than 90 mg. per 100 ml. in whole blood or 105 mg. per 100 ml. in plasma), she is overtly diabetic. If the fasting blood sugar is normal, the condition of gestational diabetes may be diagnosed by the 2-hour oral glucose tolerance test (OGTT).

2. Indications for OGTT

a. Family history of diabetes

b. Glycosuria

c. History of large fetus (more than 4,000 g.)

d. Previous stillbirth

e. Preeclampsia

f. Obesity

g. Excessive weight gain during pregnancy

h. Recurrent urinary tract infection or candidiasis

i. Grand multiparity

3. Performance of OGTT

a. Load the patient's diet with carbohydrate for 3 days preceding the test.

b. Test in the morning after an overnight fast.

c. Draw a fasting blood sugar.

d. Administer a 100-g. glucose load.

e. Obtain blood specimens at 1, 2, and 3 hours after glucose load.

4. Interpretation of OGTT

a. Normal values—

Fasting	90 whole blood
	105 serum
One hour	165 whole blood
	185 serum
Two hour	145 whole blood
	165 serum
Three hour	125 whole blood
	145 serum

b. Chemical diabetes may be diagnosed if at least two values are exceeded other than the fasting blood sugar. If the fasting sugar is elevated, the patient may be considered to be an overt diabetic in need of insulin. A normal OGTT at 13 weeks may be abnormal at 28 to 32 weeks and should be repeated.

5. The intravenous glucose tolerance test is only occasionally used due to high false-negative rate (up to 50 per cent). Fifty ml. of 50-per-cent glucose is administered intravenously over a 4-minute period. It is considered normal if the fasting and 2-hour levels are in the normal range.

CLASSIFICATION OF DIABETES

White System

The most widely used classficiation is the White system upon which a rigid delivery schedule was superimposed.

1. Class A. Chemical diabetes (abnormal glucose tolerance test)

2. Class B. Adult onset of diabetes (elevated fasting blood sugar) of less than 10 years duration

3. Class C. Diabetes of 10 to 19 years duration or onset from ages 10 to 19; no vascular disease present

4. Class D. Diabetes of more than

twenty years duration or onset before 10 years of age; vascular lesions, benign retinopathy, calcified leg vessels

5. Class E. Calcification of iliac or uterine arteries

6. Class F. Diabetic nephropathy

7. Class R. Retinal neoangiogenesis

Functional Classification

For purposes of modern management with intrauterine surveillance and careful blood sugar control, a simpler, more functional classification might be made:

1. Diet-Controlled (Non-Insulin Dependent) Diabetes. Those diabetics whose blood sugar can be controlled with diet. This group roughly correlates with Class A, including only patients with normal fasting blood sugars.

2. Insulin-Dependent Diabetics. Those patients who require insulin for blood sugar control (all patients with elevated fasting blood sugars). For prognostic significance, this group may be broken down into two subgroups.

a. No evidence of renal or retinal vascular disease—this group will usually present no problems beyond sugar control; for the fetus, the risk of growth retardation is small, although macrosomia may occur if blood sugars are high.

b. Evidence of renal or retinal vascular disease—likely to have additional problems beyond sugar control (retinal hemorrhage, renal failure, and intrauterine growth retardation).

MANAGEMENT OF OBSTETRICAL PATIENTS WITH DIET-CONTROLLED DIABETES

1. With careful management, perinatal mortality should be within the normal range for intrauterine pregnancy.

2. Once identified by OGTT, these patients are placed on a diet designed to maintain 2-hour postprandial blood sugars at no more than 150 mg. per 100 ml. and fasting levels below 100 mg. per 100 ml. If this cannot be accomplished with a diet providing at least 1,800 to 2,000 calories per day, the physician should recognize the need for insulin and treat the patient accordingly. For specific diets, a nutritionist should be consulted or the ADA diets may be used.

3. In addition to the routine antepartum laboratory testing, obtain:

a. Fasting and 2-hour postprandial blood sugars at 2-week intervals until delivery

b. Urine culture and sensitivity upon diagnosis

c. If blood sugars are within the acceptable range, no special attention is given to glycosuria.

Testing of Fetal Condition

1. Ultrasonography. Obtain initial measurements as early as possible (preferably by 20 weeks gestation) for accuracy of dating the pregnancy. Repeat every 4 to 6 weeks to assess fetal growth and detect macrosomia.

2. Estriol Determinations (Plasma or Urine). Begin once weekly at approximately 30 weeks to provide a baseline. Repeat twice weekly from 32 to 36 weeks, three times weekly from 36 weeks to term, and daily from 40 weeks.

3. Contraction Stress Testing (CST). Weekly from 35 to 36 weeks unless suggested by low estriols or abnormal growth pattern before that time

4. Nonstress Testing (NST) is coming into more general usage now and may be used in place of the CST. It should probably be done twice weekly because of its simplicity and followed with a CST if nonreactive.

5. Amniocentesis. For L/S ratio or other fetal maturity studies, before anticipated elective delivery

Timing of Delivery

1. If blood sugar control is good and fetal parameters indicate no jeopardy, the physician may await spontaneous

delivery, even beyond 40 weeks gestation.

2. Induced delivery should be preceded by amniocentesis with L/S ratio or other fetal maturity studies.

Planned Delivery

1. If delivery is easy (ripe cervix or repeat cesarean section), and all fetal indicators are favorable, deliver by induction or repeat cesarean section, when the L/S ratio is more than 2.5.

2. If delivery is not easy (unripe cervix, no cesarean section planned), and estriol levels are falling or low but the CST is negative, postpone delivery until the L/S ratio is 2.0, or the CST becomes positive. CST's should be performed daily under these circumstances.

3. If estriol levels are falling or low and the CST is positive, delivery regardless of condition of cervix or fetal L/S ratio. Preferably, attempt induction, but perform cesarean section if necessary.

Conduct of Labor or Cesarean Section for the Diet-Controlled Diabetic

With the exception of mandatory electronic fetal monitoring in labor, these may be conducted in the same fashion as for normal patients.

MANAGEMENT OF OBSTETRICAL PATIENTS WITH INSULIN-DEPENDENT DIABETES

As will be obvious from protocols below, the pregnant insulin-dependent diabetic should be managed by physicians skilled in the management of diabetes mellitus, and at hospital centers familiar with their problems.

1. Prenatal Visit Schedule. Unlike nondiabetic prenatal patients, diabetics should be seen at least biweekly during the first half of pregnancy and weekly during the second half.

2. Diet and Insulin. Strict control of blood sugar (fasting blood sugar below 100 and 2-hour postprandial less than 150) should be attempted through careful regulation of diet and a mixture of short- and long-acting insulins. This should be done in concert with an internist who is interested in both diabetes and pregnancy. Weight gain should be as for a normal pregnancy. Acetonuria and ketosis should be avoided.

3. Laboratory Testing

a. Routine prenatal tests

b. Fasting blood sugar and 2-hour postprandial sugars weekly

c. Glucose panel* early in pregnancy (for determination of insulin needs) and at least once in the third trimester.

d. Creatinine clearance should be done early in pregnancy and at least once, preferably twice, in each trimester subsequently.

e. Urine culture and sensitivity early in pregnancy and again in the third trimester.

f. Urine for sugar and acetone—three or four plus sugar or presence of acetone signals the need for blood sugar and carbon dioxide content determination.

g. Retinal exam—for baseline early in pregnancy and again in the third trimester.

Fetal Status Testing

1. Ultrasonography. Obtain by 20 weeks gestation and 4- to 6-week intervals thereafter to detect intrauterine growth retardation or macrosomia. If there is evidence of vascular disease secondary to diabetes, do ultrasonography at 3-weekly intervals.

2. Estriol Levels. Optimally begin once weekly at 28 weeks gestation, biweekly at 30 weeks, triweekly at 32 to

*This consists of measuring blood sugar levels at the following times: a) fasting, b) 2-hour postprandial (10 A.M.), c) prior to lunch (12 N.), d) 2-hour postprandial lunch at 2 P.M., e) prior to dinner (6 P.M.), f) 2-hour postprandial dinner (8 P.M.), and g) at about 10 P.M..

33 weeks, daily from 35 to 36 weeks. In diabetics who have vascular disease, begin daily estriol levels at 32 weeks.

3. Contraction Stress Test. Weekly from 32 to 33 weeks. Twice weekly or more frequent nonstress testing may be substituted as long as the result is reactive.

4. L/S ratio or other amniotic fluid tests of fetal maturity are performed prior to planned elective delivery. Initial attempts are likely to be rewarding at 36 to 37 weeks gestation.

Timing of Delivery

1. Spontaneous Delivery. May be awaited until 38 or even 40 weeks if all parameters of fetal well-being (ultrasonogram, estriol levels, CST) are reassuring, especially if the L/S ratio is less than 2.0.

2. Planned Delivery

a. If tests of fetal well-being are all within normal limits, planned delivery may be attempted when the L/S ratio is more than 2.0 or perferably 2.5.

b. If any one test of fetal well-being is ominous, but the remaining are in normal limits, delivery may be postponed until the L/S ratio is more than 2, but extremely careful surveillance in the form of daily nonstress or stress testing and estriols should be maintained.

c. If both estriol levels and CST indicate fetal jeopardy, immediate delivery should be performed, by whatever route is obstetrically indicated. A sudden drop in insulin requirements of 50 per cent or more is generally accepted as an ominous sign and an indication for delivery.

Conduct of Labor and Cesarean Section

1. Patients with good outpatient control should be admitted to the hospital for several days to 2 weeks before planned delivery for even better surveillance and control. Patients in poorer control may need earlier hospitalization.

2. All preparations for labor or cesarean section should be made as for nondiabetic patients, with the following additions:

a. The dosage of long-acting insulin should be reduced to one-half or one-third on the morning of delivery, with additional needs being met by short-acting insulin.

b. An infusion of 5-per-cent glucose in water should be started on the morning of delivery and continued at the rate of 100 to 125 ml. per hour during labor or surgery. If more fluid is required it should be in the form of salt solutions.

c. Urine sugar should be monitored at 2- to 4-hourly intervals. Levels of 3+ or 4+ should be checked with blood sugars to rule out renal glycosuria.

d. Intrapartum fetal monitoring is absolutely mandatory.

Common Indications for Cesarean Section in Diabetes

1. Fetal macrosomia, especially in milder diabetics

2. The need for early delivery in the face of a virtually uninducible cervix. Long inductions with their metabolic drain on the diabetic mother and fetus are currently in some disfavor.

Anesthesia for Delivery

1. If delivery is vaginal, local infiltration or pudendal block is preferred. Epidural and spinal anesthesia may be used, but the physician must meticulously watch for hypotension. If there is associated fetal distress, conduction anesthesia should be avoided.

2. For cesarean section, either general or nonemergency conduction anesthesia is appropriate. If cesarean section is for fetal distress in labor, general anesthesia should be used.

Postpartum Management

1. Because of the removal of the placental hormones and the fetus as metabolic stresses upon the mother, diabetes of all classes tends to become much less severe immediately after delivery.

2. Chemical diabetics usually revert to normal in the postpartum period and remain so.

3. Insulin requirements for other diabetics decrease markedly and may remain low for up to several weeks. For this reason, the mother should be managed on a reduced dosage of long-acting insulin (one-half to two-thirds the prepregnancy dose) or with no long-acting insulin until urine testing reveals a need for it.

4. In place of a fixed insulin dose, urine sugar and acetone should be checked q.i.d. for several days to weeks until stabilization occurs. Urinary glucose should be covered with short-acting insulin, usually according to the standard scale:

4 + sugar—15 units of insulin
3 + sugar—10 units of insulin
2 + sugar— 5 units of insulin
0–1 + sugar—no insulin

Five units of insulin should be added for 3+ acetonuria.

Neonatal Complications

The infant born to the diabetic mother faces the following risks more commonly than other newborns:

1. Respiratory distress syndrome, even in the face of an L/S ratio of greater than 2.0. The reason for this is unknown.

2. Hypoglycemia. Because sugar but not insulin crosses the placenta, the fetus may suffer beta-cell hypertrophy. When the constant supply of sugar is suddenly withdrawn (delivery), the neonate runs the risk of insulin shock.

3. Congenital Anomalies. The rate of congenital anomalies is at least doubled in insulin-dependent diabetics, and may be much higher in those with vascular disease or nephropathy. Many of these are forms of congenital heart disease.

21. Pregnancy Complicated by Medical Illnesses

David H. Fields, M.D.

BASIC PRINCIPLES

1. Almost any disease that can occur in a nonpregnant woman may also affect a pregnant woman.

2. When that happens, it is important to consider several things:

a. How does pregnancy affect the disease?

b. How does the disease affect pregnancy?

c. How does pregnancy affect the diagnosis and treatment of the disease?

d. How do the diagnosis and treatment affect the pregnancy?

3. Medical illnesses in pregnancy should be handled jointly by an internist (or subspecialist) expert in the particular disease and an obstetrician alert to the needs of pregnancy.

HEART DISEASE

Basic Principles

1. As detailed in Chapter 2, many of the normal cardiovascular accommodations to pregnancy would be suggestive of heart disease in a nonpregnant woman. These include the following signs and symptoms:

a. Tachycardia

b. Apparent enlargement of the heart with displacement of the PMI outward

c. Systolic murmurs

d. Third heart sounds

e. Dyspnea

f. Dependent edema

2. Because these "abnormal" findings are normal, the diagnosis of heart disease during pregnancy must be made before pregnancy or must be based on different criteria. Suggested criteria[1] from 20 years ago have essentially not been changed.

a. A diastolic or continuous murmur

b. Unquestionable cardiac enlargement

c. A loud, harsh systolic murmur

d. Severe arrhythmia (atrial fibrillation or flutter or advanced heart block)

3. Most of the physiologic studies determining risks at various stages of pregnancy (by measuring cardiac output) failed to account for aortocaval compression by the growing uterus and falsely predicted that cardiovascular volume and strain peaked in the early third trimester and then declined.

a. In fact, they continue to rise until the end of pregnancy, although more slowly after about 32 weeks.

b. There is an additional strain immediately postpartum, precipitated by contraction of the postpartum uterus with injection of several hundred ml. of blood into the vascular tree.

4. The management of most heart disease during pregnancy is directed at:

a. Predicting and combating the development of congestive heart failure

b. Protecting the mother against progression of her heart disease, especially valvular problems

c. Protecting the fetus against hypoxic insult

5. Maternal prognosis is roughly pro-

1. Burrell, C. S., Metcalfe J., *Heart Disease and Pregnancy*, Boston, Little & Brown, 1958.

portional to the severity of congestive heart failure.

6. Fetal prognosis is proportional to the severity of hypoxia.

Functional Classification of Heart Disease

The New York Heart Association has formulated a widely accepted classification for heart disease (outside of pregnancy) based on functional capacity rather than etiology or physical findings. "Symptoms" as used below refers to angina, dyspnea, palpitations, or severe fatigue.

1. **Class I.** Patients with no symptoms of heart disease on ordinary activity
2. **Class II.** Patients who are comfortable at rest, but have symptoms on ordinary activity
3. **Class III.** Patients who are comfortable at rest but have symptoms on minimal activity
4. **Class IV.** Patients who have symptoms at rest

Management of Heart Disease

1. In general, a plan of management for the pregnant woman with heart disease may be based on her functional classification in the nonpregnant state, since this will likely predict her ability to withstand the increase in cardiovascular work required by pregnancy.

2. All pregnant cardiacs should be managed in conjunction with a cardiologist.

Antepartum Management

1. Class I and Class II Cardiac Disease

a. Patients should be seen at least biweekly in the first six months of pregnancy by both obstetrician and internist, and weekly thereafter.

b. Adequate rest, usually at least 10 hours of sleep at night and a midafternoon nap, as well as after meals, should be encouraged.

c. Work should be limited to light housework or employment as tolerated WITHOUT symptoms.

d. Dietary restriction may be minimal, with exhortation to avoid excessive amounts of salt. If the patient is without symptoms on an unrestricted diet and on no medications, this regime may continue.

e. Since even mild respiratory infections are likely to provoke decompensation, they should be avoided, even to the point of not seeing people who have colds. Symptoms such as cough, shortness of breath, or increasing fatigue should be reported immediately and thoroughly investigated by the physician.

f. Since anemia increases cardiac work and is so common in pregnancy, it should be avoided if possible.

g. Careful attention to avoid cardiac decompensation is essential. If symptoms or signs of congestive failure occur, immediate hospitalization with aggressive therapy is mandatory. (see "Management of Acute Cardiac Decompensation").

h. Antepartum fetal jeopardy is proportional to the degree of maternal hypoxia. If there is no evidence of this, no special testing is necessary.

2. Class III Cardiac Disease

a. Consider therapeutic termination of pregnancy. Patients who have symptoms on minimal exertion while not pregnant are at grave risk for decompensation during pregnancy which is associated with maternal mortality rate of up to 15 per cent.

b. For Class III cardiacs who continue pregnancy, bedrest and close observation throughout pregnancy are preferred. Constant care by a cardiologist is necessary.

c. Salt-restricted (2 to 3 g. of sodium) diets help avoid congestive failure.

d. Continue all cardiac medications in appropriate dosage. These patients, who are in borderline failure before pregnancy, are already receiving various medications which may include:

(1) digoxin (Lanoxin)

(2) a diuretic such as hydrochlorothiazide (Hydrodiuril) or furosemide (Lasix)

(3) an anti-arrhythmic agent such as procainamide (Pronestyl) or quinidine.

e. Hospitalize at the first signs of worsening condition and continue hospitalization until after delivery. Once congestive failure has occurred during pregnancy, it will almost inevitably recur unless exceedingly meticulous management is undertaken.

f. Institute antepartum fetal evaluation during the third trimester if the mother is hypoxic at all, since chronic hypoxia predisposes to intrauterine growth retardation.

(1) Ultrasonography—begin at 24 to 28 weeks and repeat every 3 to 6 weeks.

(2) Estriol (or placental lactogen) determination—begin at 30 weeks gestation and obtain weekly.

(3) Nonstress or stress testing—weekly from 32 to 34 weeks gestation.

g. While early termination of pregnancy for fetal jeopardy may be necessary, it is usually not indicated for maternal disease. Long, hard, induced labors or cesarean section may be more strenuous for the mother than continuing pregnancy.

3. Class IV Cardiac Disease

a. Advise termination of pregnancy in the first trimester. These patients are in frank congestive failure before pregnancy. The strain of gestation and delivery carries a high mortality rate.

b. If the patient insists on continuing pregnancy, hospitalization for the entire pregnancy, with management using digoxin, diuretics, salt restriction, and other aids to cardiac control is mandatory.

Management of Delivery

1. Admission to the hospital before the onset of labor for Class I and Class II cardiacs is encouraged, although patients who have tolerated the entire pregnancy without incident may not require this. Class III and Class IV cardiacs almost always find themselves hospitalized before delivery for management of congestive failure.

2. While labor does involve cardiovascular strain, abdominal delivery is far more stressful, both intra-operatively and postoperatively. Vaginal delivery should be the rule, with cesarean section only for obstetrical reasons in all classes of cardiac disease.

3. The following orders should be written for labor:

a. Vital signs every 15 mins.

b. Bedrest, sitting or semi-Fowler's position.

c. I.V. fluids—D_5W at 50 to 60 ml. per hour

d. N.P.O.

e. Continuous electronic fetal monitoring

f. Nasal oxygen at 3 to 5 L. per min.

g. A Fleet's enema may be given if necessary.

h. More intensive care with monitoring of digoxin, diuretics, and oxygen status may be necessary for Class III and Class IV cardiacs.

4. Analgesia and sedation should be kept mild. The usual combinations of a narcotic and a tranquilizer may be used in reduced dosage.

5. If necessary, epidural anesthesia may be used. Every effort must be made to avoid hypotension since this may precipitate cardiac decompensation. Spinal anesthesia should be avoided for this reason.

6. Prophylactic low forceps may be used to shorten the second stage. Unless cardiac decompensation occurs, second stage labor is preferable to midforceps delivery.

7. Local or pudendal block anesthesia is preferred for vaginal delivery. If cesarean section becomes necessary, balanced general or well-performed epidural (be wary of hypotension) anesthesia is acceptable.

8. Avoid ergot alkaloids for management of the third stage as they may raise venous pressure.

9. Treat acute cardiac decompensation as it develops, although this is more likely postpartum.

Postpartum Management

1. While Class I and Class II cardiacs who have tolerated pregnancy well to this point usually encounter no problems, some may go into failure in the postpartum period. Therefore the same careful surveillance is necessary for several days postpartum.

2. Class III and Class IV cardiacs frequently need intensive care and management of severe congestive failure in the postpartum period, especially during the first 48 to 72 hours.

3. In all cases, avoid the use of ergot alkaloids unless necessary for postpartum hemorrhage.

4. Hypotension and infection still represent serious threats and careful attention for signs of either is mandatory in all cases.

Treatment of Acute Cardiac Decompensation (Pulmonary Edema)

1. Elevate the patient's head; sitting upright is best.

2. Morphine, usually 10 to 15 mg. I.M. q.2-4h., decreases anxiety, tachypnea, and pulmonary congestion. In acute pulmonary edema, a smaller dose (4 mg.) may be given intravenously to start.

3. Oxygen, 100 per cent by positive pressure if necessary, relieves hypoxia.

4. Perform rapid digitalization using digoxin 0.25 mg. stat and q.6h., up to a total dose of 1.0 mg., for the patient who has not previously received digoxin. For patients already digitalized, small additional doses of digoxin or ouabain may be required.

5. Furosemide (Lasix) in doses of 40 to 80 mg. by intravenous push may be life-saving.

6. Aminophylline, 500 mg. slowly I.V. and q.4h., relieves bronchospasm.

7. Rotating tourniquets will provide an immediate decrease in cardiac load by cutting down venous return.

8. Phlebotomy is rarely necessary, but may be used in addition to rotating tourniquets. Not more than 500 ml. of blood should be withdrawn.

Specific Additions to Management for Specific Diseases of the Heart

1. Rheumatic Heart Disease

a. More than one half of all heart disease in pregnancy is on the basis of rheumatic heart disease. Therefore, most of the management schema presented above have been developed largely in the treatment of rheumatics.

b. Antibiotic prophylaxis is indicated throughout pregnancy for all patients who have evidence of rheumatic valvular heart disease. This may be done with benzathine penicillin (Bicillin) 1,200,000 units I.M. monthly or penicillin V 250 mg. P.O. b.i.d. For the penicillin-allergic patient, sulfadiazine 1 g. P.O. O.D. or erythromycin 250 mg. P.O. b.i.d., will suffice.

c. In addition, wider coverage is indicated for delivery. Current recommendations are for broad-spectrum coverage with a combination of either penicillin and streptomycin or ampicillin and gentamicin, begun during labor and continued for one to two days after delivery.

d. Be especially watchful for the development of mitral stenosis. While other rheumatic lesions are comparatively benign during pregnancy, mitral stenosis tends to become progressively more symptomatic, with pulmonary edema a constant threat especially in the immediate postpartum period.

e. Valve repair or replacement may be attempted during pregnancy in cardiacs who do not respond to medical therapy. The fetal and maternal mortality risks of this procedure are not small and must be weighed against the alternatives.

f. Anticoagulation is reserved for the patient with a valve replacement. Since coumarin anticoagulants cross the placenta (and may be teratogenic in the first trimester), subcutaneous administration of heparin is the method of choice.

2. Congenital Heart Diseases

Increasingly common in women of childbearing age, this category includes a number of discrete lesions, including, in order of decreasing frequency, atrial septal defect, pulmonary stenosis, coarctation of the aorta, tetralogy of Fallot, aortic stenosis, and Ebstein's anomaly.

a. *Atrial Septal Defect*

(1) Even if the defect is large, with a significant left-to-right shunt, pulmonary hypertension with reversal of the shunt and cyanosis does not usually occur until after the childbearing years.

(2) These patients usually tolerate pregnancy well. Fetal loss is not overwhelming unless the mother is cyanotic.

(3) Antibiotic coverage for delivery may not be necessary, but the benefits would seem to outweigh the risks.

b. *Patent Ductus Arteriosus*

(1) Usually diagnosed in childhood because of the "machinery murmur," patent ductus has frequently been repaired before adulthood.

(2) If the defect is small, the left-to-right shunt will not reverse itself for years. If the defect is large, pulmonary hypertension may occur earlier with reversal of the shunt and cyanosis.

(3) If there is no cyanosis, pregnancy is well tolerated. If on the other hand, the mother is hypoxemic, fetal loss is very high. Early abortion, prematurity, and an increased incidence of fetal anomalies are results of chronic hypoxia.

(4) Sudden systemic hypotension may lead to acute reversal of the shunt with cardiovascular collapse. Avoid conduction anesthesia and be alert for postpartum hemorrhage.

(5) Prophylactic antibiotics are probably indicated for delivery.

c. *Ventricular Septal Defect (VSD)*

(1) Usually, patients who survive to childbearing age have small VSD's. These are associated with left-to-right shunts of varying degree and no particular problems during pregnancy.

(2) If the VSD is larger and a right-to-left shunt with pulmonary hypertension has developed, pregnancy is very poorly tolerated.

(3) Fetal loss in the face of pulmonary hypertension and cyanosis is high.

(4) The warnings about hypotension as given for patent ductus arteriosus, apply as well to VSD's if pulmonary hypertension has resulted.

(5) Again, the need for antibiotic coverage for delivery is controversial.

d. *Pulmonary Stenosis*

(1) A relatively common defect, this lesion causes symptoms proportional to the degree of stenosis.

(2) If it is severe with symptoms of dyspnea and syncope, surgical correction is indicated.

(3) If it is not severe, pregnancy is usually well tolerated.

(4) Antibiotic therapy is definitely indicated for coverage of delivery, even after surgery.

e. *Coarctation of the Aorta*

(1) Usually the lesion is near the ligamentum arteriosum, which may remain as a patent ductus arteriosus.

(2) It is usually asymptomatic and

discovered during a workup for hypertension.

(3) Major complications in pregnancy are rupture, bacterial infection, and congestive heart failure. Rupture during pregnancy is most likely to occur in the late antepartum period or in the puerperium, not during labor.

(4) Surgical repair during pregnancy is controversial but probably not indicated, since maternal and fetal survival do not appear to be increased.

(5) Antibiotic prophylaxis is indicated throughout pregnancy and during delivery.

(6) Vaginal delivery is preferred, unless abdominal delivery is necessary for obstetric reasons.

f. *Tetralogy of Fallot*

(1) The syndrome of ventricular septal defect, pulmonary stenosis, right ventricular hypertrophy, and overriding aorta is the most common cause of cyanotic heart disease beyond infancy.

(2) Because of cyanosis, the fetal loss rate is high, the rate depending on the degree of cyanosis. This has been roughly correlated with hematocrit. If the cyanosis is severe enough to result in hematocrit over 65 per cent spontaneous abortion is a virtual certainty.

(3) For those who do not abort, vaginal delivery is safe.

(4) Antibiotic coverage for delivery is indicated.

g. *Aortic Stenosis*

(1) Unless the stenosis is very severe, pregnancy is well tolerated.

(2) There is no particular increase in fetal risk unless maternal congestive failure occurs.

(3) Antibiotic prophylaxis is definitely indicated.

h. *Idiopathic Hypertrophic Subaortic Stenosis*

(1) This rare condition is characterized by hypertrophy of the ventricular system such that outflow obstruction occurs with increased cardiac output, as with exercise.

(2) Treatment consists of a B-adrenergic blocking agent, propranolol (Inderal). Although several theoretical risks may be suggested, in practice, none have been noted.

(3) Pregnancy and vaginal delivery are well tolerated.

Other Heart Diseases

1. Other forms of heart disease, such as coronary ischemic heart disease, are very rare.
2. Most of these patients are elderly and hypertensive.
3. Pregnancy is poorly tolerated, with a high fetal and maternal mortality.

PULMONARY DISEASE

Basic Principles

1. The diagnosis and treatment of the most commonly occurring pulmonary diseases of young women are largely unaffected by the presence of pregnancy.
2. With a few exceptions, pregnancy is largely unaffected by the course of, or treatment of, most pulmonary diseases of young women.

PNEUMONIA

Basic Principles

1. In or out of pregnancy, by far the most common cause of pneumonia is Diplococcus pneumoniae.
2. Pregnant women, however, do seem to be somewhat more susceptible to viral pneumonia, developing it more often and more severely than nonpregnant women.
3. The diagnosis of pneumonia hinges upon clinical suspicion leading to the chest radiograph. This is unchanged by

the presence of pregnancy. A chest radiograph may be performed with abdominal shielding without endangering the fetus at any stage of pregnancy.

4. The radiologic pictures of the various pneumonias are unchanged by pregnancy.

5. The major risks to pregnancy posed by pneumonia are:

a. A decrease in ventilatory capacity in more severe cases, and

b. High fevers

Management

1. Once the diagnosis of pneumonia is made, the management is essentially the same as out of pregnancy.

2. Hospitalization, followed by treatment with an appropriate antibiotic, most often penicillin (or erythromycin in penicillin-allergic patients) usually leads to rapid resolution of pneumococcal pneumonia.

3. The treatment for viral pneumonias, as in nonpregnant women, is largely supportive, with attention to the prevention of high fever and hypoxia.

ASTHMA

Basic Principles

1. Asthma is a chronic bronchospastic disease which frequently coincides with pregnancy.

2. Unless there is severe chronic hypoxia, it does not exert much effect on the course of pregnancy, not does pregnancy appear to affect asthma in any consistent way.

3. The major therapeutic regimes for asthma, with one exception, do not appear to have adverse effects on pregnancy.

Management

1. Asthma in pregnancy is managed in the same fashion as asthma in the nonpregnant patient.

2. Hydration, epinephrine, and bronchodilators such as aminophylline are indicated and safe for treatment of acute attacks.

3. The bronchodilators commonly used on a chronic basis between attacks may be continued in pregnancy, with the exception of those that contain iodides (Elixophyllin-KI, Isuprel compound elixir, Quadrinal).

4. Avoid iodide-containing medications because they cross the placenta and may cause fetal goiter.

5. When necessary, corticosteroids have been used to control asthma without a statistically proven ill effect on the fetus.

TUBERCULOSIS (TB)

Basic Principles

1. Screening for tuberculosis using the Tine or Mantoux test should be part of every prenatal evaluation.

2. If the test is positive, indicating previous exposure to TB, a chest radiograph should be taken to rule out disease.

3. If the chest radiograph shows evidence of disease, a full diagnostic workup, including sputum cultures, should be obtained to distinguish old from active disease.

4. A patient whose Tine or Mantoux test has converted from negative to positive within the last year, but who has no evidence of active disease, is termed a "converter."

5. This elaborate screening has been devised because there is a definite tendency for TB, which is not uncommon in the prenatal population, to activate during pregnancy.

6. Pulmonary tuberculosis has no effect upon pregnancy unless the mother has far-advanced lung disease with respiratory decompensation, or unless there is hematogenous spread of the organism.

7. Congenital tuberculosis is rare, but

neonatal infection is a real possibility if the mother has positive sputum.

Management

1. Active Disease

a. If active TB is diagnosed in a pregnant patient, therapy is initiated immediately. This consists of:

(1) Hospital isolation until sputum cultures turn negative

(2) Isoniazid (INH) 300 mg. daily

(3) Para-aminosalycylic acid (PAS) 12 g. daily

(4) Streptomycin 1 g. daily

(5) Two other drugs, ethambutol (15 mg./Kg. O.D.) and rifampin (600 mg. O.D.) have been shown to be highly effective and safe for treating nonpregnant patients. In fact the combinations of INH and ethambutol, and INH and rifampin, have replaced PAS and streptomycin regimes in nonpregnant patients. Both of these drugs are currently recommended for treatment of resistant cases in pregnancy and are under investigation for safety for the fetus. Their use should be initiated in the postpartum period.

b. Therapy should be continued as follows:

(1) INH—for 18 months (24 months in far advanced disease)

(2) PAS—until delivery, then switch to ethambutol

(3) Streptomycin—until sputum cultures turn negative and sensitivity of the organism to both other drugs is demonstrated. No longer than 3 months.

(4) If the mother has active disease at the time of delivery, the infant should be isolated from her until she has received at least three weeks of therapy. The infant should be treated prophylactically under these circumstances with INH.

2. Inactive Disease, Never Treated, and Converters

a. Until very recently, women in both of these categories were treated with INH therapy alone begun during the pregnancy, and continued for one year. However, recent recommendations of the Center for Disease Control have altered this because of reports of teratogenicity from INH.

b. Therapy is now withheld from pregnant women without active disease, and begun in the postpartum period.

Obstetric Management

1. This is unchanged from normal obstetric management unless the mother has far advanced disease with respiratory decompensation.

2. In case of respiratory embarrassment, heavy sedation should be avoided and maternal and fetal oxygen status should be carefully monitored.

RENAL DISEASE

INFECTION

Basic Principles

1. During pregnancy there is a tendency toward mild hydroureter and hydronephrosis with increased urinary stasis.

2. In addition, asymptomatic bacteriuria (a urinary colony count of 100,000 per ml. with no symptoms of infection) is present in up to 7 per cent of pregnant women.

3. Overt infection in the form of pyelonephritis or cystitis will occur in 20 to 40 per cent of women with asymptomatic bacteriuria, while its incidence in women without asymptomatic bacteriuria is under 2 per cent.

4. Pyelonephritis, as manifested by fever, chills, and flank pain, and verified by urine culture, is usually caused by E. coli. It also more often involves the right kidney.

5. Acute pyelonephritis carries a significant risk of prematurity. Asymptomatic bacteriuria has been suggested,

but not proven, to be a cause of prematurity.

6. Many patients who have asymptomatic bacteriuria or pyelonephritis are found to have chronic pyelonephritis, if investigated.

7. Urinary infections are found in greater than normal percentages of pregnancies complicated by

a. Diabetes
b. Preeclampsia
c. Sickle trait

Management

See Table 21-1. Preferred Antibiotics for Urinary Tract Infection.

ACUTE GLOMERULONEPHRITIS

Basic Principles

1. This is extremely rare, with an incidence of approximately one per 40,000 pregnancies.

2. The diagnosis is based on the occurrence of hematuria, proteinuria, oliguria, and hypertension two weeks after Group A B-hemolytic streptococcal infection, and is confirmed by elevated antistreptolysin O (ASLO) titers and low serum complements. Renal biopsy is not indicated in pregnancy.

3. During the third trimester, it may be virtually clinically indistinguishable from preeclampsia; ASLO titers and serum complement levels will aid in diagnosis if there is persistent hematuria.

4. The disease is self-limited and usually runs its course in two weeks, unless chronic disease occurs.

5. Reported fetal loss varies from very high to normal.

Management

1. Therapy is exactly the same for pregnant and nonpregnant women: supportive.

a. Control blood pressure using diazoxide, hydralazine or α-methyldopa.

b. Restrict fluid to output plus insensible loss.

c. Restrict salt.

d. Treat presumed streptococcal infection with penicillin.

2. If the disease persists beyond three to four weeks, termination of pregnancy may be advisable.

CHRONIC GLOMERULONEPHRITIS

Basic Principles

1. Chronic glomerulonephritis is actually a collection of diseases, most of unknown origin, resulting in progressive glomerular destruction.

2. Primary symptoms are varying degrees of proteinuria, impaired renal function, and hypertension.

3. The prognosis for pregnancy depends on the severity of the disease:

a. If there is severe hypertension (greater than 160/100) or severely impaired renal function (creatinine clearance under 60 ml./min., BUN greater than 25 mg. per 100 ml., creatinine greater than 1.5 mg. per 100 ml.), the prognosis for pregnancy is poor with a high incidence of fetal loss.

b. If renal function is normal and hypertension is absent or mild, the prognosis for pregnancy is good.

4. The maternal danger from chronic glomerulonephritis is primarily related to the high incidence of superimposed preeclampsia.

Management

1. Manage jointly with a nephrologist.

2. Test renal function frequently, using creatinine clearance as the yardstick.

3. If renal function begins to decrease, terminate pregnancy.

4. Control hypertension using antihypertensive agents and diuretics if necessary.

5. Restrict dietary salt and protein in proportion to the kidney's ability to ex-

Table 21-1. **Preferred Antibiotics for Urinary Tract Infection**

	Agent	*Dosage*	*Possible Pregnancy-Related Effects*
For asymptomatic bacteriuria	Sulfasoxizole (Gantrisin)	1 g. P.O. q.i.d.	When used late in pregnancy competes with bilirubin for binding by albumin and glucuronyl transferase
	Nitrofurantoin (Macrodantin)	50–100 mg. P.O. q.i.d.	May precipitate hemolytic anemia in presence of G-6-PD deficiency
	Ampicillin	500 mg. P.O. q.6h.	Decreases urinary estriol excretion
	Oral cephalosporin (any)	500 mg. P.O. q.6h.	May decrease urinary estriol excretion
For pyelonephritis	Ampicillin	1–2 g. I.V. q.6h.	Decreases urinary estriol excretion
	Parenteral cephalosporin	500 mg.–2 g. q.6–8h. (depending on specific agents)	May decrease urinary estriol excretion
For infection resistant to above agents	Gentamicin (Garamycin)	3–5 mg./Kg./day I.V. in 3 doses 60–80 mg. I.V. q.8h.	May be ototoxic or nephrotoxic to both mother and fetus
	Kanamycin (Kantrex)	500 mg. I.M. q.12h.	May be ototoxic or nephrotoxic
	AVOID TETRACYCLINES AND CHLORAMPHENICOL DURING PREGNANCY BECAUSE OF SEVERE FETAL SIDE EFFECTS.		

crete them, as measured by BUN, serum creatinine, and urinary sodium and protein levels.

6. Correct severe anemia with packed-cell transfusions. Iron and folate therapy are generally unrewarding.

7. Severe electrolyte, *p*H, and azotemic abnormalities may require dialysis.

DIABETIC NEPHROPATHY

Basic Principles

1. Characterized by azotemia, hypertension, and proteinuria, diabetic nephropathy usually only coincides with childbearing age in the juvenile-onset diabetic, because it takes so long to develop.

2. Even in those cases where it does occur in women of childbearing age, it is rarely so severe that creatinine clearance is lower than 60 ml., per minute. At this level of function or greater, renal disease usually has little impact on pregnancy.

3. The presence of diabetic nephropathy does decrease the fetal prognosis because it is usually accompanied by:

a. More brittle diabetes.

b. Generalized vascular disease, including uteroplacental circulation

4. Maternal condition in pregnancy may be worsened by two factors associated with diabetic nephropathy:

a. The likelihood of renal parenchymal infection is increased.

b. There is a high incidence of superimposed preeclampsia.

5. Beyond this, pregnancy does not appear to exert any harmful effects on the kidney disease.

Management

1. Usually, because it is relatively mild, diabetic nephropathy needs no special care.

2. Rather, diabetes complicated by vascular disease in general has severe implications for the fetus, and must be aggressively managed. See Diabetes in Pregnancy.

NEPHROPATHY DUE TO SYSTEMIC LUPUS ERYTHEMATOSUS

Basic Principles

1. Systemic lupus erythematosus (SLE) is a disease of women of childbearing age.

2. SLE without renal disease tends to remit during the antepartum period and exacerbate postpartum. Pregnancy is not dangerous for the mother but fetal loss is high, much of it early abortion.

3. Nephropathy occurs in more than one-half of patients with SLE, and may be either focal or diffuse glomerulonephritis.

4. SLE with focal nephritis and minimal proteinuria behaves as SLE without nephropathy during pregnancy.

5. SLE with diffuse glomerular disease (severe proteinuria and hypertension) suggest a poor prognosis for both mother and fetus during pregnancy.

6. Diffuse lupus nephropathy may be considered a contraindication to pregnancy.

Management

1. In patients with diffuse renal disease, avoid pregnancy if possible.

2. Azathioprine (Imuran) and prednisone are the mainstays of treatment in both the nonpregnant and pregnant states.

ACUTE RENAL FAILURE

Basic Principles

1. Acute renal failure may be secondary to anything that acutely decreases renal blood flow to the point of ischemia.

2. In pregnancy, inciting incidents are usually:

a. *Hemorrhage*—placenta previa, placental abruption, postpartum hemorrhage, uterine rupture

b. *Septic shock*—septic abortion, pyelonephritis (rarely), chorioamnionitis

c. *Intravascular hemolysis*—disseminated intravascular coagulation, eclampsia/preeclampsia, mismatched transfusion

3. Most renal failure is acute tubular necrosis. If the patient survives the oliguric phase, a diuresis occurs and the disease reverses itself, usually without residual damage.

4. Renal cortical necrosis resulting from more severe and prolonged ischemia is less common and is irreversible.

ACUTE TUBULAR NECROSIS

Diagnosis

1. Suspect acute tubular necrosis when oliguria (urine volume less than 500 ml./24 hrs.) occurs after one of the insults mentioned above.

2. Distinguish it from hypovolemia by determining urine concentration, osmolality, and sodium concentration.

a. In hypovolemic oliguria, the urine is:

(1) *Concentrated*—specific gravity greater than 1.015.

(2) *Hyperosmolar*—greater than 300 mOsm./L.

(3) *Salt-poor*—sodium less than 10 mEq./L.

b. In renal failure, the urine is:

(1) *Dilute*—specific gravity 1.010 or less.

(2) *Isosmotic with plasma*—280 to 300 mOsm./L.

(3) *Rich in sodium*—sodium greater than 30 mEq./L.

Management

1. Immediate

a. Immediate volume correction at the time of the insult with plasma expanders (Ringer's lactate) and blood, are the first steps.

b. After shock, hypovolemia, or other precipitating cause has been corrected, if oliguria persists, attempt to increase urine flow with a diuretic. Furosemide (Lasix) 40 mg. I.V. q.4h. is the best agent for this.

c. If this fails to maintain urine flow and no hypovolemia exists, oliguric renal failure may be presumed.

2. Oliguric Phase

a. Obtain daily BUN, creatinine, sodium and potassium levels.

(1) BUN will rise approximately 15 mg. per 100 ml. daily and creatinine 1 to 2 mg. per 100 ml. daily until equilibrium is reached at levels dependent on ultimate renal function.

(2) Serum potassium levels may quickly rise above 7 mEq./L. The rate will depend on intake.

b. Measure input and output of fluid daily.

c. Weigh daily.

d. Replace urine water and sodium output daily, with an extra 500 ml. water for insensible loss in the absence of fever.

e. Avoid renal infection by not using indwelling catheters, if possible.

f. Avoid potassium intake.

g. Restrict dietary protein to 20 g. daily.

h. Provide adequate carbohydrates to avoid catabolism of body protein.

i. Treat hyperkalemia with exchange resins (Kayexalate) and correction of acidosis.

j. Consider hemodialysis if there is:

(1) Resistant hyperkalemia

(2) Life-threatening hypervolemia

(3) BUN greater than 120 mg. per 100 ml., or neurologic symptoms felt to be on the basis of uremia.

3. Diuretic Phase. After approximately 2 weeks, urine output begins to gradually increase and may reach several L. per day. Management at this point should include:

a. Replacement of fluid loss, now in much larger amounts.

b. Daily measurement of BUN, serum creatinine, and sodium and potassium in both the urine and serum.

c. Replacement of sodium loss.

d. Replacement of potassium loss beginning as soon as levels fall into the normal range.

e. Liberalization of protein intake when BUN falls below 80 mg. per 100 ml.

Prognosis

1. Maternal mortality rate in acute renal failure during pregnancy may be as high as 20 per cent.

2. If the patient survives the oliguric phase, recovery is the rule with subsequent good, if not normal, renal function.

3. Future pregnancy is not usually affected.

CORTICAL NECROSIS

1. If the oliguric phase persists beyond 2 weeks, cortical necrosis should be suspected.

2. Diagnosis may be verified by renal biopsy.

3. Cortical necrosis is largely irreversible. It is usually fatal unless dialysis is instituted early.

ANEMIAS AND PREGNANCY

Definitions

1. The presence of a hemoglobin concentration less than 10 g. per 100 ml. or a hematocrit less than 30 per cent is evidence of anemia during pregnancy.

2. Hemoglobin concentrations from 10 to 12 g. per 100 ml. may be dilutional, or so-called physiologic anemia of pregnancy.

Basic Principles

1. Anything which may cause anemia in a nonpregnant woman, may also cause anemia in a pregnant woman.

2. The diagnostic workup of anemia is the same in and out of pregnancy with one basic exception: since iron deficiency is the most common cause of anemia in pregnancy and since pregnancy itself is the most common cause of iron deficiency, any microcytic hypochromic anemia in pregnancy is presumed to be secondary to nutritional iron deficiency until it fails to respond to iron supplements.

IRON DEFICIENCY ANEMIA

Mechanism

1. The normal menstruating woman frequently lives on the edge of iron deficiency although not frankly anemic.

2. Although menstruation ceases with pregnancy, the tremendous iron requirement of a normal term pregnancy (300 mg. for the fetus and 500 mg. for expanded red cell mass) virtually guarantee clinical iron deficiency in a woman not receiving supplementation.

3. This results in progressively decreasing bone marrow stores of iron.

4. A shortage of iron in the marrow leads to decreased synthesis of the heme molecule.

5. Decreased hemoglobin production leads to the formation of smaller erythrocytes.

6. Eventually, as iron stores are used up, the number of cells produced, as well as their size, decreases.

Diagnosis

1. A complete blood count done once in each trimester as part of routine prenatal care will identify the presence of anemia.

2. Overwhelmingly the most common cause of anemia during pregnancy, iron deficiency is presumed (until proven otherwise) to be the cause of any microcytic hypochromic anemia in a pregnant woman.

3. If adequate iron therapy (see below) fails to correct the anemia, further workup is indicated. This may consist of measurement of serum iron and total iron-binding capacity, bone marrow aspiration with staining for iron stores, and finally, hemoglobin electrophoresis, to rule out other causes of microcytic hypochromic anemia:

a. Chronic disease anemia
b. Beta-thalassemia minor
c. Sideroblastic anemia

4. Findings suggestive of iron deficiency are:

a. Low serum iron
b. High iron-binding capacity
c. Absence of iron stores in the bone marrow
d. Hemoglobin A on electrophoresis

5. Findings suggestive of other disease are listed below.

Management

1. Iron deficiency anemia is best treated *before* it occurs by prophylactic

Table 18-2. **Iron Studies in other Microcytic Anemias**

	Serum Iron	*Iron-Binding Capacity*	*Iron in Bone Marrow*	*Type Hemoglobin*
Chronic Disease	Low	Low	Present	A
Sideroblastic Anemia	Low	Low	Present in ring sideroblasts	A
Beta-Thalassemia	High	Low	Present	A_2 greater than 5%

administration of ferrous sulfate 325 mg. O.D. throughout the pregnancy.

2. Once anemia is diagnosed, supply iron supplementation—ferrous sulfate 325 mg. P.O. t.i.d., ferrous gluconate 450 mg. P.O. t.i.d., ferrous fumarate 325 mg. P.O. t.i.d.

3. Check the response in 10 to 14 days with a reticulocyte count. If the count is not over 3 to 5 per cent, pursue further workup as outlined above.

4. If further workup still suggests iron deficiency and rectal exam suggests that the patient is, indeed, taking her iron, consider the possibility of an absorption defect.

5. Parenteral iron in the form of intravenous or intramuscular iron dextran (Imferon) over several days to weekly is indicated if the patient cannot tolerate oral iron or appears to have an absorption defect. Total doses are calculated according to the patient's weight and hemoglobin concentration.

6. Transfusion is only indicated for anemia when it is discovered in labor, and hemorrhage or surgery is anticipated.

7. If another cause for the anemia is discovered, treat that.

Risks of Iron Deficiency Anemia

1. The risks to the mother from iron deficiency anemia are minimal, unless anemia is so severe as to result in high-output congestive heart failure or an increased risk of shock during delivery.

2. Placental changes with hypoxic effects occur at hemoglobin levels in the 8 to 10 g. per 100 ml. range.

MEGALOBLASTIC ANEMIA

Basic Principles

1. Folic acid, present in the blood as tetrahydrofolic acid, participates in many reactions, including DNA synthesis, as a coenzyme. In this capacity it is an essential participant in the production of nuclear material in red-cell synthesis. Folate deficiency results in an inability of the red cell to undergo fission within the marrow, with retarded development and the persistence of megaloblasts. Similar effects occur in the maturation of neutrophils and platelets, and folic acid deficiency is characterized by a pancytopenia.

2. Adequate intake of folic acid is supplied by a diet rich in eggs, milk products, and leafy vegetables. Absence of these items, combined with the increased daily needs of pregnancy, frequently result in folate deficiency.

3. Within three weeks, on a folate-deficient diet, blood levels begin to drop. In five weeks, hypersegmented neutrophils are seen in the marrow. By 18 weeks, the marrow is frankly megaloblastic and the patient is anemic.

4. Except in cases of severe long-term deprivation, or tremendously increased needs (especially twin gestation, epileptics taking diphenylhydantoin, and chronic hemolytic anemia), clinical evidence of folate deficiency does not occur until the third trimester.

5. It also commonly occurs in the postpartum period in nursing mothers, precipitated by the production of breast milk which is extremely high in folic acid content.

Diagnosis

1. Most commonly this is first detected by low hemoglobin levels or high-mean corpuscular volumes found on routine blood counts.

2. Further confirmation is obtained by a peripheral smear showing macrocytosis and hypersegmented polymorphonuclear leukocytes.

3. Bone marrow aspiration reveals a megaloblastic marrow, with red cells in arrested development.

4. Although vitamin B_{12} deficiency is rare, folic acid and vitamin B_{12} deficiency anemia are clinically indistin-

guishable. Since therapy is different, blood should be drawn for determination of serum folic acid and B_{12} levels before the therapy is begun for presumed folic acid deficiency.

5. Diagnosis may be complicated by the concurrent presence of iron deficiency. In such cases, a biphasic population of red blood cells is formed, some being macrocytic and some microcytic. Red cell indices by automated counters may average out to normal, but the situation becomes clear upon seeing the peripheral smear.

Management

1. Folic acid deficiency is best treated by avoiding it.
2. Provide a diet rich in folic acid-containing foods for the average gravida.
3. Supply all patients at high risk for folic acid deficiency with some supplemental folate. Most prenatal vitamins contain 0.8 mg. folic acid, an amount adequate for almost all needs. If uncertainty still exists, folic acid tablets, 1 mg. daily will eliminate any question of deficiency. Conditions which expose the pregnant woman to a greater likelihood of folate depletion include:
   a. Twin gestation
   b. Chronic hemolytic anemia, especially sickling disease
   c. Epilepsy with diphenylhydantoin (Dilantin) therapy
   d. Malabsorption states
   e. Acute infection
4. Consider the possibility of concurrent iron deficiency anemia and supply iron supplements.

Risks of Folic Acid Deficiency Anemia

1. Severe anemia, with high-output congestive failure threatening the mother and hypoxia affecting the fetus, is the most common danger.
2. Although there has been much speculation about the adverse effects of folate deficiency in pregnancy, most usually increased risk of preeclampsia and placental abruption, these are unproven.

OTHER ANEMIAS IN PREGNANCY

Vitamin B_{12} Deficiency

1. "Pernicious anemia" as a cause of megaloblastic anemia is rare in pregnancy for two reasons:
   a. Intrinsic factor defects are rare in women of childbearing age.
   b. Untreated Vitamin B_{12} deficiency usually causes infertility.
2. The diagnosis is made by measurement of serum Vitamin B_{12} levels.
3. The treatment is parenteral Vitamin B_{12}.

Glucose-6 Phosphate Dehydrogenase (G-6-PD) Deficiency

1. Due to an autosomal recessive enzyme deficiency found in a small percentage of black women, this results in hemolysis of red blood cells when they are exposed to oxidizing agents.
2. Common agents which may result in acute hemolysis are:
   a. Aspirin and phenacetin
   b. Nitrofurantoin (Furadantin, Macrodantin)
   c. Quinine and primaquine
   d. Sulfa drugs
   e. Vitamin K
3. Diagnosis is made by G-6-PD assay. However, since levels of this enzyme are lowest in old red blood cells (these are lysed during the crisis) and higher in newly formed cells, levels may approach normal immediately after hemolysis.
4. Since G-6-PD levels are lowest in old red blood cells and higher in newly formed cells, each hemolytic crisis is self-limited to cells whose enzyme content has fallen below critical levels.

Other Hemolytic Anemias

1. Any of the causes of hemolytic anemia may present during pregnancy.

2. A standard hematologic workup is necessary to identify the cause of hemolysis, followed by specific treatment.

HEMOGLOBINOPATHIES

Basic Principles

1. Hemoglobinopathies are hereditary disorders of hemoglobin production, resulting in the formation of abnormal hemoglobin (e.g., S, C, A_2).
2. When present in heterozygous forms, there is usually enough normal hemoglobin produced that pregnancy is well tolerated.
3. Homozygous hemoglobin abnormalities are usually either fatal in childhood, or severely debilitating in adulthood, and associated with an increase in maternal and perinatal morbidity and mortality.
4. Diagnosis is by hemoglobin electrophoresis for identification of abnormal hemoglobins.

SICKLE CELL ANEMIA (SS DISEASE)

Basic Principles

1. Production of hemoglobin S as the sole hemoglobin results in sickle cell anemia, occurring in approximately one in 500 blacks.
2. This results in hemoglobin levels that usually vary from 7 to 10 g. per 100 ml., and in red blood cells which sickle under hypoxic conditions, causing sludging in capillaries in all organ systems. These "sickle crises" result in intense pain and sometimes infarction in affected organs.
3. The major maternal complications of SS disease in pregnancy are:
   a. Severe anemia, frequently in the 7 to 8 g. per 100 ml. range.
   b. Frequent crises, with a high incidence of drug addiction because of pain
   c. Folate deficiency anemia
   d. Frequent pulmonary and urinary infections, especially pyelonephritis
4. Because of severe anemia, recurrent crises, and a higher risk of infection, especially pulmonary and urinary, sickle cell anemia carries a poor prognosis for pregnancy. Fetal loss is approximately 50 per cent.
5. Similarly, pregnancy worsens sickle cell disease. Anemia becomes more severe, crises more frequent, and infection more likely.

Management

1. Antepartum Management

a. Supplement the diet with folic acid (1 mg. O.D.) to avoid megaloblastic anemia.

b. Carefully screen increasing anemia, urinary tract infection, and pulmonary complications.

c. Avoid the tendency to attribute all symptoms to "crises" and seek other causes for pain or fever.

d. Transfuse with packed red cells for signs of congestive failure secondary to anemia or for hemoglobin levels below 6 g. per 100 ml.

e. Several studies are in progress evaluating exchange transfusions with normal red cells to reduce levels of cells containing hemoglobin S. Initial results indicate that, in the near future, exchange transfusion may eliminate most of the maternal and fetal complications of sickle cell anemia during pregnancy.

2. Management of Labor

a. Maintain intensive fetal and maternal monitoring.

b. Administer continuous oxygen by nasal cannula or mask during labor and delivery. Consider hypoxia as something to be avoided at all costs.

c. Avoid general anesthesia if possible.

d. Be alert for crises during labor and immediately postpartum.

SICKLE CELL TRAIT

Basic Principles

1. When the mother is heterozygous for the production of hemoglobin S, half of her hemoglobin is Type A. This is sufficient to prevent sickling under all conditions except severe hypoxia.

2. The only problem associated with sickle cell trait and pregnancy is an increased incidence of bacteriuria and symptomatic urinary tract infection.

Management

Standard prenatal management with special attention to the possibility of urinary tract infection is appropriate for pregnancies complicated by sickle cell trait.

SICKLE CELL-HEMOGLOBIN C DISEASE (HEMOGLOBIN SC)

Basic Principles

1. This rare condition is characterized by production of types S and C hemoglobin, instead of the normal A hemoglobin.

2. Having a tendency to both anemia and sickle crises, these patients have basically the same risks in the antepartum period as do those with SS disease.

3. Management during all stages of pregnancy is essentially the same as for sickle cell anemia.

B-THALASSEMIA

Basic Principles

1. This non-sickling hemoglobinopathy is characterized by the production of A_2 hemoglobin.

2. The homozygous form or B-thalassemia major (Cooley's anemia) is usually fatal in childhood and not a factor in pregnancy.

3. The heterozygous form, or B-thalassemia minor, is characterized by a mild anemia, which may be severely microcytic and hypochromic and may be confused with iron deficiency anemia at first.

4. The prognosis for pregnancy is excellent with no appreciable maternal or fetal morbidity, other than anemia with hemoglobin in the range of 8 to 11 g. per 100 ml.

5. No special management is required beyond awareness of the anemia and vigilance for infection which may aggravate it.

ENDOCRINOPATHIES

HYPERTHYROIDISM

Basic Principles

1. After diabetes, hyperthyroidism is the most common endocrinopathy associated with pregnancy. Most thyrotoxicosis during pregnancy is due to Graves' disease, rather than toxic nodular goiter. Graves' disease is a diffuse condition of the thyroid gland with overproduction of thyroxine related to a 7s-immunoglobulin, long-acting thyroid stimulator (LATS).

2. In addition to resulting in maternal hyperthyroidism, LATS crosses the placenta and may cause fetal thyrotoxicosis and goiter formation.

3. Milder degrees of hyperthyroidism are probably not related to increased perinatal morbidity, and indeed, because of the masking effects of pregnancy, may not even be diagnosed. More severe forms, however, predispose the mother to "thyroid storms" and probably result in increased fetal loss.

4. Clinical signs of hyperthyroidism may be confused by pregnancy:

   a. Weight loss of hyperthyroidism may be offset by the weight gain of pregnancy.

   b. Mild tachycardia may result from the increased cardiac demands of pregnancy.

c. Pretibial edema may result from hydrostatic changes of normal pregnancy.

d. Exophthalmos and extremity tremors are rarely the result of pregnancy.

5. Hyperthyroidism should be suspected in pregnant women who:

a. Fail to gain weight during pregnancy while consuming an adequate diet.

b. Have an elevated pulse rate

c. Are extremely "high-strung," especially those with a fine tremor of the hands or feet

d. Have exophthalmos. Exophthalmos, the most familiar sign of thyroid disease, is not medically reversible.

6. During pregnancy, placental estrogen production results in increased production of the $\alpha 2$ globulin, thyroid-binding globulin. The thyroid gland, in order to maintain "normal" levels of free thyroxine, increases total thyroxine output. This affects the normal thyroid gland and tests to evaluate it in the following ways:

a. There is a mild enlargement of the entire gland.

b. Iodine uptake increases substantially.

c. Total serum thyroxine and PBI levels increase up to 30 per cent.

d. T_3 resin uptake decreases up to 30 per cent.

e. Free serum thyroxine levels and the free thyroxine index remain unchanged.

7. Laboratory diagnosis of hyperthyroidism during pregnancy is complicated by the above changes because measurement of free thyroxine is expensive and difficult and radioactive iodine uptake studies forbidden. However, hyperthyroidism may be diagnosed if:

a. Total serum thyroxine is elevated beyond 16 μg. per 100 ml.

b. T_3 resin uptake rises into the normal range.

c. Calculation of the free thyroxine index (total $T_4 \times T_3$ resin uptake) is significantly elevated.

8. "Thyroid storm" is an acute exacerbation of hyperthyroidism with extreme fever (up to 106°F), severe tachycardia, congestive heart failure, dehydration, and cardiovascular collapse. Maternal mortality approaches 25 per cent. Immediate treatment for this medical emergency revolves around propranolol and hydration (see below).

Management

The treatment for hyperthyroidism may be medical or surgical or both.

1. Medical management is indicated especially during the first and third trimesters when surgery poses the threat of inciting abortion or premature delivery. It is also indicated to control disease and shrink the gland prior to surgical procedure.

2. Surgical management is preferred when medical control is difficult or inconstant, and should be performed during the late first, second, or early third trimester.

MEDICAL MANAGEMENT

1. Propylthiouracil (PTU) is the agent of choice for medical therapy. It blocks the synthesis of thyroxine, and is therefore without effect for one to several weeks until stores of the hormone have been exhausted. A similar agent, methimazole (Tapazole) may be teratogenic.

a. Administer PTU 100mg. orally t.i.d. until symptoms remit and serum thyroxine begins to fall. The best clinical signs are the resting pulse rate and the presence or absence of tremor.

b. Once initial control is established, decrease dosage as much as possible to avoid fetal goiter. This is usually to the range of 50 mg. P.O. t.i.d.

c. If control is not established on 300 mg. daily, higher doses may be used.

d. Be alert for complications of PTU therapy, most usually skin rashes and agranulocytosis. A falling white blood cell count requires immediate termination of therapy and careful observation.

e. Taper PTU therapy within several weeks of delivery to avoid fetal hypothyroidism at birth.

2. PTU crosses the placenta and may cause fetal goiter by blocking fetal thyroxine production. Compensatory fetal overproduction of thyroid-stimulating hormone would then result in hypertrophy of the gland.

3. Some physicians have advocated concurrent administration of PTU and thyroxine to prevent fetal goiter. Thyroxine crosses the placenta poorly and is unlikely to prevent fetal goiter. Conversely, it increases maternal PTU requirements and interferes with thyroid studies. It probably should not be used.

4. Propranolol (Inderal), a B-adrenergic blocking agent, has been suggested as alternate therapy for hyperthyroidism in pregnancy.

a. It blocks the "hyper" actions of thyroxine such as tachycardia, and decreases the likelihood of "thyroid storm." It does not affect the production of thyroxine.

b. If used, the initial dosage is 40 mg. t.i.d., increased 10 mg. t.i.d. every 2 to 3 days until adequate control of side effects occurs.

c. Adverse fetal effects of long-term intrauterine exposure to propranolol have not been noted, but have not been adequately ruled out yet.

d. Propranolol is the drug of choice for the treatment of "thyroid storm." See below.

Management of "Thyroid Storm"

This is a medical emergency. Therapy designed to control the extreme B-adrenergic symptoms until hyperthyroidism can be treated, is as follows:

a. Propranolol 1 to 2 mg. I.V. then 40 mg. P.O. q.6h. to control tachycardia

b. Institution of high doses of PTU therapy to prevent further thyroxine production

c. Massive immediate fluid replacement to combat dehydration.

d. Hypothermia blankets and other cooling agents to reduce fever.

SURGICAL MANAGEMENT

1. Partial thyroidectomy is the preferred treatment for patients who respond poorly to medical therapy.

2. While suggested by some as the therapy of choice, the morbidity and mortality risks are such that medical therapy, if effective, is preferable.

3. If performed, surgery is best done toward the middle of pregnancy, when uterine irritability is least.

4. The major complications of thyroid surgery, other than the actual risks of surgery and anesthesia, are subsequent hypoparathyroidism and recurrent laryngeal nerve paralysis. Both are extremely difficult to treat.

5. Thyroid replacement is necessary postoperatively.

HYPOTHYROIDISM

Basic Principles

1. Hypothyroidism, due to any one of many etiologies, is relatively rare in pregnant women.

2. Severely depressed thyroid function results in a high incidence of infertility and early abortion.

3. Diagnosis during pregnancy is complicated by changes in thyroid function discussed under hyperthyroidism.

4. Management consists of thyroid replacement with either USP thyroid, thyroxine or triiodothyronine (Cytomel).

CUSHING'S SYNDROME

Basic Principles

1. Adrenal hyperfunction complicating pregnancy is uncommon, and frequently due to adrenal tumor.

2. Diagnosis in pregnancy is complicated by the fact that many of the major signs (obesity, hypertension, abnormal glucose tolerance, increased pigmentation) occur in normal pregnancy.

3. Suspicion should be especially aroused if any of the following signs appear:
    a. Moon facies
    b. Centripetal obesity
    c. Fat deposition over the upper thoracic vertebrae
    d. Purple striae

4. Laboratory testing, as well, is altered. While in the nonpregnant state the basis of diagnosis is an elevated morning plasma cortisol, this occurs during normal pregnancy. The diagnosis, therefore, must depend on a test of adrenal function by dexamethasone suppression.

5. The fetal prognosis in pregnancy complicated by Cushing's syndrome is poor. In one series, 25 per cent of pregnancies aborted, 25 per cent resulted in a stillbirth, and 50 per cent in premature delivery.

Management

Because of the likelihood of a tumor as a cause for the disease and the poor prognosis, prompt surgical diagnosis and correction seems to be the therapy of choice.

ADRENAL INSUFFICIENCY (ADDISON'S DISEASE)

Basic Principles

1. Adrenal insufficiency may be secondary to chronic disease, most commonly in the past, tuberculosis; or it may be the result of previous adrenalectomy for hyperfunction.

2. Before the use of replacement steroids, Addison's disease resulted in infertility. With adequate replacement, however, a woman with adrenal hypofunction may become pregnant and carry to term.

3. The diagnosis during pregnancy is complicated by the fact that the major symptoms, fatigue, nausea and vomiting, weight loss, and increased skin pigmentation, may either be mimicked or masked by pregnancy.

4. Laboratory diagnosis, when the disease is suspected, is by measurement of plasma cortisol levels, which should be low, even during pregnancy.

5. The major danger associated with adrenal insufficiency in pregnancy is the development of acute Addisonian crisis at times of severe stress, especially soon after delivery. This is a risk in the previously diagnosed patient who receives inadequate replacement to cope with the puerperium, and may be the presenting episode in a previously undiagnosed patient.

6. Addisonian crisis is a medical emergency whose symptoms are: fever, nausea and vomiting, and shock. It may be due to the stress of the puerperium combined with the withdrawal of placental steroidogenesis, or to superimposed infection. It should always be in the back of one's mind as a possibility, in cases of puerperal shock, especially those which do not respond immediately to adequate blood and fluid replacement.

Management

1. For previously diagnosed Addison's disease, therapy during pregnancy is relatively straightforward. The normal replacement therapy (hydrocortisone acetate 37.5 mg. daily, or prednisone 7.5 mg. daily plus a mineralocorticoid) need not be changed from nonpregnant levels.

2. During labor and delivery, supplemental steroids are necessary (e.g., hydrocortisone 100 mg. IV. q.8h. for the length of labor) to avoid adrenal crisis.

3. Additional doses of cortisone should be continued until the third day of the puerperium, or if puerperal infection occurs.

4. *Management of Adrenal Addisonian Crisis*
    a. Hydrocortisone 100 mg. I.V. immediately followed by an additional 100 mg. in 1,000 ml. normal saline over 4 hours.
    b. Fluid replacement with 2 to 3 L.

of normal saline over the first 12 to 14 hours, since decreased intravascular and extravascular volumes may approach 20 per cent of normal

c. Potassium replacement as necessary

d. Broad-spectrum antibiotic coverage, instituted immediately, even if a source of infection cannot be found

e. Blood replacement with packed red cells, if hemorrhage has precipitated the crisis

f. Vasopressors as necessary, after (a) through (e) have been performed.

22. Surgical Disease in Pregnancy

Hugh R. K. Barber, M.D.

BASIC PRINCIPLES

1. In addition to obstetric complications, the pregnant patient can have any surgical disease that occurs in the nonpregnant state. The obstetrician must make the decision on what constitutes the best management of the pregnancy. The surgeon should think as an obstetrician and the obstetrician as a surgeon.
2. The plan of treatment is the same as in the nonpregnant patient.
3. If signs and symptoms indicate that a surgical emergency exists, especially if there is progressive deterioration, surgical exploration should be carried out even though a firm diagnosis has not been made.
4. An outline for differential diagnosis of the acute abdomen in the pregnant woman is:
   a. Conditions requiring immediate operation
   b. Conditions not requiring immediate operation
   c. Nonsurgical conditions presenting as an acute abdomen
5. Physical appearance of the patient often provides valuable clues:
   a. With peritonitis—lies quietly on her back with knees drawn up.
   b. With appendicitis—pulls up the right hip and knee in order to relax the psoas muscle.
   c. With pancreatitis—lies on her side with knees, hips, and back flexed.
   d. With ureteral stone—rolls around in pain.
6. The abdomen should be divided into quadrants and the symptoms, signs, and physical findings evaluated by visualizing the structures in each quadrant as:
   a. *Right Lower Quadrant.* Appendicitis, twisted ovarian cyst, Meckel's diverticulum with inflammation, regional enteritis, stone in the ureter
   b. *Left Lower Quadrant.* Twisted ovarian cyst, stone in the ureter, regional enteritis, large bowel obstruction
   c. *Right Upper Quadrant.* Acute cholecystitis, acute pyelonephritis, pancreatitis
   d. *Left Upper Quadrant.* Spleen, pancreatitis, appendicitis, diabetic crisis

ACUTE APPENDICITIS

Basic Principles

1. Early in the course the patient may not look ill.
2. Persistent pain in RLQ aggravated by walking. Point of tenderness is usually higher than McBurney's point. In retrocecal appendicitis the point of tenderness may be lateral to McBurney's point.
3. A high retrocecal appendicitis may be difficult to differentiate from cholecystitis or kidney disease.
4. If the clinical picture points to appendicitis, a few white cells in the urine should not keep the responsible physician from making the diagnosis of appendicitis.
5. Clumps of white cells and a great number of white cells strongly suggest the presence of pyelonephritis either as a concurrent problem or the main pathologic entity.

6. Most series have a 60 to 70 per cent correct preoperative diagnosis.

7. The mortality from appendicitis is the mortality of delay.

Diagnostic Signs and Studies

1. Nausea and vomiting are present.
2. Moderate abdominal distention may be present with progression of the disease.
3. Temperature usually ranges from 100 to 101°F.
4. A progressive rise in the white blood count with a shift to the left is significant.
5. Pulse rises steadily.
6. There are no characteristic x-ray findings in appendicitis, but x-ray studies may be necessary in the differential diagnosis.

Helpful Adjunctive Procedures

1. Nasogastric tube
2. Indwelling urinary catheter
3. Coagulation studies
4. N.P.O.
5. Intravenous fluids

Management of Acute Appendicitis by Trimesters

1. First Trimester (Appendix in its Usual Position)

a. If possible and practical, remove the appendix.

b. If there is a generalized peritonitis and it is possible and feasible, the appendix should be removed. Antibiotics and appropriate fluids, plasma, and electrolytes should be administered. Appropriate antibiotics will depend upon the culture reports.

c. If an abscess makes it impossible or impractical to remove the appendix, it should be drained and antibiotics started.

2. Second Trimester (Appendix at the Iliac Crest)

a. In localized appendicitis, the appendix should be removed without drainage.

b. In the presence of generalized peritonitis, the appendix should be removed and antibiotics, fluids, plasma, and electrolytes instituted.

c. In the presence of a localized abscess, it is better to drain unless the area of the appendiceal-cecal junction is intact. If the appendix can be removed in toto, it should be done.

3. Third Trimester (Appendix between the Iliac Crest and the Liver)

a. In localized appendicitis, the appendix should be removed without drainage.

b. In the presence of generalized peritonitis, the appendix should be removed and antibiotics, fluids, plasma, and electrolytes instituted.

c. In the presence of a localized abscess, it is better to drain all cases. If the appendix can be removed in toto, it should be done. Antibiotics should be given.

d. If there is a large abscess, it should be drained. After the peritoneum has been closed, an extraperitoneal Cesarean section should be carried out if further childbearing is desired. If the uterine wall is part of the abscess, a Cesarean hysterectomy is indicated with drainage. Antibiotics should be given.

ACUTE CHOLECYSTITIS

Basic Principles

1. Is a rare complication of pregnancy.

2. Since the gallbladder is not displaced in pregnancy, the signs and symptoms are similar to those in the nonpregnant state. The diagnosis is usually made on clinical signs and symptoms, but a past history of gallbladder attacks is helpful in confirming the diagnosis.

3. In the third trimester the appendix is often displaced into the right upper

quadrant and may make an accurate diagnosis difficult, if not impossible.

4. Onset is usually characterized by biliary colic accompanied by nausea, vomiting, and less often by chills. Subcostal pain may radiate to the back and fever up to 101°F may be present. Palpation of a tender gallbladder is a helpful diagnostic finding in acute cholecystitis.

5. Leukocytosis may increase progressively.

6. The disease may subside spontaneously.

7. Cholelithiasis may complicate pregnancy, but is usually not diagnosed until the postpartum period. The following factors predispose to the increased incidence of gallstones in the pregnant patient:

   a. Increased bile stasis

   b. Elevation of the amount of cholesterol in the bile

   c. Biological changes within the bile salts and acids

8. Close observation of the patient's course is mandatory, with frequent reexamination and evaluation, since progressive infection, necrosis, gangrene, and perforation are not infrequent and demand surgical intervention.

9. Conservative therapy is initially followed. If the patient does not repond to conservative treatment within 12 to 36 hours, particularly if the white blood count continues to increase, fever is higher and tenderness persists or gets worse, operation is indicated.

Diagnostic Signs and Studies

1. The clinical signs and symptoms are discussed above.

2. Oral cholecystogram. Nonvisualization may represent failure of the diseased gallbladder to concentrate.

3. The oral cholecystogram test is not valid in the presence of jaundice, vomiting, diarrhea, or associated liver disease.

4. Intravenous cholangiography may outline the bile ducts as well as the gallbladder.

Helpful Adjunctive Procedures

1. Nasogastric tube
2. Indwelling urinary catheter
3. Intravenous fluids
4. Antibiotics

Helpful Points In Evaluating The Patient

1. Liver usually functions normally in pregnancy.

2. Serum cholesterol may rise to 500 mg. in the last trimester.

3. In the third trimester, serum albumin and gamma globulin decrease, and alpha and beta globulins increase. May account for the abnormal cephalin flocculation and thymol turbidity tests seen in the third trimester.

4. The serum alkaline phosphatase rises in pregnancy and peaks in the third trimester. The increase is due primarily to a heat-stable fraction which arises from the placenta, while the hepatic phosphatase remains normal.

5. Serum transaminase and lactic dehydrogenase remain normal in pregnancy, but may be elevated during labor and shortly thereafter.

6. Jaundice of pregnancy may represent bile stasis and is often hormonally mediated, primarily by estrogens. This type of jaundice is more common in the last trimester, disappears spontaneously in the postpartum period, and tends to recur in subsequent pregnancies.

7. Jaundice may also occur as the result of drug reaction (carbon tetrachloride, tetracycline, chloroform, phenothiazine, halothane), hemolytic anemia, or with liver damage resulting from pregnancy toxemia, idiopathic fatty liver, acute hepatitis, or transfusion reaction.

8. The bromosulphalein is elevated and the serum glutamic oxaloacetic

transaminase and alkaline phosphatase may be elevated.

9. If the patient has had this problem in previous pregnancies, this diagnosis is then highly probable.

PERFORATED GASTRIC ULCER

Basic Principles

1. Problems relating to the intestinal tract during pregnancy are often delayed.
2. Since the acute abdominal problems complicating pregnancy are sometimes difficult to differentiate from exaggerated normal pregnancy symptoms, and because the classic signs are often changed by the enlarged uterus, one must be aware of the different clinical pictures produced by pregnancy.
3. Cardiospasm occurs in pregnancy with varying degrees of severity. It may have an insidious or sudden onset. Cardiospasm is due to an imbalance of the parasympathetic innervation, resulting in an inability of the sphincter of the esophagus to relax, as well as decreased peristaltic activity.
4. Heartburn and epigastric distress are common in pregnancy, making the diagnosis of peptic ulcer difficult.
5. The gastric acid curves (both free and total) decrease considerably with the low point in the 6 to 10 week group. This gradually increases to near normal at term.
6. There is an increased gastroesophageal reflux and a delayed gastric emptying time.
7. The digestion and absorption of the small bowel remains unchanged. There is a decrease in peristalsis of the large bowel.
8. In general, pregnancy has no direct effect on pre-existing gastrointestinal disease. Most changes reported are psychologically oriented.
9. Perforation and hemorrhage may occur and cause serious complications. Each of these complications occur almost exclusively in the third trimester.
10. The accepted treatment of peptic ulcer is medical management.

Diagnostic Signs and Studies

1. Previous history of ulcer disease.
2. Typically, pain is of sudden onset and is severe. Pain may be referred to one or both shoulders, usually the right because of subphrenic irritation.
3. There is nausea but usually no vomiting.
4. Examination reveals a rigid, silent abdomen, although in some instances bowel sounds may be heard.
5. There may be diminished liver dullness due to escape of gas into the peritoneal cavity.
6. In delayed cases, after 12 hours or more, the features of peritonitis with paralytic ileus are present and the patient is extremely toxic and oliguric.
7. Other conditions with which perforated ulcer is confused, are acute perforated appendicitis, acute pancreatitis, and myocardial infarction.
8. X-ray film of the abdomen in the upright position may show free gas below the diaphragm. This sign is not present in one-third of the patients.

Helpful Adjunctive Procedures

1. Nasogastric tube
2. Intravenous fluids
3. Antibiotics
4. Semi-Fowler's position
5. Indwelling urinary catheter

Treatment

1. The treatment for either perforation or excessive bleeding is the same as in the nonpregnant patient, with surgery done immediately. The philosophy should be to attack the life-threatening complication first and to deal with the pregnancy after this is controlled. More than half of the mothers will be lost after

perforation or hemorrhage from a peptic ulcer.

2. Cesarean section is reserved for obstetrical indications, but occasionally it may be in the best interest of the patient to empty the uterus by Cesarean section at the time of laparotomy in order to technically facilitate the control of bleeding from the ulcer.

3. The fetal survival is directly related to depth and length of shock, as well as the amount of peritonitis.

INTESTINAL OBSTRUCTION

Basic Principles

1. May occur in pregnancy and occasionally presents difficulty in diagnosis. Vomiting secondary to bowel obstruction in early pregnancy may be regarded as the usual emesis associated with gestation. The pain of obstruction coming on late in pregnancy may be mistaken for the onset of labor. A careful history and physical examination will avoid both these errors.

2. The usual case of intestinal obstruction is secondary to a volvulus or an adhesive band. Adhesions in the pregnant as well as the nonpregnant patient constitute the single most frequent factor in producing intestinal obstruction.

3. Intestinal obstruction occurs more commonly in the third trimester than in the first trimester. It may be related to the pulling of the growing uterus on adhesions, causing bands that can obstruct the bowel.

4. The presence of a scar on the abdomen, colicky abdominal pain which is intermittent, vomiting which is frequent and copious, distention, and obstipation indicate an intra-abdominal pathologic complication, especially an intestinal obstruction.

5. Auscultation at the time of pain reveals loud, metallic, high-pitched peristaltic rushes. The frequency and severity of the rushes decrease as the bowel gets quiet. This may take 6 to 8 hours or more after the start of obstruction. On auscultation there is a change from the high-pitched, frequent rushes to a subdued kind of sound described as a tinkling or sounds like water going down a drain.

6. X-ray studies which show air and fluid levels on an upright film will serve to confirm the diagnosis.

7. As the time interval of the obstruction lengthens the clinical picture changes.

8. The changes that occur are:

a. Fluids and electrolytes pour into the bowel. The circulating blood volume decreases. The hemoglobin and hematocrit increase due to the shift of fluid to the extracellular space.

b. The glomerular filtration rate (GFR) is decreased secondary to the diminished extracellular fluid and the abdominal distention.

c. The urinary output drops with an increase in the specific gravity of the urine. The urea nitrogen, sulfates, and phosphates increase in the plasma.

d. The diaphragm is elevated secondary to abdominal distention. Carbon dioxide retention follows and a respiratory acidosis compounds the metabolic acidosis produced by the above mechanisms. Atelectasis complicates the problem.

Roentgenographic Studies

1. Fluid levels in small bowel or stepladder effect of fluid levels indicate obstruction of small intestine.

2. Thickness of wall of the intestine indicates fibrinous exudate.

3. A very large, ovoid, distended, isolated loop of bowel usually indicates a volvulus.

4. A distended cecum is a dangerous sign in bowel obstruction. The ileocecal valve is competent, causing it to distend.

Perforation may occur if the obstruction is not rapidly relieved.

5. If the diagnosis remains uncertain after correction of the fluid and electrolyte imbalance and the passage of a nasogastric tube, further studies are indicated.

6. Contrast studies will clarify the diagnosis, using a contrast medium of one-half gastrografin and one-half barium. A minimum of radiation exposure should be used and all efforts taken to protect the fetus. The mixture can be followed either to the point of obstruction or to its entrance into the large bowel. This mixture is liquid enough to cause an obstruction, and if there is an obstruction, it will promptly pass when the obstruction is relieved surgically.

Helpful Adjunctive Procedures

1. Gastrointestinal decompression with a long tube
2. Intravenous fluids
3. Antibiotics
4. Sigmoidoscopy and barium studies in chronic obstruction
5. Enemas to remove feces and prepare the bowel for elective surgery when chronic obstruction of the large bowel is present
6. Indwelling urinary catheter

Management

1. The surgical management of intestinal obstruction is the same as in the nonpregnant state. Vascular impairment of the obstructed bowel must be avoided if the fetus is to be saved. Surgical intervention for intestinal obstruction should be performed earlier than might be done in a nonpregnant patient.

2. Necrotic bowel requires resection.

3. Obstruction of the colon may require colostomy. The obstructing mechanism must be identified and relieved.

LARGE BOWEL OBSTRUCTION ASSOCIATED WITH PREGNANCY

Basic Principles

1. There are three times that this complication occurs, i.e., between the fourth and sixth months, near term, and shortly after delivery.

2. Was first described following delivery and was due to mechanical obstruction by the postpartum uterus.

3. In the postpartum period the patient may have a slow onset of lower abdominal pain followed by progressive increase in abdominal distention. The pain increases as the distention increases. If the ileocolic valve is incompetent, the small bowel may become distended.

4. It is important to rule out an unrecognized carcinoma or a volvulus.

5. A flat plate of the abdomen often shows a distended bowel from the cecum to the pelvic brim on the left side.

6. Examination usually reveals a palpable, slightly tender cecum and high-pitched sounds on auscultation during the pain.

Management

1. By placing the patient in the knee-chest position and by gently pushing the uterus away from the bowel, considerable gas may escape with relief of symptoms. In this position a tube may be threaded up the bowel. If the patient improves after this type of management, it is acceptable to treat the patient conservatively.

2. The management is to insert a Levine tube in the stomach, a tube threaded up the sigmoid from below, and intravenous fluids.

3. In about 48 to 72 hours the signs and symptoms regress and the patient improves. If the symptoms are not relieved, however, and progressive deterioration with a rising pulse, increase in

the white blood count with a shift to the left, increasing distention, and localized tenderness develops, the diagnosis of volvulus with compromise must be considered and surgical intervention undertaken.

PARALYTIC ILEUS ASSOCIATED WITH PREGNANCY

Basic Principles

1. Is not uncommon.
2. The cause is not definitely known but may be due to the relaxed abdominal muscles, a decrease in the size of the uterus, and hormonal effects.
3. The abdomen is often markedly distended with feeble or absent bowel sounds and there is no pain.
4. Vomiting is not unusual. The patient looks well. The physical signs are minimal.
5. The condition clears within 24 to 48 hours without treatment.

MESENTERIC VASCULAR OCCLUSION

Basic Principles

1. May be either venous or arterial blood supply.
2. Often presents with acute colicky pain and is not infrequently associated with vomiting and diarrhea which may be bloody.
3. Early there may be no signs of peritoneal irritation, and tenderness on deep palpation may be the only finding. Bowel sounds may be present early in the development of the occlusion. Gradually the tenderness increases and the infarcted bowel may be felt as a mass.
4. Mesenteric venous thrombosis results in loss of blood into the intestinal wall, lumen, and peritoneal cavity with the rapid onset of shock.
5. Mesenteric arterial occlusion may also result in shock if massive.
6. Arterial occlusion without infarction may produce symptoms of intestinal angina in which abdominal pain follows meals and steatorrhea.
7. The signs of peritonitis occur after gangrene and perforation of the bowel.
8. A rising pulse rate and leukocytosis indicate progression of disease.
9. Flat plate of the abdomen usually shows nonspecific dilated loops of small and large intestine.

Helpful Adjunctive Procedures

1. Nasogastric tube
2. Intravenous fluids
3. Antibiotics
4. Abdominal paracentesis (serosanguineous fluid)
5. Arteriograms
6. Indwelling urinary catheter

Management

1. Exploratory laparotomy
2. Bowel resection as determined on opening the abdomen

PANCREATITIS

Basic Principles

1. Is a rare complication of pregnancy.
2. Is seen with increasing frequency among heavy users of diuretics such as chlorothiazides, as well as in patients with gallbladder disease, alcoholism, dietary indiscretion, chronic adrenal steroid therapy, trauma, and hyperparathyroidism.
3. Pain is severe, constant, epigastric, and often radiates to the back. Vomiting may be profuse. The patient looks sick.
4. The abdomen reveals generalized tenderness and moderate distention. Bowel sounds are diminished or absent. The usual signs of tenderness between the stomach and the spleen, elevation of the diaphragm, and low-grade fever may be present.

5. Shock, rapid pulse and cyanosis may be present.
6. Unexplained erythematous, painful subcutaneous nodules may be present.
7. The incidence is higher among primigravidas than among multiparas.
8. It occurs in all trimesters but is most common in the third trimester and postpartum periods.
9. The diagnosis should be considered in any acute abdomen accompanied by protracted vomiting, electrolyte imbalance, increased serum amylase, and hypocalcemia, and elevated urinary diastase. Occasionally glycosuria is present.

Roentgenographic Studies

1. Flat plate of the abdomen may show nonspecific ileus.
2. Chest film may show fluid at the base of the pleural cavity.

Helpful Adjunctive Procedures

1. Nasogastric tube
2. Intravenous fluids
3. Calcium intravenously
4. Antibiotics
5. Indwelling catheter

Management

1. Treatment is medical.
2. Surgery is indicated if it is impossible to establish a firm diagnosis, with pseudocyst, recurrent attacks, and occasionally when unexplained persistent diabetes is present.
3. The pancreatic bed should be carefully and adequately drained.
4. Dramatic recovery has been reported after the delivery of the baby. Therefore, after viability of the fetus, induction of labor or Cesarean section has a place in the management of these patients.

ULCERATIVE COLITIS

Basic Principles

1. Is an unpredictable disease in pregnancy. In patients who are labile with swings between exacerbation and remission, the exacerbation rate in pregnancy is 50 to 60 per cent.
2. Most of the cases are diagnosed prior to pregnancy and the problem then is merely how to manage them during pregnancy. If the patient has been in remission for two or more years, there is an excellent chance that she will be symptom-free during her pregnancy.
3. Gastrointestinal symptoms in the presence of a history of ulcerative colitis should be suspect until reactivation of the disease has been ruled out.
4. In those having the disease for the first time in pregnancy, the symptoms and signs are similar to those in the nonpregnant state. The symptoms are abdominal cramps accompanied by a diarrhea that is often bloody. Fever and tachycardia are common. A monoarticular, migrating arthritis is often present.

Diagnostic Signs and Studies

1. Can often be made on sigmoidoscopy, which demonstrates the beefy red, edematous bowel with ulcerated areas in which grayish, necrotic tissue and slough are seen.
2. X-ray studies are usually not needed to confirm the diagnosis, but should be done if considered necessary.
3. The diagnosis is often confirmed by response to medical treatment.

Management

1. The primary treatment is medical. It includes a low residual diet, antispasmodics, sulfa and steroid therapy.
2. Surgery is indicated if the medical regimen fails or if hemorrhage or peritonitis is present.
3. Total colectomy with terminal ileostomy is the treatment that must be carried out; the perineal removal of the rectum and anus may be delayed. By-passing ileostomies, various drainage procedures, and other halfway measures done

to avoid colectomy or protocolectomy are to be condemned. These procedures are followed by a stormy postoperative course and in more than two-thirds of the reported cases result in a stillborn fetus and a maternal death.

REGIONAL ILEITIS

Basic Principles

1. May occur for the first time during pregnancy.
2. Most often the diagnosis has been made prior to pregnancy.
3. Symptoms developing during pregnancy are not different from those seen in the nonpregnant state.
4. Often present with a malabsorption syndrome including anemia, hypoproteinemia, and clotting defects due to malabsorption of vitamin K.
5. The disease may mimic an atypical appendicitis or inflamed Meckel's diverticulum.
6. The chronic form may be confirmed by x-ray studies.
7. The acute form is often not diagnosed until laparotomy has been carried out.

Management

1. Prompt surgery is indicated if there is intestinal obstruction, perforation with peritonitis, or localized abscess.
2. The surgery should consist of short-circuiting operation or intestinal resection.
3. The pregnancy should be preserved, if at all possible.

23. Gestational Trophoblastic Neoplasms

Hugh R. K. Barber, M.D.

DEFINITION

Gestational trophoblastic neoplasms initiated a new concept of interconnection of such disease processes as choriocarcinoma, invasive mole, and hydatidiform mole. The term "gestational trophoblastic neoplasms" is used to define the spectrum of disease that has at one extreme benign hydatidiform mole and at the other highly malignant choriocarcinoma. Not only do these diseases form a spectrum but to understand and adequately manage a patient with one of these conditions requires knowledge of the entire group.

BASIC PRINCIPLES

1. Hydatidiform moles occur in a ratio of 1 to 2,000 normal pregnancies in the United States and 80 per cent are benign. In certain geographic areas such as Asia, the incidence may be as high as 1 in 60 to 1,000 normal pregnancies.
2. It is higher in patients in the very low economic status, and poor diet has also been noted to be associated with an increased incidence.
3. Approximately half of the patients with metastatic trophoblastic disease and 75 per cent of patients with nonmetastatic trophoblastic disease develop these tumors as sequelae to molar pregnancy.
4. Approximately 20 per cent of patients with moles require additional treatment.
5. Recurrent molar pregnancy is four to five times higher than the risk of the first.
6. When a urinary HCG excretion greater than one million international units (IU) per 24 hours is encountered in association with an enlarged uterus and vaginal bleeding, the diagnosis is almost always molar pregnancy. However, a higher percentage of patients with molar pregnancy have urinary HCG levels in the normal range for a single fetus, which makes this test relatively nonspecific.
7. In addition, approximately one-half of hydatidiform moles will be found in uteri that are small for dates. Therefore, the diagnosis should not be disregarded if the uterus is small or normal sized for dates.

HISTOPATHOLOGY

1. This is a conceptus most often lacking an intact fetus, showing swelling of the villi.
2. Three changes are found in the villi and are typically identified with hydatidiform mole. These are:
    a. Trophoblastic proliferation of both the cytotrophoblast (Langhan's cells) and syncytiotrophoblast
    b. Hydropic changes in the stroma
    c. Absence of blood vessels
3. Several authors have studied the degree of trophoblastic proliferation associated with the villi of hydatidiform mole in an attempt to predict the likelihood that a patient will develop persistent malignant disease.
4. The conclusion is that the likelihood of malignant sequelae developing is increased in patients whose trophoblastic cells showed increased proliferation and anaplasia.
5. Unfortunately, metastatic chorio-

carcinoma has developed from the most benign-appearing mole. It is therefore imperative that serial gonadotropin assays be obtained in all patients who have had a hydatidiform mole.

CLINICAL FEATURES

1. There is a higher incidence of hydatidiform mole below the age of 20 and above 40 years.

2. Vaginal bleeding occurs in virtually all patients and is generally noted at between 6 and 8 weeks following the missed period. The bleeding may range from dark brown (prune juice) to bright red and may lead to marked anemia.

3. More than half of the patients have uterine enlargement beyond the expected gestational age. When the uterus enlarges it does so rapidly and at a nonuniform rate.

4. The uterus feels boggy and despite its size no fetal parts can be felt.

5. Amniotic fluid is absent and ballottement cannot be elicited.

6. Massive enlargement of the ovaries may occur because of theca-lutein cyst formation. Molar pregnancy should be suspected when these cysts are detected. The cysts regress after delivery of the mole.

7. Uterine size is consistent with gestational dates in approximately 35 per cent of the patients and smaller in 10 to 15 per cent.

8. About 20 per cent of patients with molar pregnancy develop signs of preeclampsia which include hypertension, edema, and/or albuminuria. Rarely does eclampsia occur in association with molar pregnancy. Since this occurs in the first or early second trimester at a much earlier time than toxemia is seen, it should alert the physician to the possibility of this diagnosis.

9. Hyperemesis occurs in approximately 30 per cent of the patients. Interestingly, urinary estrogen levels were not necessarily elevated in this group. Therefore, nausea and vomiting was apparently due to some other cause.

10. About 1 in 10 patients develop some clinical and laboratory evidence in the form of elevated serum-protein-bound iodine tests accompanied with tachycardia and enlarged thyroid glands.

11. Hyperthyroidism in molar pregnancy is due to the production of trophoblastic cells of molar thyrotropin, which is similar to the hormone isolated from the pituitary gland and the placenta.

12. When this clinical state occurs, the patient must be given antithyroid therapy prior to the institution of anesthesia in order to avoid thyroid storm. This condition may be subtle and not recognized until after the patient is given general anesthesia at the time of evacuation.

13. In summary, the clinical signs of hydatidiform molar pregnancy present as follows: vaginal bleeding 100 per cent, uterine enlargement 50 per cent, hyperemesis 30 per cent, toxemia 20 per cent, hyperthyroidism 10 per cent, and trophoblastic emboli 2 per cent.

DIAGNOSTIC STUDIES

1. CBC and hematocrit
2. Urinalysis
3. A quantitative HCG test that is sensitive and reliable is most important. Detailed discussion under laboratory tests.
4. Ultrasonography is playing a significant and increasingly valuable role in the diagnosis of molar pregnancy.
   a. May be employed in uteri smaller than 14 weeks size.
   b. Is employed if there is an equivocal amniogram as well as a method chosen before amniography.
   c. The diagnosis can be made as early as 8 weeks apparent gestation.
   d. At this time a gestational sac is not visualized and the pattern described

as a snow storm is pathognomonic for molar pregnancy.

e. Currently the multilayered ultrasound screening as well as the gray mode has made ultrasonography the best method of diagnosing a mole.

ROENTGENOGRAPHIC STUDIES

1. Flat plate of the abdomen
2. Amniography

a. If the uterus is above the symphysis, a radiopaque dye can be injected transabdominally into the uterine cavity.

b. A single flat plate of the abdomen and perhaps lateral or oblique films are obtained within 5 minutes of the time of injection.

c. The x-ray appearance of molar pregnancy is that of a moth-eaten or honeycomb pattern.

3. Arteriography is discussed under nonmetastatic trophoblastic disease.
4. Chest radiograph
5. Brain and liver scan as indicated
6. Transaminase studies including an SMA-12
7. Type and crossmatch for at least 1,000 ml. of blood.

TREATMENT

1. When a definitive diagnosis of a molar pregnancy is made, evacuation should be carried out without waiting for spontaneous passage of the mole. Evacuation is best accomplished by suction curettage even though the uterus may be 20 weeks or more in size.
2. A Pitocin infusion should be running prior to the start of the evacuation. Accumulated old blood as well as fresh bright blood may gush out at first, but continued suction will remove the mole and control the bleeding.
3. After the uterus is evacuated, sharp curettage should be carried out and these curettings should be sent to the laboratory as a separate specimen.
4. In patients of advanced age or parity, total hysterectomy with or without salpingo-oophorectomy (depending on the age) is the procedure of choice for treatment of molar pregnancy, leaving the mole in situ.
5. Some advocate prophylactic chemotherapy prior to evacuation of the molar pregnancy. Since there is toxicity associated with chemotherapy, the prophylactic method is not universally accepted.

a. However, it should be considered in the high-risk group, unreliable patients who may avoid follow-up, and in parts of the world where gonadotropin follow-up may not be available or where the incidence of trophoblastic complications following a molar pregnancy may be greater than they are in the United States.

b. The regimen employed is a single 5-day course of dactinomycin, at a daily dosage of 12 μg./Kg., starting 2 to 3 days before evacuation. This reduces the 15 to 20 per cent rate of persistent trophoblastic disease following a hydatidiform mole to 1 or 2 per cent.

c. Since hepatitis may occur in these patients because of increased use of blood, some prefer methotrexate, 15 to 25 mg. intramuscularly or intravenously per day for 5 days.

d. If hepatitis develops and additional therapy is required, dactinomycin can then be given.

e. Methotrexate should not be given in the presence of impaired hepatic or renal function, since the toxicity may be overwhelming.

COMPLICATIONS OF TREATMENT

1. It is noted that embolization may occur before, during, or following evacuation, regardless of the method used.

a. Typically, the patient develops cyanosis, tachypnea, tachycardia, dyspnea, and in some severe cases, signs of right heart failure.

b. Supportive treatment should include oxygen, sedation, and digitalis for cases of right heart failure and is usually adequate.

c. Parenteral cortisone is helpful in severe cases of pulmonary edema.

d. Signs of embolization generally subside spontaneously within 72 hours. This complication is not associated with a higher incidence of pulmonary metastases.

2. Disseminated intravascular coagulation may also arise and should be treated immediately.

FOLLOW-UP

1. The prime objective is detection of persistent malignant disease following molar pregnancy in the individual patient.

2. The protocol for postevacuation follow-up must be carefully observed to detect persistent or recurrent disease.

3. The HCG assay must be recorded at evacuation and then weekly thereafter. If the HCG level becomes normal on three consecutive assays it can be done at monthly intervals for 6 months. If the titer remains within normal limits after 6 months, it can be discontinued and repeated after 6 months. During this time pregnancy should be avoided.

4. A chest radiograph is taken at the time of evacuation and at 4 and 8 weeks.

5. If the HCG level plateaus, or rises, or if metastases appear, treatment should be instituted without delay.

6. The pill serves a twofold purpose in that it prevents pregnancy and suppresses the secretion of pituitary gonadotropins.

NONMETASTATIC TROPHOBLASTIC DISEASE (INVASIVE MOLE, CHORIOADENOMA DESTRUENS)

Basic Principles

1. The hydatidiform mole invades the myometrium.

2. It retains its villous structure and is usually confined to the uterus.

3. The villi may metastasize to the vagina, parametrium, and even to the lungs and brain.

4. The invasive mole may be of this condition from the beginning or follow an apparently simple mole.

Clinical Features

1. After evacuation of a mole there may be no symptoms or signs for weeks or months. Then episodes of irregular bleeding occurs, usually accompanied by pain.

2. On examination the uterus is enlarged and cystic ovaries may be felt.

3. The presenting symptoms may be dysuria from local extension, or dyspnea with or without pleuritic pain, or headache and visual disturbances due to cerebral metastases.

Diagnostic Signs and Studies

1. It may be impossible to differentiate from choriocarcinoma.

2. HCG is usually elevated.

3. Curettage reveals a friable, hemorrhagic growth with villi present.

4. The histologic structure is usually benign even in cases with metastases.

5. Arteriography has a role in diagnosis but it is limited. In those patients failing to achieve complete remission with systemic chemotherapy, arteriography may demonstrate a focus of trophoblastic disease deep in the myometrium.

Treatment

1. There are dangers which make it imperative that active therapy be instituted.

a. Hemorrhage may occur and be fatal.

b. There may be extension to the parametrium, resulting in intra-abdominal hemorrhage.

c. Extension of growth with embolization occasionally is a complication.

The pulmonary and cerebral manifestation may be serious and require urgent treatment.

d. There may be progression to choriocarcinoma.

2. Chemotherapy should be employed as for choriocarcinoma.

3. In older women or with great parity, total hysterecomy is often chosen as the best therapy.

4. Since operative procedures in these patients may result in the dissemination of viable tumor cells, surgery should be carried out on the third day of a 5-day course of chemotherapy.

5. The follow-up is essentially the same as outlined for hydatidiform mole.

CHORIOCARCINOMA

Caution: Choricocarcinoma—A Diagnostic Problem

Gestational trophoblastic disease is a great masquerader. It is an enigma. The symptoms may appear as nongynecological. In patients in whom a diagnosis cannot be established or in whom the primary site of the tumor cannot be determined an HCG should be obtained. Since choriocarcinoma has been reported in the postmenopausal years it is no longer advisable to limit the HCG assay to those in the childbearing years. It is important that physicians who care for women consider the possibility of choriocarcinoma in a variety of medical conditions where the cause is not apparent, such as brain tumor, cerebral vascular accident, gastrointestinal bleeding, or a mass in the region of the liver.

Basic Principles

1. Is a rare disease. Incidence is roughly 1 in 14,000 pregnancies in the United States. In Hong Kong it is 1 in 114.

2. It usually follows immediately after a mole, abortion, or a normal pregnancy.

3. It may appear many years after the last pregnancy. Cases have been reported as occurring after the menopause.

Histopathology

1. Villus Formation. Villus formation is almost universally absent.

a. The tumor consists of masses of syncytium and cytotrophoblast.

b. It invades and destroys the surrounding tissues and causes gross hemorrhage owing to its ability to erode blood vessels.

c. The cells are irregular with hyperchromic nuclei.

d. Mitotic figures are frequent.

e. The syncytial masses are usually fenestrated.

2. High-Risk Metastatic Disease

a. Constitutes 20 per cent of all cases

b. Gonadotropin excretion (HCG) over 100,000 IU/24 hours

c. Duration of disease over 4 months from the termination of the antecedent pregnancy or the onset of symptoms

d. Metastatic disease in multiple sites, including the liver or brain or both, as well as metastases to the small bowel.

3. Low-Risk Metastatic Disease

a. Constitutes 80 per cent of all cases

b. Gonadotropin excretion (HCG) under 100,000 IU/24 hours

c. Duration of disease under 4 months from the termination of antecedent pregnancy or the onset of symptoms

d. Metastatic disease to the lungs or vagina or both

Clinical Features

1. These are variable.

2. The primary uterine growth may cause hemorrhage or even cerebral symptoms.

3. Metastases may give rise to respiratory or cerebral symptoms.

4. Hemoptysis may occur.

5. Irregular uterine bleeding may be present.

6. There may be pulmonary shadows on x-ray examination.
7. HCG titer may be high.

Treatment

1. Method of single-agent chemotherapy for patients in the low-risk group (good prognosis). Metastatic trophoblastic disease as published by Lewis and Hammond:

a. *Repetitive 5-day Courses.* Methotrexate, 15 to 20 mg. I.M. q.d., or actinomycin D, 10 μg. to 13 μg/Kg. I.V. q.d.

(1) Consider hysterectomy during first course of chemotherapy if further reproduction is not desired.

(2) Minimum interval between courses—7 days.

(3) Maximum interval between courses—14 days (unless laboratory values are too low)

(4) Consider oral contraception for pituitary suppression.

b. *Signs to Look For.* Continue repetitive 5-day courses of the same drug until

(1) HCG titer drops to normal pituitary range—cease treatment.

(2) HCG titer "plateaus" elevated,
(3) HCG titer rises tenfold,
(4) New metastases appear,
} Change to alternate drug.

c. *Oncolytic Effect.* Monitor oncolytic effect by weekly HCG titers, chest radiographs, and pelvic examinations.

d. *Treatment Safety Factors (Done Daily During Treatment, Less Frequently Between Courses).* Do not start, continue, or resume a dose of medication if:

(1) White blood count less than 3,000/cu. mm.

(2) Polymorphonuclear leukocytes less than 1,500/cu. mm.

(3) Platelets less than 100,000/cu. mm.

(4) Significant elevations of BUN, SGOT, or SGPT

e. *Duration of Course.* Treatment is terminated when HCG titer is within normal pituitary range. Three consecutive normal weekly HCG titers for diagnosis of remission.

f. *Follow-up*

(1) HCG titers monthly for 6 months, bimonthly for 6 months, then every 6 months thereafter.

(2) Physical, pelvic exams, chest radiographs, blood survey every 3 months for 1 year, every 6 months thereafter

(3) No pregnancy for 1 year

g. *Success Rate.* Total patients cured—98 per cent.

2. Method of triple-agent chemotherapy for patients in the high-risk group (poor prognosis). Metastatic trophoblastic disease as published by Lewis and Hammond:

a. The management is similar to that outlined under the single-agent chemotherapy but this includes three drugs and x-ray therapy.

b. The drug regimen is given in combination of methotrexate, 15 mg. intramuscularly, actinomycin D, 10 μg/Kg. intravenously, and chlorambucil, 10 mg. orally.

c. Each drug is given daily for 5 days (triple therapy).

d. The interval between treatment should be longer than 10 days but shorter than 21 days.

e. After two or three courses of such combination chemotherapy, treatment is altered to single-agent therapy with actinomycin D at a dosage of 13 μg intravenously for 5 days.

f. This change is necessary because of cumulative toxicity from the combination chemotherapy.

g. If cerebral or hepatic metastases have been demonstrated, immediate institution of whole-brain or whole-liver irradiation of 2,000 rads (total dose) should be given simultaneously with combination chemotherapy. Cortisone should be given to reduce the cerebral edema secondary to the radiation therapy.

h. Total patients cured—47 per cent.

Contraindications to Initiation and Continuation of Therapy

Laboratory Contraindications

WBC	<2,500/mm³
Total poly count	<1,500/mm³
Platelet count	<100,000/mm³
SGOT level	>50 units
BUN	Rising

1. Clinical
- a. Leukemia
- b. Thrombocytopenia
- c. Hepatocellular disease

2. Judgment Decisions
- a. Stomatitis
- b. Maculopapular rash
- c. GI disturbances
- d. Alopecia
- e. Vulvitis
- f. Conjunctivitis

3. Sequential chemotherapy is not without its toxic manifestations.

a. Leukopenia and thrombocytopenia are the main signs of marrow damage. Both are reversible if the danger is appreciated and precautions taken.

b. *Other Systemic Side Effects.* Stomatitis, skin rash, alopecia, gastrointestinal disturbances, and conjunctivitis may be treated symptomatically.

c. They rarely if ever determine whether a course is to be initiated or continued.

d. Life-threatening toxicity should be treated vigorously. Reverse isolation, infusions, antibiotics, fresh white cell and platelet transfusions, and supportive therapy as needed. All other therapy should be immediately discontinued.

Laboratory Tests

1. HCG is the best method to evaluate and follow the progress of a patient with gestational trophoblastic disease. Delfs has asserted that between days 60 and 100 of normal pregnancy, there is no level of chorionic gonadotropin, however high, that could not be caused by a normal pregnancy or some variation thereof.

2. Higher HCG levels may also be associated with multiple gestation or toxemia of pregnancy. A continued rise in HCG levels after the fourteenth week of pregnancy is the best evidence of a molar pregnancy which can be obtained by using HCG assays.

3. Routine immunoassays available in most hospital laboratories are not sensitive enough to monitor the progress of the patient. The Pregnosticon tube test is capable of a minimal detectable level of HCG of 700 to 750 IU/liter. The Gravindex is capable of a minimal detectable level of HCG of 3,500 IU/liter.

4. Patients with gestational trophoblastic disease usually have gonadotropin titers initially in excess of 1,000 IU/24-hour urine required to give a positive test.

5. Approximately 25 per cent of patients with malignant trophoblastic disease have gonadotropin titers in excess of pituitary level but below that required for a positive pregnancy test.

6. Radioimmunoassay is a hundred times more sensitive than either the immunoassay or bioassay methods, being able to detect approximately 0.01 IU/ml.

a. β-subunit portion of the HCG molecule represents only HCG and only minimally crossreacts with human pituitary LH.

b. The β-subunit assay, since it is specific for HCG, enables those using it to measure HCG down to zero rather than down to levels consistent with normal pituitary LH.

7. Serum leucine aminopeptidase, human placental lactogen, and estrogens are of little assistance in differential diagnosis or monitoring the progress of treatment.

Indications for Surgery

1. Evacuation of molar pregnancy.
2. Diagnostic D and C for persistent localized disease.
3. Treatment of surgical emergencies.
4. Total hysterectomy in the patient over 40 years of age or with high parity.

Reasons for Gestational Trophoblastic Disease Receiving Attention Disproportionate to its Incidence

1. Unique Responsiveness to Chemotherapy

a. Virtually all patients with nonmetastatic disease can be cured with most retaining reproductive function.

b. 80 to 90 per cent of the patients with metastatic trophoblastic neoplasms can be cured when appropriate treatment is given.

2. Consistent Production of Human Chorionic Gonadotropin (HCG)

a. Human placental chorionic tissue, whether normal, molar, or choriocarcinomatous in nature, produces HCG when viable and growing.

b. This consistent production by molar or choriocarcinomatous tissue of a "tumor marker" allows it to be useful in diagnosis, management, and follow-up of patients.

3. Origination in Fetal Tissue

a. Because the placenta is fetal in origin, one-half of its genetic material comes from the father and is therefore potentially foreign to the maternal host.

b. Since there is no other human malignancy in which the host of origin differs from that of the host, this unique characteristic has attracted much attention.

Gestational Trophoblastic Treatment Centers

1. Gestational trophoblastic disease is probably handled best in a center. HCG is available and is accurate. The technique of chemotherapy and the management of side effects and toxicity are understood. Supporting consultative assistance and laboratory and ancillary services are available. Unless these services are locally available, the patient should be referred to a center. Resistant disease should be referred without delay.

2. If there is any indecision or lack of confidence by the responsible physician, the patient should be referred to a center. Inadequate treatment may convert a low-risk patient with an excellent chance for cure to a high-risk patient with a decreased chance for cure. All high-risk patients should be referred to a center. When drug toxicity reactions occur, the patient is a candidate for treatment at a trophoblastic center.

24. Gynecologic Endocrinology

Sherwin A. Kaufman, M.D.

Although gynecological patients can exhibit any endocrinopathy found in both men and women, the female patient possesses a unique, overtly responsive mechanism which readily informs the physician of the possible presence of endocrine disorder, i.e., alteration of the regular menstrual pattern.

ABNORMAL PATTERNS OF MENSTRUATION

1. Amenorrhea. Absence of menses

a. *Primary.* Menstruation has never occurred.

b. *Secondary.* Menstruation has occurred but has stopped.

2. Oligomenorrhea. Less frequent menstruation, occurring at intervals longer than 5 to 6 weeks

3. Polymenorrhea. More frequent menstruation, occurring at intervals of less than 3 weeks

4. Hypomenorrhea. Menses at regular intervals (approximately every 28 days) but with significantly reduced amount of flow; the number of days of flow is of the same duration or less than the patient's usual menses.

5. Hypermenorrhea. Regular menses of approximately 28-day intervals that last the usual 4 to 6 days but are excessive in amount.

6. Menorrhagia. Menses may come at regular intervals, but bleeding is either profuse, excessive in duration (8 days or more), or both.

7. Metrorrhagia. Unexpected bleeding between menstrual periods which, if prolonged, may manifest itself as totally irregular menses.

Normal menstrual function requires an intact pituitary-ovarian-uterine axis, which in turn may be influenced by the thyroid, adrenals, and the hypothalamus.

THYROID FUNCTION IN GYNECOLGY

HYPOTHYROIDISM

Basic Principles

1. Clinical Features. Diminution of cephalic, pubic, axillary, and eyebrow (lateral aspect) hair. These changes are obvious only with marked diminution of thyroid function.

2. Dry Skin. Occasionally can resemble hyperkeratosis and may be sallow in color.

3. Pretibial Edema

4. Intolerance to cold and **tolerance** to heat

5. Symptoms. Tendencies toward lethargy, obesity, constipation, bradycardia

6. Thyroid Gland. May be normal in size or enlarged

7. Deep Tendon Reflexes. Delayed return

8. Laboratory Tests

Tests	Results
a. BMR	Outmoded
b. PBI (protein-bound iodine)	Low, but too subject to iodine intake to be of practical value

	Tests	Results
c.	T_3 (triiodothyronine) by resin uptake or RIA (radioimmunoassay)	Low
d.	T_4 (thyroxine) by RIA	Low
e.	T_7 (free thyroid index)	Low (indirect confirmation of T_3 and T_4)
f.	Glucose tolerance	Flat or increased

Management

1. Sodium *l*-Thyroxine (Synthroid; T_4). Start with small doses and increase at 2-week intervals to an average maintenance dose of 0.1 to 0.2 mg.

2. Instead, one can give sodium liothyronine (Cytomel; T_3), 25 mcg. with increments of 12.5 to 25 mcg. at 5-day intervals to 100 mcg. (U.S.P. thyroid is obsolete).

3. If the adrenal reserve is low, administer prednisone, 2.5 mg. b.i.d. to t.i.d. as a means of protecting the adrenals, and start with a lower initial dose of thyroid.

4. Combined T_3 and T_4 medication may also be used, and at times yields better therapeutic results than either one alone.

5. The PBI is of no value in following the patient's response to therapy once thyromimetic drugs have been started.

HYPERTHYROIDISM

Basic Principles

1. Clinical Features

a. *Weight loss*, with increased appetite; warm, moist skin; hair thin, fine, and does not hold a permanent.

b. *Eye Signs.* May include exophthalmus, lid lag, conversion defect, widening of palpebral fissure.

c. *Enlarged Thyroid Gland.* Invariably palpable unless substernal in position

d. *Palpitation*

e. *Nervousness*

f. *Intolerance to heat*

g. *Diarrhea* and/or *frequent bowel movements*

2. Laboratory Tests

	Tests	Results
a.	PBI	High, but too subject to iodine intake to be of practical value
b.	T_3 by uptake or RIA	High
c.	T_4 by RIA	High
d.	T_7	High
e.	Glucose tolerance test	Decreased
f.	Pituitary thyrotropic-stimulating hormone (TSH) by RIA	Decreased in hyperthyroidism (and in hypothyroidism secondary to hypopituitary or hypothalamic function). Increased in hypothyroidism.

Management

1. Medical. Antithyroid drugs such as methimazole and propylthiouracil are commonly used, as follows:

a. Methimazole, 10 mg., q.i.d., with dosage decreased at a rate of 5 mg. daily at 4- to 6-week intervals, providing adequate control has been achieved.

b. Propylthiouracil, 100 mg., q.i.d., and decrease by 50 mg. daily at 4- to 6-week intervals. The same regime is followed as for methimazole.

c. In conjunction with pregnancy and the use of antithyroid drugs, the patient should always receive liothyronine, 100 to 150 mcg. per day (according to tolerance), to prevent the possibility of hypothyroidism developing in the fetus (though there is no accurate information regarding the crossing of thyroid hormone through the placenta). The combined administration of the antithyroid drug with T_3 supplies the fetus with appropriate thyroid hormone, yet controls the hyperthyroid state of the mother. Similar combined therapy is indicated in all children with hyperthyroidism treated medicinally. Indeed, any patient with an enlarged thyroid or receiving antithyroid therapy should receive T_3 concomitantly.

d. ***Cautions.*** Drug reaction, including pruritus as well as urticaria, does not necessitate stopping therapy, inasmuch as these may subside with continuous treatment. Depression of WBC below 3,500, however, requires immediate cessation of the drug. Arthralgia and significant and generalized malaise may be an expression of drug toxicity; in such cases, cessation of therapy may be necessary.

2. Surgical

a. Ablation of the thyroid gland by surgery is indicated in toxic nodular goiter or in patients less than 40 years old who might wish to maintain their reproductive function and who are allergic to, or develop untoward reaction to, medical management, and/or are so unreliable with oral medication as to make medical management impractical.

b. It should be pointed out that a considerable number of surgically treated patients may show some measure of decreased parathyroid function after a thyroidectomy. This may be detected only after tests such as ethylenediaminetetraacetic acid (EDTA) in which depletion of blood calcium by this chelating agent may result in poor restoration of blood calcium. This is in contrast to the relatively small number of patients who develop frank hypoparathyroidism after medical treatment. The importance of detecting partial but not absolute hypoparathyroidism is that blood calcium levels below 8.5 mg per 100 ml. may not always be associated with tetany but can lead to the development of the signs and symptoms of minimal calcium deficiency, such as depression, atonia of the gut, and cataract formation.

3. Radioactive Iodine

a. Destruction of the gland with radioactive iodine (RAI) is not to be considered in any pregnant female.

b. In addition, 2 to 3 per cent a year of all patients treated with RAI become hypothyroid; thus permanent hypothyroidism may occur in a significant number of patients so treated. For this reason, medical management is preferred.

c. Unreliable patients or those exhibiting adverse effects to medical management may require RAI if surgery is refused or deemed unwise.

ADRENAL DYSFUNCTION IN GYNECOLOGY

Adrenocortical disorders in gynecology may present serious problems in diagnosis and treatment. However, it is important to recognize these problems if there is to be successful management.

HYPOADRENOCORTICOIDISM

Basic Principles

1. Clinical Features

a. Asthenia

b. Hypotension, including postural hypotension

c. Increasing pigmentation of exposed areas of the body

d. Decreased or absent pubic and axillary hair

e. Mucosal membrane pigmentation

f. Occasional vitiligo

g. Occasional craving for salt

h. Weakness and general debilitation, with weight loss, anorexia, and diarrhea., These are common, characteristic clinical signs of adrenal insufficiency.

i. Patients with *secondary adrenal insufficiency* show the stigmata listed above, except that increased pigmentation abnormalities are rarely present.

2. Laboratory Tests	*Results*
a. Glucose tolerance	*Oral test.* Flat curve; with possible hypoglycemia at the third or fourth hour. (The I.,V. test can be dangerous to the patient because of the tendency to marked hypoglycemia.)

	Tests	Results
b.	Water tolerance test	The patient cannot excrete water load, so that the volume of the hourly morning specimens never exceeds the overnight specimen. The total amount excreted is less than one-half of the amount consumed.
c.	Sodium	Serum, low. Urine, high.
d.	Potassium	Serum, high. Urine, low.
e.	Serum hydroxysteroids	Low. No diurnal variation.
f.	17-Ketosteroids (urinary)	Low. (Also decreased by ingestion of meprobamate, reserpine, and estrogens.)
g.	17-Hydroxysteroids (urinary)	Low. (Also decreased by ingestion of aspirin, Dilantin, estrogens, and barbiturates.)
h.	Metopirone test	No response
i.	ACTH test	Primary adrenal insufficiency—no response Secondary adrenal insufficiency—adequate response

j. *Caution:* ACTH may produce adrenal collapse in patients with secondary adrenal insufficiency. One must also be on guard for possible anaphylactic reactions with certain ACTH preparations.

Management

1. Glucocorticoid
Hydrocortisone, 10 mg. t.i.d. or prednisone, 2.5 mg. t.i.d.

2. Methylprednisolone. Methylprednisolone should not be used; it may be ineffective or actually aggravate the symptoms of adrenal insufficiency.

3. Mineralocorticoid
Fluorohydrocortisone acetate, 0.1 mg. daily.

Note: This steroid may produce excess sodium retention and should be watched for increased body weight and blood pressure as well as edema. Such untoward effects subside when the steroid is discontinued. The adrenal-insufficient patient is markedly sensitive to the sodium-retaining effects of the mineralocorticoid.

4. The dose of the medication used (e.g., glucocorticoid) should be augmented during stress.

CONGENITAL ADRENOGENITAL SYNDROME

1. If present at birth, the adrenal hyperplasia gives rise in the female to pseudohermaphroditism.
2. In female children, growth is at accelerated rate.
3. Body hair growth may be excessive.
4. Masculine muscle development and torso; narrow hips
5. Secondary female sexual characteristics absent
6. Clitoral enlargement.
7. *Laboratory Tests* / *Results*

Laboratory Tests	*Results*
17-Ketosteroids	Elevated
Pregnanetriol	Elevated
17-Hydroxysteroids	Normal or low
Metopirone test	Marked increase in pregnanetriol and ketosteroid excretion
Glucose tolerance	Increased

POSTPUBERTAL ADRENOGENITAL SYNDROME

Basic Principles

1. May vary from normal feminization to marked masculinization.
2. Body hair growth may be minimal or marked.
3. Clitoris may be normal or slightly enlarged.
4. Menstrual abnormalities are common, chiefly amenorrhea or anovulatory irregular menses.

5. *Laboratory Tests* — *Results*

Laboratory Tests	*Results*
17-Ketosteroids	Elevated
Pregnanetriol	Normal or elevated
17-Hydroxysteroids	Normal
Metopirone test	Marked increase in pregnanetriol and 17-ketosteroids (only occasional increase in 17-hydroxysteroids)
Glucose tolerance	Increased
Sodium	Normal
Potassium	Normal

Management

1. Therapy is the same for both the congenital and postpubertal syndromes and includes the use of any one of the following preparations:

Prednisone, 2.5 mg., t.i.d.
Hydrocortisone, 10 mg., t.i.d.
Medrol, 2 mg., t.i.d.
Triamcinolone, 2 mg., t.i.d.
Dexamethasone, 0.25 mg., t.i.d.
Betamethasone, 0.3 mg., t.i.d.

2. A repeat 17-ketosteroid is obtained 2 to 4 weeks later. If the levels are normal or low, the dose of corticoid is reduced to twice a day, and then further decreased, depending upon 17-KS excretion.

3. The congenital type must be treated for life.

4. Postpubertal adrenogenital syndrome may be discontinued in most patients after several months of treatment, with a permanent cure expected. (If therapy is discontinued in the congenital type, however, there is a marked increase in pregnanetriol.)

NEOPLASTIC ADRENOGENITAL SYNDROME

1. The clinical picture is the same as in the congenital adrenogenital syndrome except that the clinical changes appear so suddenly that defeminization is obvious and sudden in onset in the adult.

2. Increased hair growth, clitoral enlargement, decreased breast size, and oligomenorrhea terminating in amenorrhea are symptoms.

3. *Laboratory Tests* — *Results*

Laboratory Tests	*Results*
17-Ketosteroids	Elevated: moderate to marked
Pregnanetriol	Normal
17-Hydroxysteroids	Normal
Glucose tolerance	Normal
Sodium	Normal
Potassium	Normal
Metopirone test	No abnormal increase in steroid excretion
Visualization by arteriography, intravenous urography, venography, etc.	To demonstrate presence of tumor

4. The adrenogenital syndrome in children is more likely to be caused by an adrenal tumor than by hyperplasia, and the tumor is commonly malignant. (In adults, such a tumor is more often benign).

5. Sometimes the differential diagnosis between hyperplasia and tumor can only be settled by surgical exploration.

CUSHING'S SYNDROME

Basic Principles

Usually due to adrenocortical hypersecretion; occasionally associated with pituitary adenoma.

1. Clinical Features. Characteristic buffalo obesity with dorsocervical fat hump, thin arms and legs, muscle wasting, skin atrophy, presence of striae, and hypertension.

2. *Laboratory Tests* — *Results*

	Laboratory Tests	*Results*
a.	17-Ketosteroids	Normal or low
b.	17-Hydroxysteroids	Elevated
c.	Pregnanetriol	Normal or low
d.	Glucose tolerance	Decreased
e.	Serum sodium	Increased
f.	Urinary sodium	Decreased
g.	Serum potassium	Decreased
h.	Urinary potassium	Increased

i. Radiographs	Osteoporosis is common, especially in the vertebrae. Sella turcica rarely enlarged. Delayed bone age in children with retarded growth.

3. Provocative Tests

a. *Dexamethasone.* Blood hydroxysteroid is *normally* suppressed below 5 mcg. per 100 ml. in A.M. after 1.0 mg. of dexamethasone at 11:00 P.M. In patients with Cushing's syndrome the blood hydroxysteroid after dexamethasone is above 12 mcg. per 100 ml. (A urinary dexamethasone suppression test may be done instead, giving 0.5 mg. q.i.d. for 2 days, and then collecting a 24-hour urine on the morning of the second day; the 17-hydroxysteroids should normally drop at least 50 per cent from previous values).

b. *ACTH Stimulation.* Marked increase in blood and urinary 17-hydroxysteroids.

c. *Metapirone.* Marked increase in blood and urinary hydroxysteroids and 17-ketosteroids.

4. Further Differential Diagnosis

a. In females, Cushing's syndrome must be differentiated from masculinizing syndromes such as occur with adrenogenitalism or arrhenoblastoma and other virilizing ovarian tumors.

b. Cushing's syndrome is characterized by muscle weakness, whereas adrenogenitalism is characterized by muscular strength.

c. Urinary 17-ketosteroids are markedly elevated in adrenal carcinoma, while they tend to be within normal range with simple adenoma.

d. Urinary 17-hydroxysteroids are generally significantly elevated in all three types: adrenal neoplasia, adenoma, or hyperplasia.

Management

The prognosis may be poor unless the disease is arrested, with complications resulting from hypertensive cardiovascular disease. If tumor is present, it should be removed surgically. For hyperplasia, bilateral total adrenalectomy with appropriate adrenocortical replacement therapy is indicated when clinical response does not occur to more conservative measures such as pituitary irradiation.

OVARIAN DYSFUNCTION

Basic Principles

1. The two basic functions of the ovaries are to produce estrogen and progesterone, and to form ova.

2. Ovarian function is dependent upon pituitary stimulation.

a. Pituitary follicle-stimulating hormone (FSH) promotes follicular development.

b. Both FSH and LH (luteinizing hormone) from the pituitary are necessary for normal estrogen secretion and menstrual function.

c. Ovulation is triggered by a midcycle surge of LH, which is also required for the formation and maintenance of the corpus luteum and the secretion of its hormones, including progesterone.

3. Pituitary function is, in turn, dependent upon hypothalamic stimulation.

a. Hypothalamic LH-releasing hormone (LH-RH) has been synthesized; it is believed to release both LH and FSH.

b. The midcycle LH surge has been attributed to feedback by the chief ovarian estrogen (estradiol), perhaps mediated by LH-RH release from the hypothalamus.

4. The goal in the evaluation of gonadal-pituitary function is to determine whether the insufficiency is due primarily to ovarian inadequacy or to selective pituitary insufficiency of gonadotropic hormones. Several diagnostic proce-

dures may be undertaken to determine the functional state of the ovary.

Testing Ovarian Dysfunction

1. Progesterone Test. Progesterone in oil (100 mg.) is given I.M., or 10 mg. oral medroxyprogesterone acetate (Provera) may be given twice a day for 7 days, in order to determine whether the patient with **amenorrhea** will menstruate.

a. Normally, menstruation should take place within 2 weeks if the patient has adequate proliferative phase (estrogen) function, since progesterone cannot cause endometrial shedding unless there has been prior stimulation with estrogen.

b. The failure of menstruation to occur after the progesterone test would indicate inadequate estrogen secretion, possible pregnancy, or persistent corpus-luteal function.

c. No other progesterone preparations should be used for this test because of (1) pain at the site of injection (aqueous suspension); (2) prolongation of effect (Delalutin or Depo-Provera); (3) inherent estrogenic activity of agents such as contraceptive pills.

2. Vaginal Smear. An atrophic vaginal smear suggests complete ovarian insufficiency. A cornified or partially cornified vaginal smear indicates that there is at least some estrogen production, even if there is no ovulation (in cases of amenorrhea). The patient with the atrophic smear will not menstruate after progesterone, while the one with a cornified smear most probably will.

3. Pituitary Gonadotropin Assay. The FSH and LH levels may be obtained either by urinary or blood (radioimmunoassay) samples. A high gonadotropin level suggests primary ovarian inadequacy (premature menopause) and has a poor prognosis for fertility. A low gonadotropin secretion implies either pituitary insufficiency or hypothalamic disorder and, with appropriate treatment, the prognosis is good.

4. Estrogen Assay

a. With ovarian hypogonadism, there is a low serum estradiol by radioimmunoassay.

b. With primary ovarian failure the FSH and LH are high.

c. With secondary ovarian insufficiency, both the serum estradiol and serum gonadotropins (FSH, LH) are low.

d. Although early follicular phase levels of estrogen may normally be low, estradiol levels that are repeatedly lower than normal follicular phase levels by radioimmunoassay are indicative of ovarian insufficiency.

e. In contrast to estradiol, which is almost exclusively secreted by the ovaries, serum estrone values are of less value since they may also be formed peripherally from adrenocortical androstenedione.

5. Chromatin Pattern. In patients with immature or poor secondary sexual development and primary amenorrhea, a chromatin-negative pattern points toward gonadal dysgenesis. A positive chromatin pattern combined with a high FSH points toward ovarian dysgenesis or agenesis. *Note*: Whenever FSH values are inappropriately high (as in premature menopause or ovarian dysgenesis), it is also important to get a karyotype determination. If a Y chromosome is found, a testicular component within the gonad is suspected, and the patient should have a prophylactic gonadectomy before neoplastic changes occur. A blood assay for H-Y antigen may also be helpful in detecting testicular tissue, even in cases where the karyotype is apparently normal.

6. Clinical Stigmata

a. *Hypothalamic-Pituitary (Secondary) Amenorrhea of Short Duration.* No specific clinical stigmata apparent. Pregnancy should always be considered.

b. *Hypothalamic Amenorrhea of*

Long Duration. This may be associated with:

(1) Major weight gain or loss (including anorexia nervosa).

(2) Stopping oral contraceptives (post-pill amenorrhea)

(3) Psychological factors; severe emotional stress

(4) Infertility; occasionally pseudocyesis

(5) Postpartum (Sheehan's syndrome)

(6) Excessive prolactin secretion, with or without galactorrhea (Serum prolactin level will clarify.)

c. *Primary Ovarian Failure*

(1) In the previously menstruating woman this occurs naturally as menopause or, if at a relatively early age, as premature menopause.

(2) *Ovarian Dysgenesis (Turner's Syndrome)*

Absent secondary sexual characteristics

Short stature

Webbed neck

Cubitus valgus

Normal bone age, as a rule

Normal thyroid function

High FSH

Cardiovascular abnormalities and abnormalities of the terminal or middle phalanges of the fourth or fifth fingers

Negative chromatin pattern—absent Barr bodies on buccal smear

(3) *Prepubertal Ovarian Insufficiency (Without Dysgenesis).* Eunuchoid build, usually excessively tall.

(a) Public and axillary hair may be diminished

(b) Secondary sexual characteristics show poor development.

Management

1. General Principles

a. In the absence of local or systemic disease, tumor, congenital abnormality, or specific hormonal imbalance, amenorrhea per se requires no treatment unless the patient desires to become pregnant. However, since absence of menstruation may be emotionally disturbing to some women who may feel sexually inadequate or abnormal, and since absence of menstruation for a porlonged time may predispose to endometrial hyperplasia, it is generally prudent and helpful to induce artificial menstrual cycles.

b. Before hormonal therapy is begun, there should be an attempt to correct any dietary excesses or deficiencies, and to relieve unfavorable emotional and environmental situations. Often such measures alone will result in the spontaneous resumption of menses.

c. The patient may be given conjugated estrogens (Premarin) 1.25 mg. b.i.d. or t.i.d. for 21 days, or ethinyl estradiol (Estinyl) 0.05 mg. in the same manner. Medroxyprogesterone acetate (Provera) 10 mg. b.i.d. is given during the third (last) week of estrogen administration. Most patients will menstruate within 10 days of such therapy, which may then be repeated either monthly or every few months.

d. Failure to menstruate after such estrogen-progesterone administration (rare) indicates endometrial failure, with generally poor prognosis. Before drawing that conclusion, however, one should try giving the progesterone parenterally instead of orally for the rare patient who does not absorb the oral medication well.

e. For those patients who desire to become pregnant, where amenorrhea or faulty ovulation is the chief problem, the use of clomiphene citrate (Clomid) 50 mg. for 5 days starting on the fifth day of an induced menstrual cycle, is often helpful in inducing ovulation and thus spontaneous menstruation. The dosage of Clomid may have to be increased according to the response, or lack of it, as determined by the basal temperature graph, endometrial biopsy, and pelvic examinations to detect any tendency toward cystic ovaries. In those infertility patients where pituitary insufficiency is the background cause of the ovarian problem, human menopausal gonadotropins (HMG) have been highly successful in inducing ovulation.

2. Turner's Syndrome

a. Conjugated estrogens (Premarin) 1.25 mg. b.i.d. may be given daily without interruption.

b. Provera 10 mg. b.i.d. is given for a week, beginning on the first day of each calendar month.

c. If the estrogen dose is not sufficient to adequately develop the patient, it may be doubled, and the Provera dose increased to 30 mg. per day. Ethinyl estradiol (Estinyl) may be substituted for the conjugated equine estrogens in doses of 0.05 mg. twice a day.

d. Estrogens should *not* be started unless the patient has reached her full growth potential or she is too upset about her lack of secondary sexual characteristics and does not care whether she grows any more.

e. Since fertility is virtually absent in such cases, hormonal substitution therapy is all that can be offered.

f. However, it should be kept in mind that ovarian tumors (dysgerminomas, embryonal cell carcinomas) arise more often in dysgenetic ovaries. Tumor development is especially frequent when mosaicism is present, particularly in 45, X/XY individuals. For this reason, preventive oophorectomy should be done if the karyotype shows a Y chromosome.

3. Prepubertal Ovarian Insufficiency

This condition is treated only if the patient is excessively tall. High-dosage estrogen is given in an effort to close her epiphyses, thus preventing further growth. At the same time, progesterone is given to deciduate the endometrium monthly. Premarin may be given, 2.5 mg., two tablets twice daily. Provera 10 mg. t.i.d. may be given once a month for a week, during which time the patient does not take Premarin.

4. Uterine Agenesis

a. *Basic Features.* A normal-appearing female with good feminization. Cyclic changes occur in the vaginal smear, but with no menstruation. There is failure to menstruate after treatment with progesterone alone or with estrogen. The vaginal introitus is shallow.

b. *Management.* This is a congenital phenomenon caused by absent or rudimentary development of the uterus. Hormonal therapy is not indicated. If the vaginal introitus is too shallow for sexual intercourse, surgical correction of the vaginal defect is indicated.

5. Testicular Feminization Syndrome

a. *Basic Principles*

(1) A normally developed female, but with pubic or axillary hair diminished or absent (short vaginal tract).

(2) Negative chromatin pattern

(3) The patient may have bilaterally palpable inguinal masses or hernias.

(4) The vaginal smear may show evidence of diminished estrogenic activity.

(5) the pituitary FSH may be high.

(6) These patients cannot be masculinized with androgens, nor do they menstruate after progesterone alone or in combination with estrogen.

(7) Vaginal dilatation may have to be performed in order to produce an adequate vaginal introitus.

(8) Some patients may have a rudimentary uterine-like structure.

b. *Mangement*

(1) These patients must have their testes removed at about age 17 to 18 to prevent anaplastic changes from occurring.

(2) Replacement therapy with estrogen is necessary when such surgery is performed.

(3) It is unwise to tell the patient or family that "testicles" or other male features are present, since the mere knowledge of the presence of any features of the opposite sex may cause profound emotional problems.

PITUITARY DYSFUNCTION

Basic Principles

1. The anterior pituitary secretes many important hormones:
   a. Follicle-stimulating hormone (FSH)
   b. Luteinizing hormone (LH)
   c. Thyrotropic, or thyroid-stimulating hormone (TSH)
   d. Prolactin (PRL)
   e. Growth hormone (GH)
   f. Adrenocorticotropin hormone (ACTH)
2. The concentration of circulating hormone from the target gland (e.g., ovary, thyroid, adrenal) exerts a negative feedback control on the secretion of its corresponding tropic hormone, the effect being at the level of the hypothalamus, the pituitary, or both.
3. Each pituitary hormone is regulated by hypothalamic hormones via the secretion of both stimulating and inhibiting factors.
4. A hypothalamic hormone with LH-releasing activity (LH-RH) (LRF) has been isolated and synthesized. This LH-RH is capable of releasing not only LH but also FSH. Normally, a midcyclic high estrogen peak is believed to trigger a midcyclic burst of LH-RH, causing LH and FSH secretion.
5. There are now radioimmunoassays for pituitary hormones such as FSH, LH, TSH, GH.

HYPOPITUITARISM

Sheehan's Syndrome

1. Basic Principles

a. Sheehan's syndrome specifically refers to postpartum hemorrhage associated with pituitary necrosis.

b. The clinical features of Sheehan's syndrome are precisely the same as those seen when the pituitary gland has been destroyed after the initiation of gonadal function.

2. Clinical Features

a. Diminished or absent axillary or pubic hair

b. Premature aging of skin

c. The breasts are usually well formed and do not atrophy

d. Cephalic hair is thick and coarse

e. Pelvic examination shows atrophic vaginal mucosa and a markedly hypoplastic uterus and cervix, with the adnexae usually not palpable.

3. Laboratory Findings

a. Thyroid and adrenal function tests are low.

b. FSH is low.

c. 17-ketosteroids low

d. 17-hydroxysteroids in blood or urine low; no diurnal fluctuation

e. Glucose tolerance (oral)—flat curve

f. Metopirone—no response

g. ACTH—good adrenal response

h. Blood—hypochromic anemia that may be associated with a bleeding tendency

4. Therapeutic Response

These patients will show evidence of ovarian stimulation following the use of gonadotropins in tests for ovarian function.

5. X-ray Findings

a. Sella turcica. Normal in Sheehan's syndrome, but may be markedly enlarged from a pituitary tumor or craniopharyngioma in patients with hypopituitarism not following pregnancy.

b. Osteoporosis of the skeletal system generally noted in long-standing disease.

6. Management

a. *Complete Replacement Therapy.* This is done with thyroid and glucocorticoids.

b. *Ovarian Replacement Therapy.* Premarin 2.5 mg./day or Estinyl 0.1 mg./day administered continuously. Provera 10 mg., b.i.d. for 7 days, at monthly intervals.

c. *Alternative Treatments.* Instead of oral gonadal steroids, one could give, parenterally, Depo-Estradiol, 10 mg., at 3 week intervals, or Delestrogen, 20 mg., at 3 week intervals. Progesterone in oil, 100 mg., is then given I.M. at monthly intervals.

Amenorrhea With Persistent Lactation (Galactorrhea)

1. Basic Principles

a. May be postpartum (Chiari-Frommel syndrome) or unrelated to pregnancy (Forbes-Albright or Del Castello's syndrome)

b. Inappropriate lactation may also be caused by drugs, such as opiates, diazepines, tricyclic antidepressants, phenothiazines, and reserpine derivatives.

c. Excessive estrogen (e.g., birth control pills) can lead to galactorrhea via hypothalamic suppression.

d. Lactation is also associated with hypothyroidism and, less frequently, from stresses associated with surgery and anesthesia.

2. Laboratory and X-ray Findings

a. Almost all patients with galactorrhea have an elevated prolactin assay (> 20 ng./ml.).

b. Polytomography of the sella turcica for pituitary tumor

c. Thyroid function tests for hypothyroidism

d. *Note*: Even with no demonstrable pituitary tumor, a patient with a markedly elevated prolactin level may be harboring a small functional microadenoma that will eventually be radiologically detectable. Such patients should have periodic radiologic, endocrinologic (prolactin), and ophthalmologic (visual field) examinations with this diagnosis in mind.

3. Management

a. The treatment of choice for galactorrhea is a relatively new, nonhormonal compound, bromergocryptine. The usual dose is 2.5 mg. b.i.d. or t.i.d. daily for 3 to 6 months, if needed. Spontaneous menses may occur within a few weeks.

b. Contraception (other than birth control) is advisable during this therapy.

c. For patients wishing to conceive, the drug is discontinued. Should amenorrhea (anovulation) with or without galactorrhea recur, clomiphene citrate may be used to induce ovulation, in doses of 50 mg. b.i.d. for 7 to 10 days. If ineffective, Pergonal may be tried.

d. *Note:* There are no dogmatic rules concerning the treatment of small pituitary tumors, and each case must be individualized as to whether to observe periodically to detect changes, to irradiate, or to remove surgically.

MULTIGLANDULAR DYSFUNCTION

STEIN-LEVENTHAL SYNDROME

Basic Principles

1. This syndrome, also referred to as polycystic or sclerocystic ovarian disease, is not a specific entity. It is associated with a thickened, fibrotic ovarian tunica and accompanied by an ovarian follicular cystic disorder. It is still unclear whether these abnormal ovarian changes constitute the etiological basis of the "syndrome," or whether they are simply one of the effects.

2. The following are frequent findings:

a. Failure to ovulate, or only occasional ovulation

b. Menometrorrhagia is uncommon, but may occur between episodes of amenorrhea.

c. Infertility, either primary or secondary

d. Hirsutism in about half the cases

e. Thickened ovarian tunica and multifollicle cysts (*smooth white capsule*)

f. Ovaries usually, but not necessarily, enlarged.

g. Obesity may be present.

Laboratory and Other Findings

1. There are no "typical" laboratory

findings in the so-called Stein-Leventhal syndrome.

2. Efforts to determine the source of increased androgens in women with polycystic ovarian disease have been unrewarding.

a. In the 25 per cent of patients in whom 17-ketosteroids are significantly elevated, suppression by prednisone or dexamethasone (though inconsistent) would *appear* to implicate the adrenal cortex. If suppression followed the administration of estrogen, an ovarian source of androgen would *appear* to be implicated.

b. In about 50 per cent of patients with polycystic disease, there is an elevation of the plasma testosterone and androstenedione. However, the testosterone level is usually well below 200 ng./100 ml. If levels are higher than this, one should suspect an androgen-secreting adrenal or ovarian tumor.

c. Ovarian and adrenal vein catheterization studies in women with excess androgens (but without distinct elevations of urinary 17-ketosteroids) have demonstrated that:

(1) The ovary is indeed a common source of androgen.

(2) Sometimes excessive androgen can arise from *both* the ovary and adrenal.

(3) Suppression and stimulation tests appear to be of very little value in predicting the source of excess androgen.

3. Characteristically, FSH levels are low or normal while LH levels tend to be high or normal.

4. Estradiol levels are usually normal, while estrone levels are usually elevated.

5. Pelvic examination may reveal palpably enlarged ovaries.

6. Cervical mucus is typically profuse and clear, the result of unopposed estrogen production.

7. Endoscopy (either culdoscopy or laparoscopy) will confirm the presence of polycystic ovaries.

Management

1. If fertility is not desired, for a limited time, one can consider the use of Provera, 10 mg. b.i.d. for 7 days each month to deciduate the endometrium.

2. A special problem exists for those women who plan no children at all. They are bothered mainly by hirsutism and functional uterine bleeding, and there is some evidence (though inconclusive) that untreated polycystic disease may increase the potential for endometrial cancer. For these reasons, it is desirable to suppress ovarian function by giving cyclic estrogen/progesterone. Oral contraceptives containing ethinyl estradiol and mestranol help to replace endogenous estrogen and suppress ovarian androgen production. Continued use of oral contraceptives, by suppressing the pituitary, help to arrest abnormal steroid secretion.

3. When pregnancy is desired, the drug of choice to induce ovulation is clomiphene citrate (Clomid). Starting with 50 mg. daily for 5 days, from the fifth day of the cycle, the dose can be gradually increased up to 150 or even 200 mg. The aim is to achieve ovulation, as demonstrated by the basal temperature graph, endometrial biopsy, or serum progesterone. The patient must be monitored carefully by pelvic examination toward the end of each cycle, to make sure there is no overstimulation (significant cystic ovarian enlargement).

4. If several cycles of Clomid are unsuccessful in stimulating ovulation in those women desiring children, then wedge resection of the ovaries may be considered. The results are generally favorable as far as ovulation is concerned, and are further enhanced by the use of Clomid after the resection.

5. The use of Pergonal (human menopausal gonadotropin) is both unpredictable and hazardous, since women with polycystic ovarian disease are particularly prone to overstimulation.

MISCELLANEOUS ENDOCRINE IMBALANCE

HIRSUTISM

Basic Principles

1. Hirsutism is an understandably distressing symptom for any woman and thus has both medical and emotional components.

2. Excessive hair growth in the female, with the exception of that which is genetically acquired, is caused by increased androgen secretion.

a. The source of increased androgen can be the ovary, the adrenal, or both.

b. So-called idiopathic hirsutism has been ascribed to end-organ response in the skin—an aberration of end-organ metabolism of androgen by peripheral conversion of plasma precursors.

3. History and physical examination important.

a. The majority of patients with hirsutism give an onset that is postpubertal (though it may be in the teens) and gradual, slow progression.

b. A later onset and/or rapid progression suggests organic disease.

c. Oligomenorrhea or secondary amenorrhea are common.

d. Other common complaints are acne, oily skin, and infertility.

e. Virilization suggests androgenic tumors, and the findings may include baldness (occipital or temporal), increased muscular size and strength, clitoral enlargement, and deepening voice. Androgenic tumor is also suggested by defeminization, such as decreased breast size and loss of female body contours.

4. Statistically, the vast majority of women with hirsutism, irregular menses, and acne, without other clinical evidence of androgen overproduction, do *not* have ovarian or adrenal tumors, nor do they have Cushing's syndrome.

5. Although tumors are rare, when they do occur most virilizing ovarian tumors are benign or of low-grade malignancy, while most virilizing adrenal tumors are malignant, especially in children.

Laboratory Tests

1. Basic Principles

a. The commonly employed substances tested for are 17-ketosteroids, pregnanetriol (both from 24-hour urines), and plasma testosterone.

b. A urinary creatinine is also helpful to exclude major collection errors.

c. The 17-ketosteroid excretion may be influenced exogenously; it is increased by ingestion of chlorpromazine, MAO inhibitors, and penicillin; it is decreased by meprobamate, reserpine, and estrogens.

d. The Metopirone test (metyrapone) is often used for "suppression." Metopirone selectively inhibits beta hydroxylation, preventing the formation of hydrocortisone. This in turn increases ACTH secretion, with consequent adrenocortical stimulation and (normally) a rise in 17-ketosteroid (and 17-hydroxysteroid) excretion. The test consists of giving three tablets of Metopirone (each 250 mg.) q.i.d. for 6 doses, having previously obtained a urinary 17-ketosteroid and pregnanetriol value. A second 24-hour urine collection is begun with the fifth dose—that is, on the second morning of Metopirone ingestion.

Identifying Tests

1. With this background, the following tests may be used to help identify which organ may be responsible for the excessive androgen secretion.

a. *Adrenals.* 17-ketosteroid and pregnanetriol levels are obtained prior to and during administration of Metopirone, as described above. If there is no inordinate increase in the excretion of both these steroids, then the likelihood of adrenal origin of the hirsutism is remote. If there is a significant increase in

17-ketosteroids and pregnanetriol, then the adrenogenital syndrome must be considered. On the other hand, if the Metopirone test fails to induce an elevation of 17-ketosteroids and pregnanetriol, the ovaries must then be considered as a possible source of androgens. The following method may be employed to demonstrate this.

b. *Ovaries.* Prednisone, 5 mg., b.i.d. is given 4 days prior to and during the administration of HCG. HCG is administered in doses of 4,000 I.U. per day for 3 days. A significant increase in the 17-ketosteroid excretion points toward ovarian origin of the hirsutism. Failure of such an increase, however, does not rule out the ovaries as a source of androgens, and calls for additional testosterone determinations. A significant increase in testosterone levels from the blood and urine (as compared with levels before the prednisone-HCG test) suggests the ovary as a source of the hirsutism.

c. *Plasma Testosterone Levels.* They are normally 0.2 to 0.8 ng./ml. and show some elevation in most women with hirsutism and anovulation, but there is much individual variation. The reason serum testosterone is not often significantly elevated is due to decreased bound testosterone; it is the unbound fraction that produces the androgenic effect. Also, serum testosterone is elevated by estrogens, hyperthyroidism, and cirrhosis; it is lowered by progestins, hypothyroidism, and glucocorticoids.

d. *Note:* Ovarian and adrenal vein catheterization studies of women with hirsutism with normal or slightly elevated urinary 17-ketosteroids have led to the observations that (1) the ovary is a common source of androgen overproduction; (2) it is not uncommon to find that the source of androgen hypersecretion is from *both* the ovary and the adrenals; and (3) the various suppression tests do *not* really correlate well with the more direct catheterization findings in terms of pinpointing the exact source of androgen oversecretion.

Management

1. If the patient desires to conceive, the infertility takes precedence over the idiopathic hirsutism. Clomiphene citrate, with wedge resection if the Clomid fails completely, are the methods commonly employed.

2. In patients who do not desire pregnancy, hirsutism is managed by suppressing ovarian steroidogenesis with progestin administration. Any low-dose combination oral contraceptive pill given in the usual cyclic fashion will serve to suppress plasma testosterone levels *after 6 to 9 months* of treatment. This slow response to treatment should be explained to the patient beforehand.

3. If oral contraceptives are contraindicated, Depo-Provera may be used instead.

4. Although these suppressive treatments will suppress new hair growth after many months, they will not affect the hair already present. Thus the patient may wish to consider such additional methods as shaving, waxing, or depilatories at appropriate intervals, once new hair growth has ceased. For permanent hair removal, electrolysis is used.

5. The above management applies to patients whose 17-ketosteroid suppression with dexamethasone is within the normal range of 5 to 11 mg.

6. If the suppression of 17-ketosteroids is profound (e.g., to a level of 3 mg./24 hours or less), the suspected adrenal hyperplasia is treated with a glucocorticoid such as prednisone, 5 mg. daily, enough to maintain 17-ketosteroid excretion within normal range.

7. A complete lack of 17-ketosteroid suppression suggests an adrenal tumor (rare) which warrants further and separate investigation.

8. Although also relatively uncommon

(but not as rare as adrenal tumor), one must consider the possibility of an androgen-producing *ovarian* tumor if there is:

a. An enlarged ovary

b. No enlarged ovary but abnormally high testosterone levels

c. No enlarged ovary and normal testosterone levels, but no decrease in the original testosterone level after 6 months of treatment with progestational steroid suppression. One should not hesitate to do an endoscopy in any questionable case, to rule out a small ovarian tumor. When an ovary is palpably enlarged, however, an exploratory laparotomy is warranted under the special circumstances mentioned.

SEXUAL PRECOCITY

Basic Principles

1. The occurrence of menses prior to age 10 is considered precocious.

2. This may be the first symptom, although commonly there is also increased growth, followed by pubic hair and breast development.

3. Although most sexual precocities in the female are idiopathic, this diagnosis cannot be made except by exclusion with careful follow-up in an effort to uncover a slow-growing lesion in the ovary, adrenal gland, or brain.

4. History is important, since a familial occurrence makes the likelihood of tumors very remote.

5. Premature development of the female secondary sex characteristics may be seen in patients with:

a. Idiopathic causes—i.e., constitutional sexual precocity (most common)

b. Space-occupying brain tumor, particularly in the region of the third ventricle

c. Postencephalitis or meningitis

d. Cranial injury

e. Hypothyroidism

6. Other neoplasms may induce sexual precocity, including tumors of the adrenals or of the ovaries—i.e., tumors primarily associated with increased estrogenic production.

a. Feminizing tumor of the adrenals (very rare)

b. Thecal tumors of the ovary

c. Granulosa cell tumors of the ovary

d. Brenner tumors of the ovary

Clinical Features

1. Precocious development of breasts and pubic and axillary hair

2. Increase in height and weight—much above that seen in normal females of the same age

3. Premature menarche

Laboratory Findings

1. Increased estrogenic level in 24-hour urine or in blood sample.

2. Vaginal cornification

3. Low FSH in most patients; occasionally normal FSH

4. Both FSH and LH levels are indicated to ascertain gonadotropic function, and the urinary 17-ketosteroid should also be measured, as well as thyroid tests. However, parameters of thyroid and adrenal function are usually normal.

Differentiation between Neoplastic and Corticoidal Types

A vaginal smear is taken initially, followed by the administration of 100 mg. medroxyprogesterone acetate (Depo-Provera), I.M. at weekly intervals for 3 injections.

1. *Interpretation*

A change in the vaginal smear from one with normal estrogenic activity to one with marked estrogenic deficiency is not a characteristic finding in patients with adrenal or ovarian tumors, and indicates premature release of pituitary gonadotropin. If the vaginal smear (after the injections) shows secretory activity without estrogenic deficiency, then the patient must be suspected of having an ovarian or adrenal tumor. In clinical practice, however, it is important to keep in mind that if a tumor is present, it is usually palpable; therefore, thorough physical examination is most important.

Management

1. Constitutional Type (Idiopathic)

a. Treatment when no cause can be found is limited to the use of a potent progestational agent in order to inhibit gonadotropin production.

b. Administration of Depo-Provera in large doses, 400 mg. I.M. monthly for 3 months, then once every 3 months thereafter. The dosage and schedule may be modified according to the amount necessary to induce castration changes in the vaginal mucosa.

(1) This stops menstruation, thereby preventing the child from being psychologically upset by a physiologic state which is greatly advanced over the mental capacity.

(2) Breast development decreases and stops. (Pubic hair will not disappear.)

(3) Premature closure of the epiphyses is delayed by this procedure. Although the child is taller for her age, accelerated sexual development and secretion of estrogens would ordinarily cause premature closure of the epiphyses, with the result that she would eventually be much shorter than her age-mates.

(4) Because such children are not mentally capable of discerning right from wrong, they may be preyed upon by perverts and become impregnated at an early age. Depo-Provera prevents menses from occurring, and in addition may curtail any libidinous drive the patient might have.

(5) Treatment should be continued until the chronological age matches the bone age or until age 12 to 13. Hand-wrist films should be obtained every 6 months until epiphyseal closure has been demonstrated.

(6) If there is any breakthrough bleeding after starting Depo-Provera, it may be stopped by estrogen (e.g., Premarin 1.25 mg. daily for a week).

EXCESSIVE LINEAR GROWTH IN FEMALES

Basic Principles

1. The patient is frequently a daughter of very tall parents.

2. If there is no family history of tallness, a history, physical, and routine laboratory examinations are done. A hand-wrist radiograph for bone age is important. In the physical examination, the degree of secondary sexual characteristics development is most important, since the more mature her development, the less likely that any treatment will influence her eventual height.

3. In general, a girl who is 5 feet 8 inches tall or more, in whom sexual maturation or menarche has not occurred, is a possible candidate for preventive therapy. Ideally, treatment should begin therefore as early as age 9 to 10, but in any case before menses have begun.

4. Once treatment is begun, it must be continued until the epiphyses are fused, otherwise further growth will take place.

Management

1. The treatment involves the use of high dosages of estrogens, in order to close the epiphyses and inhibit growth-hormone secretion from the pituitary.

2. The estrogen best tolerated for this purpose is conjugated estrogens (Premarin). It is given in high doses (10 mg. daily, in divided doses, if tolerated, otherwise at least 5 mg. daily), for the first 25 days of each calendar month.

3. During the last five days of estrogen therapy, medroxyprogesterone acetate (Provera) 10 mg. is added, to ensure withdrawal bleeding.

4. Both the patient and the parents should be told about possible side effects such as breast engorgement, menorrhagia, or water retention.

5. If successful, epiphyseal closure occurs in 6 to 9 months. The overall growth achieved during this time will usually be less than 2 inches, and frequently less than 1 inch.

ANOVULATION

Basic Principles

1. Absence of ovulation is physiologically normal and expected during the first year or two after menarche, and again at the approach of menopause.

2. In the woman who is not interested in becoming pregnant, anovulation per se is unimportant if she has normal periods (anovulatory menses).

3. More frequently, anovulation will be accompanied by abnormal bleeding (menorrhagia, metrorrhagia) or amenorrhea. These are often associated with the development of endometrial hyperplasia from unopposed estrogen stimulation.

4. The most frequent clinical manifestation of anovulation is amenorrhea of the hypothalamic type.

a. This may occur under any stressful experience, during travel, overwork, etc.

b. Weight loss is another common cause, particularly a "crash diet." For reasons not clearly understood this may lead to a hypogonadotropic state.

c. Obesity may also be associated with anovulation, but here the amenorrhea is not usually associated with a hypogonadotropic state unless the patient has a concomitant emotional disorder.

Tests for Ovulation

1. Basal temperature chart which shows a biphasic curve

2. Vaginal smear changes, from cornified to luteal type

3. Cervical mucus

a. Clear, thin, stretchable (*spinnbarkeit*) during and preceding ovulation

b. Thick, viscid, not stretchable postovulatory

c. Ferning on microscopic examination of a dried smear from the cervix, which increases as ovulation approaches, then gradually disappears

4. Endometrial biopsy, showing secretory phase postovulatory

5. Serum progesterone by radioimmunoassay determinations

All of the above criteria for ovulation are actually measures of increased progesterone production, and the occurrence of ovulation is "presumed."

Absolute Evidence of Ovulation

1. Direct observation of the ovaries by endoscopy or at laparotomy

2. Pregnancy

Induction of Ovulation

1. Prior to attempting to induce ovulation in a woman who wishes to conceive, the couple should be normal as far as:

a. Tubal patency (Rubin test, hysterosalpingography, endoscopy if needed)

b. Semen quality

c. Postcoital (Huhner) test

d. Thyroid, pituitary, and adrenal function by tests previously outlined

2. There should be normal proliferative phase activity as evidenced by:

a. Regular menses (even though anovulatory), or occurring at irregular intervals

b. Normal (cornified) vaginal smear

c. In the amenorrheic patient, menstrual response after giving progesterone

d. Normal serum prolactin and pituitary tomogram

Management

1. Improvement of general constitutional state (environmental, lifestyle, stresses), and nutrition (obesity, under-

weight), as well as correction of any specific hormonal defect (e.g., thyroid) that may be found

2. For women who do not wish to conceive, the use of cyclic estrogen and progesterone or one of the oral contraceptives will not induce ovulation but will deciduate the endometrium at regular intervals, thus preventing the development of hyperplasia or adenomatous hyperplasia.

3. For women who wish to conceive, and in whom estrogenic and pituitary function are normal:

a. Clomiphene citrate (Clomid) 50 mg. daily for 5 days starting the fifth day of the cycle. If ovulation fails to occur, as determined by the basal temperature graph, endometrial biopsy, or progesterone levels, the dose of clomiphene may be increased by 50 mg. daily up to 200 mg. per day. the Clomid is always begun on the 5th day of a spontaneous or a progesterone-induced period, and the dosage is closely monitored by a pelvic examination about 2 weeks after completion of medication to determine if there is any evidence of ovarian cystic formation. If there is such overreaction, the drug may be stopped for the next month or two, then resumed more cautiously with smaller dose increments.

b. In some cases, induction of ovulation with Clomid is enhanced by the addition of HCG, 5,000 to 10,000 I.U. given about 3 to 5 days after the last Clomid medication.

c. Wedge resection of the ovaries may be considered in women with polycystic ovaries, when Clomid has failed to induce ovulation.

d. The use of Pergonal (human menopausal gonadotropin; HMG) is reserved for a minority of cases of infertility where all factors are normal but the anovulation is due to a very low pituitary gonadotropin secretion (FSH). The dosages of Pergonal and HCG must be worked out individually, and patient monitoring must be strict because of the tendency to complications such as ovarian cysts, ascites, and multiple births.

MENORRHAGIA

Basic Principles

1. Excessive uterine bleeding may have either an organic or functional origin; in this chapter we will assume that organic causes have been ruled out.

2. Functional uterine bleeding requires endocrine evaluation as well as hematological examination to rule out bleeding tendency.

3. Such bleeding is most prevalent in adolescence and near the menopause. In both of these situations, a common cause is anovulatory bleeding due to continued estrogen stimulation without progesterone formation.

4. The remaining causes of functional (or dysfunctional) uterine bleeding are probably due to endocrine imbalance involving the thyroid, pituitary, or adrenal glands. It can also follow estrogen (or progesterone) withdrawal.

Diagnostic Procedures

1. Laboratory blood studies
2. Endometrial biopsy
3. Rule out endocrine (thyroid, adrenal) dysfunction

Management

1. Most patients with severe functional bleeding have a proliferative endometrium, some to the point of hyperplasia. The first step if menorrhagia is associated with anemia is to stop the bleeding.

2. A potent progestational agent such as Norlutate, 5 mg., 3 to 4 tablets at once, will generally stop the bleeding promptly. The Norlutate can then be continued 5 mg. b.i.d. for the next 3 weeks. The norethindrone acetate changes the endometrium to a secretory

phase and thereby promotes endometrial shedding after it is discontinued.

3. The Norlutate can then be restarted on Day 5 of the next (induced) menstrual period (sooner if bleeding tends to be heavy again), and continued cyclically in doses of 10 mg. daily (or more, if needed), for 3 weeks at a time.

4. Anemia should be corrected by the simultaneous use of an oral iron preparation.

5. If there is specific thyroid or other endocrine dysfunction, therapy is directed toward the specific abnormality.

6. Once the patient begins having normal "periods" from the cyclic progestational agent, it can be discontinued in favor of simply shedding the endometrium at monthly intervals with *any* progestational steroid (Norlutate, Provera) in doses of 10 mg. b.i.d. for 7 days, for the next 2 to 3 consecutive months.

7. If parenteral preparations are preferred, progesterone in oil, 100 mg. I.M. is often effective in controlling bleeding.

8. Obviously, if severe bleeding is not reasonably controlled by any of these measures, the diagnosis of functional bleeding should be reassessed in favor of a previously missed organic cause, whether intrauterine pathology (D and C) or adenomyosis, and appropriate measures taken.

9. Postmenopausal bleeding can also be functional (atrophic endometrium), but in such instances it is essential to rule out uterine pathology before coming to that conclusion.

MENOPAUSE

Basic Principles

1. The menopause, which means cessation of menses, is physiological and due to ovarian senescence and decline in estrogen production.

2. It is considered definitely established after 1 year of amenorrhea, at which time there is a concurrent loss of reproductive function.

3. The broader term, climacteric, refers to a general and gradual decline in ovarian function; it encompasses a span of years during which time menopause occurs.

Symptomatology of the Climacteric and/or Menopause

1. Amenorrhea, usually preceded by irregular (further apart) menses

2. Anovulation

3. Vasomotor Symptoms. Flushes and sweating

4. Vaginal discomforts and/or dyspareunia due to atrophic vaginitis

5. Urinary discomforts due to atrophic urethritis and trigonitis

6. A host of other symptoms have often been attributed to "menopause," but because of their emotional and psychosomatic components, they could also be attributed to lifestyle factors and the multiple stresses of middle age. These include symptoms such as depression, insomnia, headache, fatigue, nervousness, backache, myalgias, etc. In any individual instance it is difficult to isolate the specific contribution that estrogen deficiency makes for two reasons:

a. When estrogen replacement therapy eliminates flushes, sweats, and atrophic vaginal discomforts, the patient will expectedly feel much better, and this may be reflected in an improvement in her vaguer emotional symptoms.

b. The possibility of a placebo effect when estrogen is given for "menopausal" symptoms.

Physical Findings

1. The physical changes most directly due to estrogen deprivation occur in the female genital tract—smaller uterus and ovaries, thin endometrium, atrophic vaginal mucosa.

2. There may also be less muscle tone and fascial strength in pelvic structures, predisposing to pelvic relaxation and atrophy.

3. Additional atrophic changes are general loss of labial subcutaneous fat, sagging of the breasts, markedly diminished cervical secretions.

4. Not all changes in the muscle, skin, and bone (e.g., osteoporosis) are due to estrogen deficiency, since there is a substantial contribution from protein catabolism, degenerative changes of aging, and muscle disuse.

Laboratory Findings

1. Decreased estrogenic activity in the vaginal mucosa, as seen on wet or stained smear, showing gradually increasing numbers of intermediate and, finally, parabasal cells.
2. Elevated FSH

Management

1. Must be individualized.
2. A careful history and physical examination are essential. One cannot properly assess the multiple, often vague symptomatology of "menopause" without knowing the patient's personal, marital, sexual, and socioeconomic history.
3. Vaginal discomforts and dyspareunia due to atrophic vaginitis are promptly relieved by the use of a local estrogenic cream, which can then be used preventatively every 2 or 3 weeks.
4. Classical symptoms such as flushes and sweats can be dramatically eliminated by oral estrogen.

   a. The lowest dose that will make the patient comfortable is preferred. Therefore, one may start with conjugated estrogen (Premarin) 0.3 to 0.625 mg. daily for 3 weeks out of 4, cyclically. Higher doses may be necessary.

   b. A progestational agent such as medroxyprogesterone acetate (Provera) 10 mg. daily is given during the last 5 days of estrogen therapy to deciduate the endometrium. This may be given every 2 to 3 months if the patient prefers to menstruate less often.

   c. Depending upon the response to treatment, medication is gradually discontinued.

5. Even though estrogen is specifically helpful for the symptoms mentioned, the benefits of estrogen therapy must be reappraised in the light of several reports which apparently relate the prolonged use of estrogen with an increased risk of endometrial carcinoma.

   a. The FDA now requires additional warnings to that effect for all estrogen products, and so it should be discussed with the patient.

   b. It may be reassuring for the patient to know that there are additional measures the physician can take to minimize the risk, whether real or potential.

      (1) A careful history and physical examination has already been stressed.

      (2) Preliminary screening of the endometrium by intrauterine Pap smears, an endometrial biopsy, or office suction-curettage are all helpful in establishing a baseline.

      (3) Thereafter, annual office suction curettage or at least an endometrial biopsy would be a meaningful follow-up for those on long-term therapy.

6. Estrogens are contraindicated in women with a history of or in the presence of cancer of the breast or endometrium, inasmuch as some of these tumors may be hormonally dependent and thus stimulated. In addition, estrogen should not be prescribed, or at least prescribed with great caution, to women with edema from cardiac decompensation, renal disease, or severe liver disease.

Estrogen Use in Prophylaxis

1. There is no satisfactory evidence that coronary disease in postmenopausal women is delayed or prevented by the administration of estrogen. However, there does seem to be evidence that the risk of heart disease is *increased* in women smokers who take oral contraceptives (which contain estrogen).
2. There are some studies favoring es-

trogen as a preventive measure and for treatment of osteoporosis. However, the dosage required is generally high (1.25 to 2.5 mg. conjugated estrogens daily), there may be a loss in beneficial effects after 6 to 9 months, and uterine bleeding may become a problem. Actually, osteoporosis is known to be a multifaceted disorder, and is also influenced by other therapeutic measures such as a high-calcium diet, vitamin D, increased fluoride intake, and a systematic exercise program.

3. In summary, estrogen replacement therapy for the menopause and postmenopause will probably continue to be a controversial subject for some time to come. The physician must therefore be familiar with both the benefits and drawbacks, and make his therapeutic decisions on an individualized basis.

PROGESTATIONAL STEROIDS

Many synthetic progestins are now available for clinical use. Some of them may be used interchangeably, others have a specific application in certain clinical entities. Their particular properties and use are listed below.

Medroxyprogesterone Acetate

1. Oral Preparation (Provera). This steroid has no androgenic or estrogenic effects. The oral preparation closely simulates progesterone in its morphological effect upon both the stroma and the glands of the endometrium.

2. Application

a. It is the only oral preparation that should be used as a diagnostic test in amenorrhea, since it would not produce a menstrual flow in an estrogen-deficient patient without previous estrogen priming. As a test for determining endometrial response in amenorrhea (not associated with pregnancy), it should be administered in doses of 10 mg., b.i.d. for 7 days.

b. *Note*: Since it is considered inadvisable to give any progestational steroids (or estrogens) during pregnancy, because of uncertain effects upon the fetus, gestation should be ruled out if there is any question after physical and pelvic examination. This can be done by a pregnancy test, the most sensitive being the blood radioreceptor assay (RRA), the more common urinary tests for HCG, or simply by having the patient take her basal temperature for two days before starting medication. Basal temperatures below 98.0° F are characteristic of a nonpregnant proliferative state.

c. Provera has been used in the past for some patients with history of habitual abortion or so-called deficient luteal phase. However, there is no conclusive evidence that this medication has been of value in either of these conditions. Moreover, as stated, there is uncertainty as to the effects on the fetus from any of the steroids, whether progestational or estrogenic, and therefore it is no longer recommended.

d. If one wishes to employ pure (nonsynthetic) progesterone, one of the few modes is by vaginal suppositories. Unfortunately, the product is not commercially available as such and must be specially made up by using progesterone powder with polyethylene glycol to give a concentration of 25 mg. per suppository. This is not only cumbersome to prepare but equally cumbersome to use, since it must be administered either as vaginal or rectal suppositories (25 mg. each) and used twice daily after ovulation until a period begins.

Parenteral Provera (Depo-Provera)

This is chiefly used in patients in whom prolonged and absolute gonadal inhibition is desired, such as in patients with sexual precocity. It should never be used in patients in whom reproduction or prompt return of menstrual function is desired, since its effects in inhibiting ovulation and menstruation may be very long lasting, even after discontinuing usage.

Norethindrone Acetate (Norlutate)

This compound is very useful in the immediate control of menorrhagia if organic causes have been ruled out (by D and C), or in the control of very heavy bleeding while awaiting other tests or procedures such as a D and C. An initial dose of 3 to 4 tablets (each 5 mg.) will usually stop bleeding within a few hours, and then the dosage can be maintained at 10 to 15 mg. daily cyclically, for functional bleeding, or until definitive diagnostic tests are carried out. Since the compound has both androgenic and progestational effects, it has a twofold effect in producing both hemostasis (androgens) and secretory alteration (progrestin).

Norethynodrel (Enovid)

1. This compound contains norethynodrel in varying dosage (2.5 mg. in Enovid-E) plus mestranol 0.1 mg. It is one of the common drugs of choice in the treatment of endometriosis, to produce a pseudopregnancy. The dosage is gradually increased to prevent both menstruation and breakthrough bleeding.

2. As one of many oral contraceptives currently available, this falls under the heading of all other oral contraceptives in that contraindications must be observed and all the potential hazards and side effects should be explained to the patient beforehand.

25. Family Planning

Hugh R. K. Barber, M.D.

The purpose of family planning is to assist individuals in achieving their reproductive goals. Family planning is population control reduced to the individual rather than to the national or global level.

BASIC PRINCIPLES

1. Demographers report that the low reproduction rate and the inordinately high death rate of the human allowed for a stable population from the beginning of time until about 1850 when the first billion population was reached.

a. From 1850, the world population has taken an incredibly sharp rise upward.

b. By 1930, in slightly less than 100 years, the population had doubled to 2 billion, largely due to the falling death rate and lowered infant mortality. Modern medicine and advances in nutrition have cut the death rates throughout the world, producing a fantastic population growth rate. Death rates for both children and adults have fallen sharply in recent years due, in some part, to successful assistance in combating such ancient killers as malaria, cholera, typhus, typhoid, and smallpox.

c. By 1960, less than half the previous time, another billion had been added. The current rate of population growth is 2 percent per year or 76 million per year. In the developing countries, where the population is increasing most dramatically, food production is rising at an average rate of 2.7 percent annually. But the present minimum food demand considered sufficient to supply adequate diets is increasing at an even faster rate—4 per cent annually. If this gap is not closed through increased food production and decreased population growth, the great majority of people will be undernourished and unschooled, economically unproductive and living in hovels.

d. Among low income, poorly educated parents surveyed, 56 per cent of their children were unplanned and 31 per cent were unwanted.

e. Over one-seventh of all children in the United States under 18 (15 per cent) are reared in proverty. Over one-fifth of the children with 5 or more children in the family (21 per cent) are being reared in poverty. Among whites, about one-ninth of all children (11 per cent) and over one-seventh of children in families with 5 or more children (15 per cent) are reared in poverty. Among blacks, over 40 per cent of all children and 44 per cent of children in families with 5 or more children are being reared in poverty.

f. It is estimated by 2000 the number could reach 7 billion (highly theoretical) people (twice the world's population today).

g. Successful planned population control or some unforeseen catastrophe could change this trend.

2. Demographers agree that the responsible parent today should plan a family of two or not more than three children, in an effort to replace, but not increase the world population.

3. Acceptance of family planning must be voluntary. Motivation will determine who will participate.

4. It has been calculated that a single exposure, at any time of the menstrual cycle, regardless of cycle regularity, carries a pregnancy risk of 2 to 4 per cent, while one episode of intercourse every five days yields a 20 per cent chance of conception in one cycle.

5. Methodology determines how. The patient's method of choice should be prescribed unless there are medical contraindications.

6. Counseling allows the contraceptive user to make and implement an informed choice. It is the most important factor influencing correct usage of the chosen method, as well as assuring good continuation rates.

7. The moral and ethical values of the patient must be respected and counseling carried out within the framework of those views.

8. Once an option has been selected, a complete physicial examination, including a pelvic examination and appropriate laboratory testing, should be carried out.

9. Follow-up visits should be outlined.

METHODOLOGY

Abstinence

1. Couples should be queried about their moral and ethical views concerning sexual practices.

2. It is important to counsel them on alternate methods of sexual fulfillment other than sexual intercourse. It is rare that this relationship will exist but it must be dealt with when it does.

3. If they elect to use contraception at a later date the couple should be counselled that it will be available to them.

Coitus Interruptus (Withdrawal)

1. The husband withdraws his penis just prior to ejaculation.

2. It is widely practiced and is probably the most commonly used contraceptive method in Europe.

3. To be successful, the man must have good self-control and be highly motivated, with a strong sense of responsibility to protect his sexual partner.

4. It is completely unsatisfactory for men with premature or early ejaculation. It is estimated that 50 per cent of all males would not be able to use this method due to an inability to control ejaculation.

5. The failure rate is approximately 15 to 25 pregnancies per 100 woman-years in all users.

6. It has no medical side effects, no cost is involved, and it is always available.

7. Since withdrawal at the time of ejaculation is unnatural, it may diminish the sexual satisfaction of the couple.

Rhythm Method (Safe Period)

1. Is based on three concepts:

a. The fertilizable life span of an oocyte is not over 24 hours after ovulation.

b. Sperm survival in the female genital tract is not over 4 days.

c. Ovulation which determines the rhythm of a cycle occurs 14 days before the menstrual flow.

2. This means the avoidance of coitus around the time of ovulation. The woman must take her temperature every morning, watching for the drop in temperature followed by a sustained rise which indicates ovulation.

3. Once the normal rhythm has been established, the woman may assume that ovulation occurs between day 12 and 14. Another day is added to allow for ovum survival, and as sperm may live for at least 3 days, coitus must be avoided from the ninth to the eighteenth day, and the seventh to twentieth day would be safer.

4. Even this semi-celibacy is unreliable because it depends too much on regularity of ovulation.

5. Failure rate is 38 per hundred woman-years of use.

Sheath (Condom, "French Letter")

1. A thin rubber sheath or a lamb's cecum is placed over the erect penis.
2. Is probably the most widely used mechanical contraceptive in the world.
3. The precautions that must be practiced with its use are:
   a. To leave a dead space in the condom from which air has been expelled to receive the ejaculate (some have a built-in receptacle)
   b. To use proper lubrication, if necessary (some are prelubricated)
   c. To effect withdrawal before cessation of the erection
   d. To grasp the ring of the sheath at the time of withdrawal to prevent it from slipping off.
4. It protects both against pregnancy and venereal disease. Therefore, it is most useful in casual intercourse.
5. In men with premature ejaculation, the condom may blunt the sensation sufficiently to prolong the intercourse time.
6. It may interfere with sensation. In older men who have difficulty in achieving full erection, it is impossible to use.
7. It may interrupt the mood, for application of the condom requires an erect penis.
8. Instruction of the partners in effective use can be aided by advising the female to apply the condom at the time of foreplay, which may offset the reduced sexual pleasure some couples say they experience.
9. It is not satisfactory in hot climates because of the deterioration of rubber.
10. The failure rate is 18 to 20 per hundred woman-years of use. The failure is due in most instances to rupture of the condom with the deposition of the entire ejaculate into the vagina.
11. The "morning-after pill" which is a high dose of estrogen for 5 days usually prevents pregnancy.

The Vaginal Diaphragm ("Dutch Cap")

1. This is a rubber diaphragm which when smeared with spermicidal cream will prevent sperms from reaching the cervical canal.
2. It must fit snugly behind the pubic bone and over the cervix into the posterior fornix.
3. The diaphragm should not be removed until at least 8 hours after the last intercourse.
4. In the early days of marriage the most satisfactory method for using a diaphragm is to insert it each night with jelly or cream before retiring and to remove it, cleanse it, and reinsert it with jelly the following evening.
5. The failure rate is 15 pregnancies per hundred woman-years of use.

Chemical Methods (Aerosol, Foams, Jellies, Creams, and Suppositories)

1. The spermicidical ingredient used is usually p-triisoprophylphenolopolyetoxy-ethanol.
2. The aerosol and jells are effective immediately, whereas the tablets require from 5 to 10 minutes to dissolve before effectiveness.
3. The advantage is that they are inexpensive, easy to use, and require no instruction.
4. The disadvantage is that the woman or man may experience local irritation from them.
5. The failure rate is between 15 and 40 per hundred woman-years of use.

Intrauterine Devices (IUD)

1. A polyethylene spiral or coil is inserted into the uterine cavity and effectively prevents conception although the mode of action is not known.
2. Ovulation is not prevented and no recognizable characteristic changes occur in the endometrium.
3. The great advantage of this method is the lack of necessity for high motivation. Once it is in place no further action is needed by the patient.
4. It should be placed in the uterus at the time of menstruation by an experienced gynecologist.

5. The disadvantages of this method are the menstrual complications which occur, i.e., excessive, profuse periods, irregular bleeding between periods, and abdominal cramps.

6. Major complications include pelvic infection, perforation, and pregnancy.

7. Medicated IUDs (those containing copper or progesterone) appear to have increased effectiveness when compared to inert plastic devices.

8. The copper IUD has two disadvantages: first, the introduction into the system of copper, a potentially toxic metal; second, the necessity for removal and reinsertion every 2 years.

9. If pregnancy occurs with an IUD in place, its removal will reduce spontaneous abortion from a rate of about 50 per cent to approximately 25 per cent.

10. Removal, if there is a pregnancy, reduces the likelihood of septic abortion.

11. If a pregnancy occurs, there is a relatively greater chance that it will be an ectopic pregnancy.

12. The failure rate is 2.3 per hundred woman-years of use.

Oral Contraception (OC)

1. These drugs are taken by mouth and permit the patient to indulge in normal coitus without the risk of conception.

2. The efficacy of the pill in preventing pregnancy is the greatest of any form of contraception short of permanent sterilization.

3. The oral contraceptives are efficacious in preventing pregnancy primarily by inhibiting the midcycle release of luteinizing hormone (LH) and therefore blocking ovulation.

4. Other changes contributing to preventing pregnancy are:

a. Changes in tubal transport

b. The nature of the endometrium and cervical mucus

5. The combination pill contains either mestranol or ethinyl estradiol and the progestin is usually norethynodrel or norethindrone.

6. The sequential-type of oral contraceptives have been removed from the market.

7. The complications reported are:

a. Thrombophlebitis

b. Cancer of the endometrium

c. Hypertension

d. Postpill amenorrhea

e. Emotional lability and depression

f. Myocardial infarction

g. Cerebral infarction

h. Gallbladder disease and benign and malignant hepatomas

8. The failure rate is less than one pregnancy per hundred years of use in combination method.

Sterilization

1. Surgical

a. This in practice means permanent interruption of the fallopian tubes.

b. Laparoscopy, laparotomy, and mini-laparotomy are used to produce sterilization in the female.

c. Most of the laparoscopic sterilizations use the standard electrocoagulation method. Although rare, bowel burn is one of the complications of this technique.

d. Nonelastic techniques include the clip or the band. The results are comparable to those with electrocoagulation.

e. The mini-laparotomy has become popular and can be carried out under local anesthesia.

f. The techniques are:

(1) Pomeroy subtotal bilateral salpingectomy (most frequently used)

(2) Madlener requires no cutting but is less reliable.

(3) Irving—at the time of Cesarean section the tubal stump is buried in the uterine musculature.

(4) Cornual resection for interim, nonpregnant uteri

(5) Aldridge—reversible sterilization, buries the fimbriated ends between the leaves of the broad ligament

g. Hysterectomy is usually reserved for the patient with concurrent uterine or pelvic disease.

h. The only certain method of surgical sterilization is to remove the ovaries.

2. Surgical Sterilization of the Male

a. Vasectomy is the only popular method of male sterilization.

b. There are few immediate contraindications. These are local infection and bleeding disorders.

c. Sperm-agglutinating antibodies can be found in the serum of over half the men undergoing vasectomy, although the titer decreases with time.

d. More serious autoantibodies may form and in extremely rare cases have produced a clinical disorder with autoimmune characteristics.

e. There is about 0.4 per cent failure rate.

f. The advantages of vasectomy over surgical methods of sterilization in the female are simplicity, safety, low cost, and high effectiveness.

Estrogens and Postcoital Contraception

1. It has been estimated that approximately 60 per cent of first sexual exposures among young, unmarried women on university campuses are unprotected, while 40 per cent of subsequent intercourse is insufficiently protected.

2. The need for some form of postcoital contraception clearly exists; the only alternatives at present are endometrial aspiration, menstrual extraction, and abortion. They are costly, have side effects, and are inconvenient.

3. The postcoital contraception (PCE) has been defined as the pharmacological inhibition of implantation after unprotected intercourse. The term *interceptives* has been used to describe the use of estrogens as a method of preventing pregnancy after intercourse.

4. Diethylstilbestrol (DES), 50 mg., ethinyl estradiol, 5 mg., or conjugated estrogens, 30 mg., will be effective if given within 72 hours of the unprotected midcycle (ovulatory) exposure and continued for 5 days.

5. The preparations are potent and have side effects that contraindicate their use. Women suffering from thrombophlebitis, hypertension, cerebrovascular accident, epilepsy, migraine, and chronic liver and renal disease should not receive estrogen as a postcoital contraception.

6. For those receiving estrogen as PCE if pregnancy occurs, abortion should be recommended because of the potentially teratogenic and carcinogenic effects reported in the offspring of mothers treated during pregnancy.

7. Since ectopic pregnancy has been reported following the use of PCE, great care must be taken when evaluating a patient complaining of abdominal pain and who is known to have been exposed to high-dose estrogen therapy.

8. It is recommended that a signed and witnessed informed consent be obtained. It should outline the known risks and limitations of high-dose estrogen therapy as well as the alternatives to treatment.

9. It must be emphasized that the use of high-dose estrogen is not a casual matter, that close observation is necessary and that her medical care is not complete until after the 6-week examination. Patients should be advised against having unprotected intercourse during or subsequent to treatment.

26. Cytology

Hugh R. K. Barber, M.D.

Cytology probably makes its greatest contribution as a screening method for the detection of cancer of the cervix in women. It is also used as a diagnostic method in detecting cancer in other organ systems. In addition, it has been employed as an index of hormonal levels.

Cytologic screening of women for cancer of the vagina, cervix, and endometrium may represent the most important advance in gynecology in this century. The technique was perfected by Dr. George N. Papanicolaou and is known as the Pap test or Pap smear.

It is estimated that two or three (some report five to seven) unsuspected cases of cervical cancer per thousand women are usually found by this method.

BASIC PRINCIPLES

1. Due to the action of estrogen and progesterone, cyclical changes occur in the vaginal mucosa which can be identified by examining a stained smear. Such smears can to some extent be used as a rough guide to the hormonal status of the patient. The phases are:

a. *Postmenstrual.* The cells are mainly of precornified type and by Papanicolaou's stain the cytoplasm is stained blue-green.

b. *Proliferative.* The rising titer of estrogen increases cornification and causes glycogen to appear in the cells. Brown deposits of glycogen appear in the pink cytoplasm. The nuclei are small and pyknotic.

c. *Secretory.* The cornified cells diminish in number. Precornified cells with folded edges make their appearance and many polymorphs are seen.

d. *Premenstrual-menstrual.* The cells are clumped and degenerate. Debris and leukocytes are present giving a "dirty" appearance to the smear.

2. Cells collected for hormonal evaluation should be taken from the anterior-lateral fornix.

3. Cytohormonal evaluation involves interpreting the intricate pattern resulting from epithelial maturation, secretory activity, cellular membrane status, inflammatory response, and many other features under endocrine influence.

4. The state of maturation which the cells of the vaginal epithelium attain at the time of their exfoliation yields the most objective and reliable information and accurately expresses this maturation.

5. The maturation index (MI) expresses the level of cellular maturation attained at the time of exfoliation, is expressed as a ratio of the precentages present of parabasal, intermediate, and superficial cells in that order. 0/55/45 represents the maturation index (MI) of a patient exfoliating no parabasal cells, 55 per cent intermediate cells, and 45 per cent superficial cells which accurately reflect their ratio on the surface of her vaginal epithelium.

6. There will be 20,000 new cases of invasive cancer of the cervix with 7,700 deaths this year. There has been a decrease in incidence of cervical cancer in the last 40 years. One of the main reasons for the relative decrease in the incidence of invasive carcinoma of the cer-

The normal cytohormonal patterns of the endocrine periods are:

Childhood—50/50/0
Perimenarchal—45/45/10
Reproductive period ovulation—0/40/60 to menstruation 0/70/33
Pregnancy—0/95/5
Postpartum—100/0/0
Postmenopausal—0/100/0 or 100/0/0
Atrophic pattern—100/0/0 followed by estrogen therapy will approach 0/50/50
Progestogens—0/100/0
Androgens—100/0/0
Cortisone—0/100/0
Ovarian granulosa-cell tumors that produce estrogen produces a shift to the right—0/0/100
Vaginal inflammation—31/35/34
Turner's syndrome—0/100/0 which may shift with age to 100/0/0
Symmond's disease—100/0/0

vix is the fact that so many lesions were discovered by exfoliative cytology before invasion.

7. Exfoliative cytology (Pap test) is primarily a screening test. Obvious lesions must be biopsied.

8. If the smears are properly taken and adequately interpreted, exfoliative cytology is accurate more than 95 per cent of the time in cases of carcinoma of the cervix.

9. On one smear there is a false-negative rate ranging up to 20 per cent. Therefore, it is important to have cytologic examinations at stated intervals.

10. The false-positive diagnosis, i.e., the presence of cells interpreted as malignant in the absence of histologic confirmation, is more frequent than the false-negative. The consequences of a false-positive result, however, are not as grave as those of a false-negative.

11. The presence of endometrial cells detected on a routine Pap smear demands reevaluation and an endometrial aspiration.

12. The routine Pap smear is not adequate to screen the endometrium. Cervical scraping would give a low yield of positive cytology for endometrial cancer. The average return would be about 50 per cent, the posterior fornix would be about 65 per cent, endocervical aspiration about 75 per cent, but with the jet washer or a similar method or the Novak suction curettage, the accuracy of diagnosis should exceed 90 per cent.

13. Collection of specimens for screening the cervix may include swabbing, scraping, or aspiration of the cervical canal. A combination gives a higher yield.

COLLECTION OF A PAP TEST SPECIMEN

1. Lubricant should not be used on the glove or speculum.

2. With the cervix visualized, a cotton-tipped applicator moistened with saline is introduced into the external cervical os and twisted. The cellular specimen is deposited on the slide by rolling but not rubbing the applicator tip against the glass surface. Rubbing may streak or break the cells.

3. The external os should be scraped with a wooden or plastic spatula. The end that is shaped to conform to the cervix is inserted in the external os. The spatula is rotated clockwise while moderate pressure is exerted on the edge in contact with the cervix. The sample is deposited on the slide by passing the tip of the spatula and its slanted edges slowly and firmly against the surface of the glass.

4. Some prefer to aspirate the cervical canal. The tip of a glass or plastic cannula with an attached rubber bulb is introduced into the cervical canal and the contents of the canal are aspirated. The fluid from the syringe is emptied onto the slide. It serves the same purpose as cervical scraping or swabbing, i.e., detection of cervical carcinoma.

5. The advantage of aspiration over

the others is debatable. A combination of aspiration and scraping enhances the sensitivity of the cytologic test for cancer detection.

6. Cytologic examination of the vaginal pool is the least reliable of the various methods used to detect cervical cancer. It usually contains a small amount of material and there is poor preservation of the representative cells.

7. The laboratory request slip, in addition to the usual identifying data, should include the following information:

a. Last menstrual period

b. Pregnancy, if present

c. Use of oral contraceptives and intrauterine devices

d. History of hormonal imbalance or dysfunction

e. Current diagnosis

f. Previous surgery, patricularly cervical surgery, i.e., conization, biopsy, etc.

g. Radiation therapy, and if so, the time of the last treatment

h. History of previous cancer

REPORTING RESULTS

1. The cytologic diagnosis may be reported using a numerical classification system, a narrative description, or both.

2. The numerical classification introduces a great deal of subjective interpretation. Therefore, many laboratories report the results as positive, negative, or borderline.

3. A numerical classification based on Papanicolaou's original five-class system or its modification is most often used to report results. Papanicolaou's classification is:

a. *Class I—Negative.* Only normal cells are present.

b. *Class II—Negative.* There are no signs of malignancy; some atypical cells are present.

c. *Class III—Doubtful.* The smear contains cells with atypical features suggestive but not diagnostic of malignancy.

d. *Class IV—Positive.* Isolated atypical cells are present.

e. *Class V—Positive.* Numerous atypical cells or cell groups are present.

ENDOMETRIAL SCREENING

1. The routine cervical-vaginal smear is less effective for detection of endometrial cancer than of cervical malignancy.

2. Screening methods employing cytology to detect endometrial abnormalities have been elusive.

3. Screening programs by cytology carried out to identify early changes in cervical abnormalities have not yielded the same results in picking up patients with early changes in the endometrium that will be at risk. The pickup rate on routine screening for the asymptomatic patient is only about 3 per cent or less of all endometrial cancers.

4. Negative cytology does not have the same accuracy in prognosticating that the development of cancer is highly unlikely, because on cytologic evaluation the preinvasive lesions are not diagnosed with the same accuracy as is obtained in cancer of the cervix.

5. It is unlikely that screening programs directed at detecting cancer of the endometrium will have a major impact on morbidity and mortality rates in the foreseeable future.

6. The cytologist can diagnose the benign or malignant endometrium with a high degree of accuracy but has trouble detecting the in-between groups with adenomatous hyperplasia, dysplasia, or cancer in situ.

7. Endometrial hyperplasia develops into endometrial cancer in only 1.5 per cent of patients. Endometrial cancer patients do not have a higher than normal

estrogen titer; therefore, there must be factors other than simple prolonged estrogen stimulation at work.

8. The most optimistic detection rate is 75 per cent.

9. A vaginal smear taken from the pool of secretion in the posterior fornix gives a relatively better chance of detection of endometrial cancer.

10. When screening for endometrial cancer, uterine aspiration or washing should be added to the routine Pap smear.

11. The rate of positive returns in asymptomatic women is low and the discomfort is significant.

12. In women who have symptoms of endometrial cancer or even if there is significant suspicion, a fractional curettage is indicated.

27. Basic and Clinical Immunology

Hugh R. K. Barber, M.D.

INTRODUCTION

1. Immunology is a relatively new discipline of medicine. Immunity has been recognized for centuries and has been termed the study of resistance to infection. However, it has now taken on an expanded role and is the property whereby the lymphoreticular system makes a memorized response to an antigenic stimulus. This may result in a state of positive reaction known as sensitization or a negative reaction known as immunologic tolerance, enhancement, or immunosuppression.

2. As a scientific discipline, *immunology* encompases immunity, dealing with the adaptive response to infective agents, *immunochemistry*, concerned with the chemical nature of antigens and antibodies; *immunobiology,* which deals with the activity of the cells of the immune system and their relationship to each other and their environment. As a biologic science, immunology includes developmental biology, genetics, biochemistry, microbiology, anatomy, and medicine. These basic concepts are fundamental for an understanding of the principles and practice of modern medicine.

3. Currently immunology and immunotherapy have contributed little to the individual treatment of a patient. However, there is great promise for the future use of the principles of immunology in clinical medicine. Therefore, a summary of the basic principles is included. On the other hand, immunology has played a key role in laboratory diagnoses. The following tests are listed—precipitation, immunodiffusion or gel diffusion test, immunoelectrophoresis, agglutination, mixed hemoadsorption, Coombs, Australian SH, complement fixation, fluorescent antibody, cytotoxic colony inhibition, migration inhibition, mixed lymphocyte culture, and radioimmunoassay tests—as those widely employed in clinical medicine.

BASIC PRINCIPLES

1. The cellular events in an immune response are fundamental in understanding the basic mechanisms relative to the development of both cell-mediated and humoral immunity.

2. The macrophage represents the keystone in the development of an immune response. The macrophage in blood is called a monocyte; in connective tissue is a histiocyte; and in the spleen, lymph nodes, and thymus is called a sinus-lining macrophage or a reticulum cell. The macrophage has a wide distribution.

3. The antigen, and more correctly, the immunogen (any substance foreign to the host), is processed by the macrophage if an immune response is to occur. The antigen is now a processed antigen.

4. Following contact of the antigen with the macrophage, the latter sends out a message in the form of an RNA or RNA-antigen complex. The uncommitted lymphocytes are transformed into lymphoblasts.

5. The transformed blast (lymphoblast) gives rise to sensitized lymphocytes as well as plasma cells.

6. The plasma cells (B cells) in turn produce a variety of immunoglobulins; five have been identified, i.e., IgM, IgG, IgE, IgA, and IgD.

7. The sensitized lymphocytes (T cells) proliferate into the so-called killer lymphocytes that have the ability to destroy cancer cells and produce lymphokines and delayed hypersensitivity.

8. The B cell must receive a stimulus from the antigen, plus one from the antigenically stimulated T cell, if it is to mature into a plasmocyte.

9. This helper function of the T cell appears to depend in a large measure on the T and B cells sharing certain products of the major histocompatibility locus.

10. When the sensitized lymphocyte comes in contact with the antigen that sensitized it, the lymphocyte is stimulated to form an immunoblast which produces at least four mediators of cellular immunity, including transfer factor (TF), lymphoctye-transforming activity (LTA), migration inhibition factor (MIF), lymphotoxin (LT), and interferon.

DEVELOPMENT OF B AND T CELLS

1. Pluripotent stem cell gives rise to a variety of cells but only two will be described. They are distinct cell types clearly separable from one another in the process of differentiation. Pluripotent cells differentiate into the precursor stem cells of all of the major hematopoietic elements.

2. Lymphoid stem cells can function as prethymic cells and are processed in the thymus under the influence of thymosin (thymopoietin) to differentiate into T cells.

3. Lymphoid precursor cells are processed by an alternate pathway in a poorly defined organ in man, but have been extensively studied in birds (in the bursa of Fabricius), in some mammals (in the fetal liver, probably under the influence of another hormone-like substance, "bursin"), and they differentiate into B cells.

4. A subpopulation of thymus-independent lymphocytes (B cells) has been detected which mediates cytotoxic reactions on antibody-coated target cells in the absence of complement and are called K cells. Sometimes they are referred to as null cells because they lack the markers characteristic of T or B cells.

5. In addition to the above three classes of lymphocytes, there is another population of circulating lymphocytes that has the chracteristics of both T and B lymphocytes. These double (D) cells represent 2 to 3 per cent of circulating lymphoid population. Their origin, function, and role in tumor immunology remain undetermined.

HUMORAL AND CELL-MEDIATED IMMUNE RESPONSES

The immune response takes two forms: A humoral response results from the transformed lymphoblast being converted to a plasma cell. It is a cell-free fluid containing antibodies which are circulating freely in the blood stream as well as other body fluids. Also, a cell-mediated immunity is carried out by sensitized lymphocytes.

The Humoral Response

1. The humoral response (B cell) is mediated by immunoglobulins.

2. It is cell-free and is made up of the immunoglobulins IgG, IgM, IgA, IgD, and IgE.

3. The cell-free antibody to have a killing or cytotoxic effect must always have a third substance, complement, present.

4. Without complement, an antibody can bind to an antigen on a cell surface but cannot damage or kill the cell.

5. The humoral response offers a de-

fense against most bacteria and some foreign proteins.

6. Bacterial vaccines inoculated into the organism result in the production of antibodies (immunoglobulins).

7. The humoral response includes B cells, K cells, and D cells.

The Cell-Mediated Response

1. The cell-mediated response (T cell) is mediated by sensitized lymphocytes.

2. In the cell-mediated immune (CMI) response, the antibody remains an integral part of the cells that produced it and is a cell-associated antibody.

3. Sensitized lymphocytes carrying such antibody are carried in the lymph to tumor cells, where their antibody combines with the antigen determinant on the surface of the tumor cell.

4. The cell-bound antibody then becomes capable of rupturing and killing tumor cells. It also produces potent mediators of cellular immunity, including transfer factor (TF), lymphocyte-transforming activity (LTA), lymphocyte blastogenic factor, migration inhibition factor (MIF), lymphotoxin (LT), and interferon.

5. The cell-mediated response is particularly important in graft rejection, eliminating viruses as well as intracellular bacteria and cancer cells.

IMMUNODEFICIENCY: NATURE'S EXPERIMENT TO DEMONSTRATE THE DIFFERENCE BETWEEN HUMORAL AND CELL-MEDIATED IMMUNITY

Any deviation in nature supplies valuable material for studying normal mechanisms. Nature has supplied such an experiment to study the role of the humoral and cell-mediated response.

Deficiency of Cell-Mediated Immunity (T Cell)

1. In the DiGeorge syndrome, there is dysplasia or hypoplasia of the thymus and often absence of the parathyroid glands.

a. The patient has no resistance to viruses or to other agents that are controlled by cell-mediated immunity such as tuberculosis, brucellosis, leprosy, fungi, and parasitic diseases.

b. They do not have the immunologic capacity to develop a delayed hypersensitivity reaction or to reject grafts of foreign tissue.

c. They can produce circulating antibodies and have the ability to respond to bacterial vaccines by developing circulating antibodies (immunoglobulins).

d. Research programs have been structured to implant embryonic thymus glands with some success.

Deficiency of Humoral Immunity (B Cell)

1. In the Bruton type of agammaglobulinemia, there is a deficiency of immunoglobulin synthesis.

2. IgG is decreased tenfold and IgA and IgM about a hundredfold.

3. These patients do not have natural circulating immunoglobulins and are susceptible to bacterial infections.

4. They do not respond to bacterial vaccines by producing an increased antibody titer (immunoglobulins).

5. The cell-mediated immune mechanism functions normally and they have the capacity to reject tissue or organ grafts and exhibit delayed hypersensitivity to the tuberculin skin tests.

6. Treatment with gamma globulin has served to help these patients resist bacterial infections.

Combined Deficiency of T and B Cells

1. In "Swiss type agammaglobulinemia," which is an X-linked disease of male children, both cell-mediated and humoral mechanisms are deficient.

2. There is a block of the stem cell mechanism. These children cannot make humoral antibodies (immunoglobulins)

or develop cell-mediated immune reactions.

3. They suffer from progressive bacterial and/or viral infections and die within the first two years of life.

4. Some highly selected patients have been treated with bone marrow that has been matched for major histocompatible antigens. The preliminary work has been promising and some success has been reported.

Other Immunodeficiencies

1. Currently, more than 30 phenotype patterns of immunodeficiency have been recognized in human beings.

2. In addition to T, B, and stem defects, other immunodeficiencies have been recorded.

3. The patient's phagocytic system may not function to adequately ingest and kill bacteria and fungi. Absence or malfunction of the complement system which normally aids in bacterial killing may give rise to serious illness.

4. Other significant immunodeficient states are hereditary ataxia telangiectasia, Wiskott-Aldrich syndrome, Chédiak-Higashi syndrome, selective IgA (immunoglobulin A) deficiency disorders, Good's syndrome, and chronic mucocutaneous candidiasis (moniliasis).

AUTOIMMUNE DISORDERS

Introduction

Clinical and experimental observations show that individuals can sometimes respond immunologically to certain of their own antigens (self-antigens). These important exceptions to the principle of self-tolerance help to analyze the fundamental mechanisms, and they are frequently associated with disease. It is often not clear, however, whether these anomalous responses cause, or are the result of, disease; hence, it is necessary to emphasize the distinction between an autoimmune response, in which an individual makes antibodies or becomes allergic to self-antigen, and an autoimmune disease, which is a pathological condition arising from an autoimmune response. Autoimmune reactions can be both antibody and cell-mediated. There is a great overlap between immunological deficiency diseases and autoimmunity.

Basic Mechanisms

1. Autoimmunity may arise whenever there exists a state of immunologic imbalance in which B-cell activity is excessive and suppressor T-cell activity is diminished.

2. This imbalance occurs as a consequence of genetic, viral, and environmental mechanisms acting singly or in combination.

3. A central mechanism in this concept involves a disturbance of the delicate balance between suppressor and helper activity of regulatory T cells.

4. Either an excess of helper-T activity or a deficiency of suppressor-T activity could lead to the development of autoimmunity.

5. The mechanisms by which such a balance may be upset are complex but may involve both viral factors and the abnormal production of thymic hormones.

6. The B cell has several different membrane receptors on its surface. There are immunoglobulin receptors for antigen and receptors for helper-T and suppressor-T cells.

7. The balance of the T-regulatory signals (helper T and suppressor T) arriving at the cell surface of the B cell would determine whether the B lymphocytes remain inactive or whether it goes into active synthesis and proliferation.

8. If the B lymphocyte represents a clone with the potential for producing an autoantibody, then this balance of sig-

nals would determine whether or not autoimmunity appears.

9. Three general autoimmune diseases are: acquired (autoimmune) hemolytic anemia (AHA), systemic lupus erythematosus (SLE), and rheumatoid arthritis (RA).

HYPERSENSITIVITY

Definition

1. Hypersensitivity is a state of the previously immunized (to alter the reactivity of a host to an antigen by exposing it to that antigen in such a way that it produces an immune response) host which results in tissue damage from an immune reaction to a further dose of antigen.

2. Hypersensitivity reactions may be antibody- or humoral-mediated as in immediate hypersensitivity, or they may be a reaction of cell-mediated immunity as in delayed hypersensitivity.

3. The term hypersensitivity implies a heightened reactivity to an antigen, but it is difficult to define all hypersensitivity reactions, particularly cell-mediated reactions, in such terms.

4. The hypersensitivity reactions have been classified into four types.

a. The first three develop as immediate reactions and are humorally mediated (type 1, anaphylactic reactions; type 2, cytolytic or cytotoxic reactions; and type 3, toxic-complex syndromes).

b. Although they are classified as immediate reactions, this may not be absolutely so.

c. Cytotoxic reactions may be delayed for hours and in the toxic-complex syndrome, serum sickness may develop after days or even weeks.

d. The humoral hypersensitivity reactions often dovetail in their responses and effects.

e. The fourth type is cell-mediated and is termed delayed hypersensitivity.

Basic Mechanisms

1. Type 1

a. Anaphylaxis occurs when the immunoglobulins of the IgE class interact with antigen, thereby causing the release of vasoactive substances which induce an immediate inflammatory response.

b. Examples: asthma, hayfever

2. Type 2

a. Cytotoxic hypersensitivity results when antibodies bind to self-antigens and destroy the host cells.

b. Examples: blood transfusion reactions, hemolytic disease of the newborn

3. Type 3

a. Immune complex hypersensitivity occurs when antigen-antibody complexes are deposited at tissue sites and a subsequent destructive inflammatory response ensues.

b. A local version of immune complex hypersensitivity in which inflammation occurs 3 to 8 hours after cutaneous administration of antigen is termed an Arthus reaction.

c. A generalized inflammatory reaction characterized by inflammation of blood vessels, joints, and kidney resulting from the formation of circulating antigen-antibody complexes, is termed serum sickness.

4. Type 4

a. Delayed hypersensitivity is an immunologic process. It is an acquired and transferable capacity which exhibits memory and specificity for the antigen. A sensitized lymphocyte reacts with specific antigens and releases lymphokines.

b. Thus delayed hypersensitivity, a form of cell-mediated immunity, differs from immediate hypersensitivity, which is mediated by antibodies.

c. Examples: contact dermatitis, tuberculin reaction, skin and allograft rejection

THE IMMUNE DEFENSE SYSTEM

The logical question is, if tumor cells possess antigens on their surface capable of stimulating a specific immune response, why does cancer continue to grow in the presence of a mechanism designated to control its growth? The explanation may be that the rate of growth exceeds the capacity of the immune response. However, from studies in animals, more specific reasons are known for the failure of the immune response to prevent the start and growth of cancer.

FAILURE OF THE IMMUNE RESPONSE

Immunosuppression

1. Many factors contribute to this. Among these factors are aging, the cancer itself, anticancer drug therapy, radiation therapy, genetic defects, neonatal thymectomy. To a lesser extent, antibiotics, anesthetics, analgesics, and hypnotics contribute to immunosuppression.
2. In reality, it is often difficult to separate the contributions of drugs and disease in bringing about this state of immunosuppression.
3. Removal of a bulk of tumor reduces the immunosuppression of the host.

Immunological Tolerance

1. In a broad sense, this represents a form of immunosuppression.
2. It can occur with exposure to an antigen during embryonic or early neonatal life before the immune system has matured. The latter then fails to recognize the antigen as nonself and is incapable of mounting an immune response.
3. Since cancer is considered to arise from a single cell clone, the tolerance theory for progress of cancer is often suggested as an explanation. Choriocarcinoma has been advanced as a prototype for this theory.
4. The host is not immunologically tolerant in general but only for that specific tumor antigen.

Acquired Tolerance

1. Was formerly called immune paralysis.
2. It is induced by injecting very small or very large doses of antigen and persists as long as that antigen remains in the body.
3. In clinical practice, acquired tolerance or immune paralysis may suppress the immune response of the host in the presence of a large tumor.
4. Following removal of the tumor mass, the host exhibits resistance to the reimplantation of that tumor.
5. The conclusion is that there was not an intrinsic failure of the immune response but that it was overwhelmed by the volume of tumor.
6. Removal of the tumor or debulking the tumor may restore the integrity of the immune response.

Immunological Enhancement

1. This results in an increased growth of the tumor in animals.
2. Animals transplanted with grafts of foreign cancer cells and then injected with antiserum against that cancer often experienced a rapid growth of the cancer rather than the anticipated rejection of the tumor.
3. Obviously, the antibodies produced against the cancer and then injected into the host with the transplanted tumor were enhancing or blocking antibodies rather than cytotoxic antibodies.
4. These antibodies formed complexes with the antigens on the surface of the tumor and blocked the killer lymphocytes from attacking the tumor. The tumor was protected from destruction.
5. Indirectly immunological enhancement has been shown to play a role in the growth of choriocarcinoma.

6. Removal of a bulk of tumor such as ovarian cancer may suppress the enhancement phenomenon and permit the killer lymphocytes to successfully attack the tumor cells.

Immunoselection

1. Cancer develops from a clone of cells.
2. The cell has tumor antigens on the surface and as the tumor grows the cancer cells have the same surface antigens.
3. During the course of many generations mutations occur and some of the cells have a greater number of antigens present and therefore stimulate a greater antibody production.
4. The cells with a greater number of antigens produce a significant number of antibodies which help to eliminate the cells with a strong antigenic component.
5. The cells that remain are those with few antigens present and the result is a colony of cells with weak antigens followed by a relatively slow growth of tumor at first.
6. It is conceivable that this may lead to tolerance.
7. After a period of time the tumor cells develop autonomy and progressively greater invasive properties.

Antigen Modulation

1. This is temporary change in antigenicity reflecting an adaptational alteration in an entire population of cells.
2. It can be stated that as soon as antibody is produced, cancer cells of certain leukemias in animals cease synthesizing antigens.
3. As a result, the immunological defense becomes ineffective.
4. In humans, this response has not been documented.

Unknown Factors

1. The tumor-bearing host may possess factors that depress the immunological reactivity in a nonspecific way or possibly may lack factors that are important for such reactivity.
2. This has been suggested by the poor response that the tumor-bearing host develops when tested for delayed hypersensitivity to a variety of antigens.
3. In vitro studies in this group have also shown a decreased ability to transform lymphocytes after stimulation with phytohemagglutinin (PHA).

IMMUNOLOGIC TESTS

1. An antigen is a substance that binds to an antibody but does not always elicit an immune response. An immunogen is a molecule that has the ability to elicit an immune response. It should be noted that substances that are immunogenic are always antigenic, but substances that are antigenic are not necessarily immunogenic. Although not correct, the expressions are currently used interchangeably.
2. Antigens stimulate the production of immunoglobulins (antibodies). There are literally thousands of antigens, each capable of producing a specific antibody. The antigens may be potentially harmful, such as a virus or bacteria, or it may be an inert protein. The antibodies produced can only combine with the antigen that is identical to it or nearly so. The antigen binding site links up with the Fab fragment on the immunoglobulin to form a complex. The reaction forms the basis for the detection of antigen-antibody by various laboratory tests.

COMMON CLINICAL LABORATORY TESTS

Immunoelectrophoresis

1. Electrophoresis. The combining of electrophoresis with precipitation in agar is a simple but exceedingly powerful method for identifying antigens in complex mixtures.

2. Technique. A glass slide is covered with an agar gel buffered at pH 8.8. Serum is placed into a well cut in the agar. A direct current is applied across the field for 1 to 2 hours.

3. Differential Migration of the Serum Components. The albumin migrates toward the anode, but due to electroendosinosis, the IgG migrates towards the cathode in agar support medium. The different serum components are not normally visible in agar but will show up if suitably stained.

After electrophoresis is carried out for 1 or 2 hours, a trough is cut longitudinally in the agar and an antiserum against the electrophoresed antigen is placed in the trough. The two components diffuse toward each other, and precipitin bands form where the antigen and antibody meet at equivalence.

4. Uses. This is a very powerful analytic technique and can show up about 30 different components in human serum, as compared to four or five by electrophoresis.

Agglutination Test

1. Bacteria and other cells in suspension are usually clumped (agglutinated) when mixed with antisera prepared against them.

2. The antigen can be made part of some particulate material such as red cell, bacterium, or perhaps an inorganic particle such as polystyrene latex that has been coated with antigen. Antibody added to the suspension of such particles combines with surface antigens and links them together to form clearly visible aggregates or agglutinates.

3. This phenomenon is referred to as an agglutination reaction.

4. The steps of the agglutination test are outlined as follows:

a. The antigen is part of the surface of some particulate material (red cell, bacterium, or polystyrene latex).

b. Antibody is added to the suspension of such particles and links them together to form agglutinates.

c. The actual test is carried out by placing dilutions of the antiserum in round bottom wells.

d. Doubling dilutions of antiserum are made up in tubes (1:2, 1:4, 1:8, 1:16, 1:32, etc.).

e. Particulate antigen is added.

f. After incubation at 37°C, agglutinate is seen in the bottom of the tubes.

g. The last tube showing clearly visible agglutination is the end point of the test.

h. The reciprocal dilution of the antiserum at the end point is known as the titer of the antiserum.

i. This measures the number of antibody units per unit volume of serum.

5. Uses are listed below:

a. The agglutination tests are employed routinely in crossmatching of blood.

b. The Widal test is used for the demonstration of antibodies to salmonella in serum specimens in patients suspected of having enteric fever.

c. It is used as a thyroid antibody test using thyroglobulin-coated cells or latex particles.

d. Its principle is used in the hormone assay which employs an agglutination inhibition test as reactions for pregnancy.

e. It is the basis for a virus infection.

f. *The immunological pregnancy test* is carried out as follows:

(1) *Control*. Red cells coated with hormone (HCG) are mixed with an antihormone antibody. Agglutination results.

(2) *Testing for the Unknown*. Antihormone antibody is added to known hormone molecules (HCG). An antigen-antibody complex is formed. The antigen-binding sites are thus blocked. The addition of hormone-coated red cells does not result in agglutination (because

the antihormone antibody has already formed a complex with the hormone molecules in the urine or serum). There is agglutination inhibition. The test can be carried out quantitatively by comparing the activity of a known standard hormone preparation with the test sample. The test is not sensitive enough to measure below 3,000 or 4,000 IU/liter.

The Coombs' Test—The Antiglobulin Test

1. The Coombs' test is a method for detecting incomplete or blocking antibodies.
2. The test exploits the ability of an antibody molecule to participate simultaneously in binding to an antigen on the red cell surface and in complexing with antibody to itself.
3. The direct Coombs' test is a test for incomplete antibodies attached to red cells.
4. The cells are washed several times and then mixed with Coombs' reagent (antihuman globulin). If incomplete antibodies are attached to the red cells, being human globulins, they will react with the Coombs' reagent, and the cells will agglutinate.
5. It has been demonstrated that the red cell antibody, probably because it is directed against an antigen situated deep in the cell wall, cannot link two red cells together for agglutination. Therefore, the addition of an antihuman globulin brings about agglutination by linking two attached immunoglobulins to one another.
6. This test is used extensively in testing the red cells of newborn babies and in investigating cases of hemolytic anemia.
7. In the indirect Coombs' test, cells of known antigenic content (Rh-positive cells) are mixed with serum suspected of containing the corresponding complete antibodies. After incubation, the cells are washed several times and Coombs' reagent is added as in the direct Coombs' test. The cells are then examined for agglutination. If agglutination occurs, it proves that the corresponding antibodies were present in the suspected serum.
8. This test is used for checking the serum of pregnant women for incomplete antibodies and in crossmatching tests prior to blood transfusions.
9. The direct Coombs' test differs from the indirect test only in that Coombs' serum is added directly to a washed erythrocyte suspension in the direct test.
10. The indirect test requires the addition of serum from one individual (prospective transfusion recipient) to a washed erythrocyte suspension from another individual (the prospective transfusion donor) before the addition of Coombs' serum to the system.

Complement Fixation (CF)

1. The ability of certain immune complexes to bind or fix the components of complement may be used as a test for antibodies if one has a known antigen or vice versa.
2. To detect the consumption of complement by the test system, indicator cells consisting of red cells coated with antibody are added. Complement is measured as an activity as are other enzyme systems and is expressed in terms of the degree of lysis of a standard suspension of optimally coated sheep red cells produced within a fixed time.
3. Sometimes an antigen-antibody reaction that is completely invisible occurs, but in the course of which all available complement is used up or fixed. This is called complement fixation.
4. That complement is no longer available or that an antigen-antibody reaction has occurred is shown by adding red cells together with a hemolytic antibody.
5. If hemolysis now takes place, it

must be assumed that there was complement available. If hemolysis does not take place, it must be assumed that there was no complement available; hence, an antigen-antibody reaction must have taken place with the original ingredient.

6. The test is performed as follows:

a. *Indicator System*

(1) Sheep red cells are coated with antibody to the sheep red cells.

(2) Complement (fresh guinea pig serum) is added.

(3) Complement reacts with anti-sheep red cell antibody.

(4) Lysis of cells occur.

b. *Positive Test*

(1) An antigen is added to a specific antibody directed against that antigen.

(2) Complement is added.

(3) The antibody reacts with antigen, and complement combines with the antigen-antibody complex.

(4) Complement is used up and is no longer available.

(5) The addition of antibody-coated red cells does not then result in lysis.

7. The complement fixation test is used in identifying the Wasserman antibody in syphilis as well as identifying an antigen such as a virus antigen.

Fluorescent Antibody Test (Coon's Test)

1. The fluorescent dye, fluorescein isothiocyanate, can be coupled onto antibody molecules by allowing the isothiocyanate group to react with free amino groups present on the antibody molecule.

2. The resulting antigen-antibody complex shows up as a brilliant yellow-green fluorescence when observed under the microscope using an ultraviolet light.

3. Rhodamine isothiocyanate is often used instead of fluorescein isothiocyanate. Rhodamine is more stable and gives a more brilliant fluorescence.

4. Because immunofluorescent staining reflects the serological specificity of the antibody employed, it is a highly specific histochemical tool.

5. The technique is more sensitive than precipitation or complement fixation techniques, and fluorescent protein tracers can be detected at a concentration of the order of 1μg. protein/ml. body fluid.

6. The Coon's fluorescent antibody test has been used for detection of antigens in bacteria, viruses, protozoa, and fungi as well as human tissue antigens.

7. There are two ways of applying the test in practice—the direct method and the indirect.

a. *Direct Method*

(1) The fluorescein-tagged antibody reacts with an antigen specific to it.

(2) The attached fluorescein-tagged antibody is visualized by use of the ultraviolet microscope.

(3) It is used as a diagnostic laboratory test to identify bacteria in tissue sections, blood, cerebrospinal fluid, urine, feces, or other clinical specimens.

b. *Indirect Method*

(1) Untagged antibody reacts with an antigen specific to it.

(2) The antibody attaches to the antigen determinant forming an antigen-antibody complex.

(3) To the antigen-antibody complex is added a fluorescein-tagged antiglobulin serum (usually purchased from one of the commercial companies) specific for the globulin of the serum.

(4) The fluorescein-tagged antiglobulin reacts with the antigen-antibody complex.

(5) It is visualized by the ultraviolet microscope.

(6) The end point is much sharper and therefore easier to read than that seen in the direct method.

(7) This method is commonly used for detection of antibodies in serum.

Cytotoxic Tests

1. Cytotoxic tests are used in combination with red cell agglutinations for studying histocompatibility antigen system in tissue typing.

2. The purpose of this test is to determine whether the permeability of the cell changes after incubation with an antibody and complement.

3. Cytotoxic antibodies have the ability to attach to a cell, activate complement components, and produce changes in the permeability of the cell membrane.

4. If the permeability of the cell membrane is changed, trypan blue will enter the cell and can be identified on microscopic examination.

5. The test has wide application but is usually chosen for work with blood leukocytes. It is less sensitive than the red cell hemagglutination test.

6. The test is performed as follows:

a. *Negative Test—No Antibody*

(1) Leukocytes react with trypan blue in the presence of complement.

(2) Dye is excluded from the cell.

(3) Antibody is not present—a negative test is reported.

b. *Positive Test—Antibody Present*

(1) Leukocytes react with trypan blue in the presence of complement.

(2) Antibody is present and forms an antibody-complement complex on the surface of the cell (antigen).

(3) Cell is rendered permeable to the dye.

(4) Dye enters the cell, proving that antibody is present—a positive test is reported.

7. A modification of this test, where eosin and trypan blue dyes are taken up by the damaged cell, employs radioactive chromium (^{51}Cr).

a. The ^{51}Cr is incorporated into the living cell after a period of incubation.

b. The addition of a specific antibody to the antigen on the surface of the cell in the presence of complement causes a change in the permeability of the cell membrane and results in ^{51}Cr leaking out of the cell.

c. This can be measured, and a judgment can be made on the titer of antibody present.

d. A cell incubated in the presence of a specific antibody directed against its surface antigen, activates complement to produce an antigen-antibody complex which damages the cell.

e. The damaged cell is not able to utilize a radiolabelled precursor for the synthesis of nucleic acids and will not form colonies when plated in vitro.

f. Tritiated thymidine is used to label the precursor for this test.

28. Diagnostic Radiology in Obstetrics and Gynecology

Hugh R. K. Barber, M.D.

BASIC PRINCIPLES

1. The use of radiology in obstetrics has almost been phased out by the increased acceptance and use of ultrasonography. Radiologic studies in obstetrics are reserved for a very rare case where ultrasound has not provided a positive diagnosis.

2. The limited use of radiology in obstetrics is a result of:

a. Fear of radiation injuries to the fetus and to the ovaries of women of childbearing age.

b. No threshold for gene mutation.

c. Estimates for doubling of the spontaneous mutation rate in man run from 10 R to 140 roentgens (R)

3. The estimated threshold doses for the human that may cause fetal damage are:

First month of pregnancy	40 R
Second month of pregnancy	90 R
Third month of pregnancy	140 R
Fourth month of pregnancy	200 R
Fifth month of pregnancy	250 R
Sixth month of pregnancy	350 R
Eighth month of pregnancy	500 R
Tenth month of pregnancy	600 R

4. X-ray pelvimetry gives 1,200 mR to the skin and 1,300 mR to the female gonads.

5. Chest film 14″ × 7″ gives a skin dose of 100 mR and 0.07 mR to the gonads.

6. Lymphocyte depression has been reported from 50 R.

7. It is suggested but not conclusively proved that diagnostic radiation in the prenatal period may result in an increased incidence of leukemia in the children so exposed.

8. Long-term studies of the delayed effects of the atomic bomb have shown a significant lag in the growth and development of children whose mothers received a radiation dose of 50 rads or more.

9. Therapeutic levels of radiation for pelvic malignancy during pregnancy have resulted in approximately one-third of the babies being born with malformations. Microcephaly was the most frequently seen abnormality.

OBSTETRICAL RADIOLOGY

ANTENATAL FETAL STUDIES

Diagnosis of Pregnancy

1. Fetal skeletal parts such as the fetal skull, vertebral column, and ribs are visible by the fifteen to eighteen week.

2. Lower-limb ossification center appears in the femur at 9 weeks; epiphysis around the knee joint at 35 to 40 weeks.

Fetal maturity

Although ultrasound is more commonly employed, occasionally a flat film of the pregnant abdomen is taken. It is used to interpret:

1. The epiphysis of the distal end of

the femur ossifies at about the thirty-fifth week of gestation.

2. The epiphysis of the proximal end of the tibia ossifies between the thirty-sixth and fortieth week, usually indicating a full-term fetus.

3. If the biparietal measurement of the infant's head is more than 8.5 cm., the infant is estimated to be over 5½ pounds.

Multiple Pregnancies

Fetal presentation and position.

Fetal Death

Fetal death is detectable on radiograph by the overlapping of skull sutures (Spaulding's sign) and by the presence of gas in the fetal circulatory system.

Abdominal Pregnancy

Malformations of the fetus. Hydrocephaly, anencephaly, lacunar skull (spina bifida), and long-bone deformities can be diagnosed.

X-RAY PELVIMETRY

Basic Principles

1. Currently 5 to 7 per cent of all deliveries involve the use of x-ray pelvimetry.

2. The purpose of pelvimetry is to help the clinician decide whether or not to perform Cesarean section.

3. Pelvimetry measures bony landmarks. It does not assess soft tissues, the moldability of the fetal head, the forces of labor, or the degree of relaxation of the pelvic ligaments.

4. Pelvimetry offers no information regarding uterine dysfunction.

5. Pelvimetry offers one set of parameters in a whole constellation of information from which the decision whether or not to do a Cesarean section must be derived.

6. Pelvimetry is not always essential to make this decision and the adroit obstetrician seldom uses x-ray pelvimetry.

Indications

1. There are no clear-cut universally accepted indications for x-ray pelvimetry. At one end of the spectrum are those who feel it has no place in the practice of obstetrics, while at the other end are those who have a record of heavy utilization.

2. There are three possible measural outcomes from x-ray pelvimetry:

a. The pelvic measurements are well within normal limits.

b. The measurements are clearly in the abnormal realm.

c. The measurements fall in the overlap at the lower limits of normal and the upper limits of the abnormal range.

3. If the obstetrician states that his management will be influenced by the findings of pelvimetry, the study is then indicated. The usual indications are:

a. Clinical Evidence of Pelvic Abnormalities

(1) Biischial diameter below 8.5 cm. in a primigravida

(2) Suspected clinical evidence of midplane contraction or other evidences of a contracted pelvis

(3) Diagonal conjugate less than 11.5 cm.

(4) Floating head at term in a primigravida

b. History of difficult forceps operation

c. A history of pelvic trauma

d. Breech presentation in a primigravida

e. An obstetric history suggestive of possible pelvic abnormality, e.g., stillbirth, hard or prolonged labor, unexplained neonatal death

f. Persistent fetal malposition

g. Lack of progess in labor with possible cephalopelvic disproportion

h. Prior to the use of oxytocin in possible cephalopelvic disproportion

4. The views commonly taken are:

a. *Erect lateral view* (taken with the patient standing) shows:

(1) Obstetric conjugate diameter, sacral angle, and the angle of inclination of the brim

(2) Antero-posterior diameter of the midpelvic cavity

(3) Antero-posterior diameter of outlet

(4) Shows the shape of the sacrosciatic notch, length and curvature of sacrum, and shape of ischial spines. The thickness and depth of the symphysis pubis can be estimated and the presenting part and its relationship to the brim assessed.

b. *The antero-posterior view* (taken with the patient lying down) shows:

(1) Transverse diameter of the outlet

(2) Interspinous diameter

(3) The general shape and symmetry of the pelvic brim can be assessed and the breadth and shape of the sacrum observed.

c. *The outlet view* (taken with the patient sitting with legs spread and leaning as far forward as possible) shows:

(1) Shape of subpubic arch. The angle may be measured by the lines joining the lower border of the symphysis pubis to the ischial tuberosities.

(2) Intuberischial diameter is measured 1 cm. above the tuberosities.

(3) Assessment of subpubic capacity. A circle 9.3 cm. in diameter is applied to the subpubic area and the distance between the symphysis and the circumference is measured. The measurement is the "waste space of Morris" and should not exceed 1 cm. The fetal head in labor, well flexed and molded, should approximate to 9.3 cm. (3¾ inches).

d. *Alternative View*. There is another view sometimes taken with the patient reclining at an angle of 60° to bring the pelvic brim into the horizontal. This gives an excellent view of the brim shape but means a high dosage of radiation for the fetal gonad in the vertex presentation (nearly twice as much as for the three other views). It is not commonly employed.

5. Because of these untoward effects and because of the difficulty of estimating the amount of radiation delivered to the maternal and fetal gonads, certain restrictions and precautions should be employed. These are:

a. Elimination of routine radiography of the abdomen for the purpose of diagnosing the presentation of the fetus or for pelvic measurements.

b. Use of obstetric radiography for significant clinical indications only.

c. Limitation of the number of exposures and use of the maximum tube distance when x-ray pelvimetry is employed.

d. Utilization of such special devices as aluminum and brass filtration, high kilovoltage, fast screens, high-speed films, light localizers, adequate cones, and limiting diaphragms to reduce the area of exposure.

e. The use of diagnostic techniques when applicable.

X-RAY CLASSIFICATION OF THE PELVIS

Basic Principles

1. The Caldwell-Moloy System introduced in 1933 classified pelves from the approach of the architectural structure.

2. X-ray films (anteroposterior, lateral, and stereoscopic) are necessary to determine the different types in this classification.

3. The portion of the pelvic cavity anterior to the longest transverse diameter was called the forepelvis and the posterior portion, the posterior or hindpelvis.

4. They divided pelves into four main groups: gynecoid (true female), android (male type), platypelloid (flat), and anthropoid (apelike).

5. Not all pelves fall definitely into one of these parent types.

6. The Caldwell-Moloy classification has now been altered to include 14 types based upon the shape of the anterior and posterior segments of the inlet.
7. With the addition of small, average, and large sizes, the Caldwell-Moloy classification includes 42 different types.

Gynecoid Pelvis (True Female)

1. The gynecoid or true female pelvis is the most common type (normal) and is approximately round (or slightly oval).
2. The transverse diameter is a little longer than the anteroposterior diameter and is considerably anterior to the sacral promontory.
3. The hindpelvis is roomy, broad, and deep, leaving the forepelvis sufficiently roomy.
4. The sacrosciatic notch is broad, showing that there is ample room for normal birth in both the anterior and posterior pelvis.
5. The pelvic arch is wide.
6. Normal birth is the rule.

Android Pelvis (Male Type)

1. The inlet of the android or male type of pelvis is heart-shaped because the sacral promontory is pushed forward nearer the widest transverse diameter, making the posterior pelvis shallow.
2. The pubic arch is narrow.
3. The sacrosciatic notch is narrow with the outlet diameter shortened.
4. This type of pelvis is a frequent cause of difficult labor.
5. The labor is difficult because of the masculine shape, angulated forepelvis, shallow hindpelvis, and narrow pubic arch.
6. Difficulties in labor arise from the pelvic brim to the outlet.

Platypelloid Pelvis (Flat)

1. The anteroposterior diameter is shortened.
2. The widest transverse diameter is relatively lengthened and lies approximately equidistant from the promontory and symphysis.
3. Both the forepelvis and hindpelvis are shortened.
4. The sacrosciatic notch appears narrowed, and the subpubic angle is usually relatively wider.
5. The fetal head enters the pelvic brim transversely in marked asynclitism.

Anthropoid Pelvis (Apelike)

1. The anteroposterior pelvic diameter is long and the transverse diameter is short, giving the inlet the shape of a sagittal eclipse.
2. Since the widest transverse diameter is so far from the promontory, the posterior pelvis is deep and the sacrosciatic notch is wide.
3. The head enters the pelvis obliquely (because of the relatively or actually short transverse diameter of the inlet).
4. The occiput frequently lies posteriorly, and not infrequently the infant may be born with the occiput persistently posterior.

PELVIC CONTRACTIONS

A contracted pelvis is one in which an important diameter is 1 cm. less than that of the normal gynecoid pelvis.

Inlet Contraction

1. The inlet is contracted if the anteroposterior diameter is 10 cm. or less or if the greatest transverse diameter is 12 cm. or less.
2. When the diagonal conjugate diameter is less than 11.5 cm., it is assumed that the anteroposterior distance is under 10 cm.
3. The most common cause of pelvic inlet contraction is probably rickets in infancy.

Midpelvic Contraction

1. Average midpelvic measurements are:

a. Interspinous (transverse), 10.5 cm.

b. Anteroposterior (lower symphysis to junction of fourth and fifth sacral vertebrae), 11.5 cm.

c. Posterior sagittal (midpoint of interspinous line to same point on sacrum), 5 cm.

d. When the interspinous is below 9 cm. and the posterior sagittal measurement is below 4 cm., dystocia with a fetus of average term size can be anticipated.

2. Accurate midpelvic measurements are possible only by radiologic methods.
3. In white women midpelvic contraction is more common than inlet contraction and leads to transverse arrest of the fetal head.

Contracted Outlet (Funnel Pelvis)

1. Are not as rare as once supposed.
2. They may occur with all types of pelves.
3. Complete perineal tears occur when funnel pelvis is not recognized.
4. When the transverse diameter of the outlet between the tuberosities of the ischium (normally 10 or 11 cm.) is 8 cm. or less, the outlet is contracted and the pubic arch (angle) is narrowed so that the baby's head cannot fit into it.
5. The head is forced back toward the tip of the sacrum.
6. If there is enough room in the hindpelvis, the head may pass the outlet.
7. When the outlet is adequate, spontaneous delivery will usually follow.
8. Forceps and a wide episiotomy may be indicated.
9. When the outlet is clearly inadequate, Cesarean section should be elected before labor or at its start.

TRIAL OF LABOR

1. Trial of labor is the term used when the outcome of labor is uncertain.
2. Usually it means that the pelvic capacity for the baby is in doubt but that with good uterine contractions and reasonable cranial molding, vaginal delivery is feasible.
3. A trial of labor is conducted in vertex presentations only and should never be used in breech presentation.
4. The term is sometimes used nowadays to mean the trial of induction of labor and if labor has not started or progressed well in some arbitrary time, e.g., 12 hours, then Cesarean section is used for delivery.
5. The conduct of a trial of labor necessitates constant vigilance, frequent checking of descent of the head, cervical dilatation, fetal heart rate, and monitoring of the labor.
6. In this group the indications for Cesarean section should be liberal.

PLACENTAL LOCALIZATION

1. Soft tissue placentography, arterial placentography, intravenous placentography, isotope placentography have been phased out with the wide acceptance of ultrasound as an alternative.
2. Thermographic localization has a poor success rate of only 50 per cent but is free of radiation danger.
3. Amniography has been reserved for certain suspected cases of hydatidiform mole in which ultrasound evaluation is not conclusive.

NONOBSTETRICAL RADIOLOGIC TECHNIQUES DURING PREGNANCY

Basic Principles

1. Routine chest radiographs should be avoided except in tuberculin-positive women or in those with signs of active chest disease. Chest film 14″ × 7″ gives 100 mR skin dose and 0.07 mR to the female gonads. Chest photofluoroscopic film gives 1000 mR skin dose and 0.7 mR to the female gonads.

2. Unless absolutely necessary, radiographs should be deferred until the second trimester. The abdomen should be adequately shielded.

3. Gastrointestinal and gallbladder studies should be deferred until the pregnancy is terminated. However, in an occasional case it will be necessary to do x-ray studies.

4. Intravenous pyelograms are difficult to interpret in pregnancy because of the gestational dilatation of the renal pelves and ureters. However, if they are indicated, the studies should be carried out. A pyelogram gives 1,200 mR to the skin and 1,300 mR to the female gonads.

5. Dental studies may be done with maximum shielding of the abdomen.

6. Bone studies associated with trauma should be done with maximum shielding of the abdomen. X-ray studies should not be ordered for the usual complaints of pubic symphysis or sacroiliac relaxations.

7. When a pregnant woman becomes ill, she deserves as complete an evaluation as if she were not pregnant.

a. If, in the considered judgment of her physician, roentgen examination might supply helpful information that could not be obtained more simply by other methods, then obviously the study should be undertaken.

b. The patient should not be denied radiologic study if there is reasonable probability of its value.

c. Prior consultation between the referring physician and the radiologist will ultimately prove of greatest benefit to the patient as well as to her baby.

RADIOLOGY IN GYNECOLOGY

Basic Principles

1. Whenever possible, radiologic studies in the female of childbearing age should be performed prior to ovulation (first half of the menstrual cycle).

2. Radiologic studies in gynecological patients have been generally related to:

a. The evaluation of an infertility problem

b. The evaluation of the preoperative patient

c. Gastrointestinal studies and cholecystograms are included in the gynecologist's area of interest as an aid to better differential diagnosis.

3. A metastatic workup of the patient with pelvic malignancy should include an intravenous pyelogram, upper and lower gastrointestinal series, and a bone survey.

HYSTEROSALPINGOGRAPHY

Basic Principles

1. Is an outpatient roentgenographic procedure requiring an aseptic technique, a radiolucent vaginal speculum, a cervical plug to prevent reflux, and media.

2. It is important to have taken a good history and to have done a thorough physical examination.

3. Excessive material exposes the patient to irritation from the medium and prevents proper interpretation.

4. Inadequate amounts result in an incomplete study.

5. Constant pressure without excessive force is maintained in the filled syringe.

6. Severe abdominal pain during the test demands termination of the test.

7. The optimum time for performing the procedure is one week after the menses.

8. Occasionally a sedative and/or an antispasmodic is indicated.

9. Indications are: evaluation of tubal patency, endocervical defects, myomas, polyps, congenital malformations of the uterus, and adenocarcinoma of the endometrium (questionable).

10. Image intensification and television fluoroscopy enable physicians to

arrive at a proper conclusion promptly, safely, and with convenience to the patient.

Technique

1. A careful pelvic examination is carried out.
2. After cleansing the vulva and perineum, a bivalve speculum is inserted into the vagina and the cervix is cleaned with antiseptic followed by aspiration of cervical mucus.
3. A cannula, with a rubber acorn tip of proper size to occlude the external os, is inserted into the cervical canal. Before inserting the cannula, the air in the cannula is replaced by a contrast medium.
4. A preliminary film is first taken.
5. For evaluation of the endocervix and uterine cavity, 1 ml. of contrast material is instilled under low pressure.
6. Small amounts of material are then instilled in increments of 1 to 2 ml., with films being taken after each increment.
7. For tubal evaluation it is necessary to instill approximately 6 to 10 ml. and in patients with an enlarged uterus and obstructed or distended fallopian tubes, even larger amounts may be necessary.
8. A 45-minute delayed film should be taken to evaluate peritoneal spill, and a 24-hour film in order to evaluate both spill and the presence of peritubal adhesions.
9. Water-soluble media rather than oil media are often chosen for evaluating the uterus. Films should be taken during and within 5 to 10 minutes after the instillation.
10. Image-intensified fluoroscopy and cineradiography adds to the information provided by the test.

Potential Errors in Technique

1. Failure to take a preliminary film, especially if the patient has had a previous test with radiopaque material
2. Failure to test the equipment, especially the patency of the cannula, prior to the test
3. Too small an acorn on the cannula will allow the contrast material to leak out
4. Failure to maintain even pressure during the instillation
5. Excessive or insufficient contrast media may result in failure
6. Failure to use an aqueous material when there is evidence of previous infection or tubal stenosis
7. Failure to take sufficient films, including laterals when necessary

Adverse Effects

Faulty technique and poor selection of patients usually are the causes of morbidity or are contributing factors in the untoward sequelae that occasionally follow hysterosalpingography.

The following complications can result from hysterosalpingography.

1. Mechanical Complications
- a. Pain
- b. Uterine perforation
- c. Tubal rupture
- d. Endometriosis
- e. Hemorrhage
- f. Shock

2. Chemical and Toxic Complications
- a. Granulomas
- b. Allergic reactions
- c. Iatrogenic thyroid dysfunction

3. Genetic Hazards

4. Intravasation
- a. Uterovenous intravasation
- b. Lymphatic structures

Interpretation of Hysterosalpingogram

1. Intrauterine Adhesions

Are detected as lacunar shadows which are single or multiple as well as large or small.

2. Infertility

a. May be related to tubal lesions as well as to congenital anomalies.

b. Tubal obstruction is almost always secondary to salpingitis.

3. Tuberculosis

a. Multiple structures, dilatations, sinus tracts may be present.

b. Tubes are obstructed, calcification is often present, and the tubes look like "pipe stems."

4. Malformations

Congenital defects or anomalies such as bicornuate uterus can be outlined.

5. Filling Defects

a. Are caused by polyps, hyperplasia, fibroids, synechiae, and adenomyosis.

b. Hydatidiform moles are easily detected.

c. Cervical canal stenosis and atresia can be demonstrated.

PELVIC ARTERIOGRAPHY

Basic Principles

1. This method of demonstrating pelvic tumors directly is based upon observation of displacement of the normal arterial system, the presence of abnormal vessels, and the formation of communications to adjacent arterial systems, attesting to the invasiveness of such a tumor.
2. It has very limited usefulness for assessing tumors of the pelvis exclusive of gestational trophoblastic disease.
3. Arteriography which is properly timed may help diagnose a molar pregnancy. There is early bilateral filling of the uterine veins in the presence of mole or choriocarcinoma, presumably on the basis of arteriovenous shunts which may be present. The test cannot be applied except in rare cases because it may expose a normal pregnancy to excessive radiation.
4. Arteriography may be useful in identifying the localized uterine disease which may be poorly responsive to systemic chemotherapy. If further reproduction is planned, arterial infusion chemotherapy may be of assistance in such an individual. Otherwise, hysterectomy should be carried out.
5. Organs of interest to the urologist that are amenable to angiography include the kidney, adrenal, and bladder.
6. In the kidney, arterial patterns characteristic of tumors, cysts, arteriovenous fistulas, or other pathologic or normal processes, such as ectopic renal cortical tissue, are seen in detail.
7. Adrenal arteriography can accurately detect adrenal tumors, adenomas, and cysts.
8. Bladder arteriography has been used to detect invasion of bladder tumors into or through the bladder muscle. The bladder is partially filled with air to give better contrast. This procedure is only occasionally useful.

INTRAVENOUS PYELOGRAM

1. Excretory urography is a term used synonymously with intravenous pyelography.
2. Is a widely used test and expression that means that the calyces, renal pelvis, ureters, and bladder are delineated by renal excretion of intravenously given iodinated contrast medium.
3. The test should be preceded by an adequate plain film (KUB).
4. Cathartics and enemas are given to prepare the bowel.
5. Fluid intake is limited for at least 8 hours prior to the examination.
6. Before administration of the contrast medium, a careful history and physical examination should be carried out. Allergic reactions should be recorded. The reaction to previous pyelographic studies should be determined.
7. Equipment and drugs necessary to treat an anaphylactic or allergic reaction should be readily available.
8. Pregnant patients should only receive a pyelogram if it is truly indicated.

9. Multiple myeloma has been considered to be a contraindication to intravenous pyelography because of the risk of subsequent acute renal failure. If carried out, the patient should be thoroughly hydrated prior to the procedure.

10. Tomography is a roentgenographic technique that focuses on a desired level within the patient. This test should be ordered at the discretion of radiologist.

11. Pyelography gives a skin dose of 1200 mR and 1300 mR to the female gonads.

29. Venereal Disease and Vulvovaginitis

Hugh R. K. Barber, M.D.

SYPHILIS

Definition

Syphilis is an infectious disease caused by the human parasite *Treponema pallidum*, which ordinarily enters vulnerable mucous (anogenital, oral) or cutaneous surfaces during sexual contact.

Basic Mechanisms

1. The primary chancre of syphilis frequently involves the vulva 3 to 4 weeks after exposure and is sometimes overlooked.

   a. It presents as a small, rounded or ovoid ulcer, with raised indurated edges and a depressed center.

   b. It is usually present on the labia, with associated edema and inguinal lymphadenitis. The initial lesion will regress in a month or so.

2. The incidence of syphilis has increased by 4 to 4.5 per cent in the past year. This may reflect the failure of the responsible physician to report cases of infectious syphilis to local health authorities so that all contacts can be adequately traced.

3. All contacts should be traced and treated even though they are asymptomatic, since they may be in the incubation period and lost to subsequent follow-up.

4. The incubation period is about 3 to 4 weeks.

5. It is accompanied by inguinal adenopathy. The glands are hard and enlarged but not tender. It is called an inguinal bubo.

6. Syphilis is a systemic disease which may be either acute or chronic and is capable of revealing itself through varied manifestations or of lying quiescent for months or years.

7. Primary syphilis is characterized by a lesion as described above.

   a. It may occur on the inner surface of the labium (minus or major), on the clitoris, cervix, or as an extragenital lesion.

   b. Diagnosis of primary syphilis is confirmed by examining the discharge from the lesion by dark field examination and watching the movements of the treponema.

8. Secondary syphilis appears in a few months, usually 2 or 3, after the primary stage. It is a systemic infection with various skin rashes, usually symmetrical and of a copper-brown color like raw ham and without irritation.

   a. Snail-track ulcers and painless shiny gray patches appear in the mouth.

   b. There may be sore throat, generalized lymph node enlargement, low fever, and malaise.

   c. The gynecologist is usually consulted because of vulvar and peri-anal condylomata—multiple round and oval-shaped, only slightly raised warts.

9. The lesions are highly infective. Dark field is positive and serological tests are positive.

10. Tertiary syphilis appears years (often many) after infection. The lesion is a localized swelling called a gumma and has the consistency of rubber.

    a. The gumma does not contain treponemata and is not infective.

    b. Gummata are irregular in distribution and may be found anywhere in the body.

c. A gumma may break down and give a punched-out ulcer.

SYPHILIS IN PREGNANCY

Basic Principles

1. There is now a significant rise in the incidence of syphilis and concomitant increase in the occurrence of congenital syphilis.
2. Effective prenatal screening of pregnant patients has removed those children whose congenital disease can be manifested at birth or in the immediate neonatal period.
3. Even before the advent of massive screening for *T. pallidum* in pregnancy, only about 10 per cent of cases of congenital syphilis were identified in the first year of life.
4. Recently there has been an increase in the maternal acquisition of syphilis in the interim period between the initial serological testing and parturition.
5. Organ pathology in congenital syphilis is not complete at the time of parturition but is a continuing organ-spirochete well into the first two years of life.
6. By the early identification of a congenital infection and the institution of appropriate therapy, the disease process may be arrested and the subsequent morbidity lessened.
7. Until the incidence of syphilis in the community is markedly reduced, the pregnant patient should be screened early and then again near parturition for evidence of infection with *T. pallidum*, especially if more than 90 days have elapsed between parturition and the initial serological test.
8. Adequate treatment of the mother during the first 18 weeks of gestation prevents infection of the baby (congenital syphilis), as the *T. pallidum* probably does not cross the placental barrier until the 19th week.
9. Treatment begun after the 18th week of gestation amounts to treatment of the baby in utero.
10. The fetus can be infected in utero with resulting abortion or stillbirth and the liveborn baby may be congenitally syphilitic.
11. The syphilitic placenta is a large, pale organ very like the placenta in hydrops fetalis, showing the microscopic changes of endarteritis and fibrosis.

Diagnosis

1. Dark field examination gives absolute diagnosis.
2. Serological tests used in the serological diagnosis of syphilis are of two main types, i.e., nontreponemal and treponemal tests.
3. *Nontreponemal Tests*

   a. Venereal Disease Research Laboratory (VDRL) test is well controlled, easily performed, and inexpensive. If VDRL is reactive, a quantitative test should be done.

   b. Other nontreponemal tests such as rapid plasma reagin (RPR) test and automated reagin test (ART) are less specific and should only be used for screening when speed is essential.
4. If a screening test (such as RPR) is positive, the more specific VDRL test should be performed for verification and a quantitation for follow-up.

   a. Conditions associated with false-positive reactions are narcotic addition, aging, leprosy, and terminal malignancy.

   b. Acute false-positive tests are seen in infectious mononucleosis, hepatitis, malaria, viral pneumonia, chickenpox, measles, and smallpox vaccination.

   c. If a false-positive reaction is suspected, it should be validated by more specific treponemal tests.
5. Treponemal tests are those employed to detect specific antibodies to *Treponema pallidum*.
6. The fluorescent treponemal antibody test (FTA-ABS) is highly specific

with only 1 per cent false-positive reactions.

a. False-positive FTA-ABS tests are limited to the group of diseases with abnormal and increased immunoglobulins such as systemic lupus erythematosus and other autoimmune diseases.

b. Most FTA-ABS false-positive tests give an atypical beading fluorescent pattern which can be differentiated from the normal homogeneous treponemal fluorescence.

c. When there is a borderline FTA-ABS test, a *T. pallidum* immobilizing test (TPL) should be performed for verification.

7. Once the diagnosis of syphilis is made, the quantitative VDRL and not the FTA-ABS test should be used for post-treatment follow-up.

Congenital Syphilis

1. The fetus can be infected in utero with resulting abortion or stillbirth, and the liveborn baby may be congenitally syphilitic.
2. If the cord blood is positive for VDRL in an asymptomatic infant, serial quantitiatve VDRL should be performed for a rise or fall of titer.
3. A falling titer indicates passive transfer of reagin from the blood of a mother who had been treated adequately before pregnancy.
4. A rising titer indicates active infection and the need for immediate treatment.
5. IgM antibodies represent fetal response to infection. A positive *IgM*-FTA-ABS test confirms active infection.

Management

1. Primary and secondary syphilis is treated with benzathine penicillin G, 2.4 million units I.M. divided into two equal doses given simultaneously.
2. Early and late latent syphilis should be treated according to whether the spinal fluid is positive or not.
3. If the spinal fluid is positive or if no spinal fluid examination is performed, aqueous procaine penicillin G (APPG), 2.4 million units, is given every 2 days for 10 treatments. Total dosage is 24 million units. Aqueous procaine penicillin results in higher penicillin levels in spinal fluid than benzathine penicillin G.
4. If spinal fluid is negative, 2.4 million units benzathine penicillin G, I.M., is divided into two equal doses and given simultaneously.
5. Late syphilis excluding neurosyphilis is treated with 6 to 9 million units of benzathine penicillin G, given according to the following schedule: 2.4 million units I.M. every 7 days on one or two separate occasions.
6. Syphilis in pregnancy under 16 weeks is treated the same according to the stage of disease as outlined above. If over 16 weeks, treatment with APPG, 2.4 million units every 2 days × 6 doses. The total dosage is 14.4 million units.
7. Treatment of infants is given as follows: small infants are treated with APPG in equally divided I.M. doses every day for 10 days for a total dose of 100,000 to 200,000 units per kilogram body weight.

Alternate Treatment When Penicillin Is Contraindicated

1. Tetracycline 0.5 g. orally q.i.d. for 20 to 30 days (total dose in early syphilis is 40 g. and in late neurosyphilis is 60 g.).
2. Erythromycin base or stearate 0.5 g. orally q.i.d. for 20 to 30 days.
3. During pregnancy, under 16 weeks, erythromycin in the same regimen as for a nonpregnant patient. Over 16 weeks, cephaloridine, 1 g. I.M. daily for 10 days in early syphilis and for 20 days in late syphilis.
4. All treated patients should be followed with serology in the first, third, sixth, and twelfth months during the first year and every 6 months during the second year.

GONORRHEA

Definition

Gonorrhea is an infectious disease caused by the gram-negative diplococcus *Neisseria gonorrhoeae*.

Basic Principles

The incubation period for gonorrhea is 3 to 10 days from infection. It is a delicate organism that does not survive easily outside the body.

2. Gonorrhea is acquired by intercourse with an infected person, though it may be spread by clothing or towels, especially in young children.
3. It is an ascending infection of the female genital tract.
4. The clinical manifestations may present with the following stages:
   a. *Stage I* (acute phase) is often of only a few days' duration. It may be accompanied by a history of urinary frequency and burning dysuria with a thick yellow discharge.
      (1) At this time the patient may have a red urethra with a purulent urethral discharge, an inflamed cervix with a profuse mucopurulent discharge from the external os, swelling or abscess of either Bartholin gland, and acute skenitis.
      (2) Many women have no acute phase, especially if the cervix is the primary source of infection.
   b. *Stage II* (chronic phase) follows the acute phase. The ascending infection (occurring during menses) moves to the upper genital tract, with involvement of the tubes, ovaries, and pelvic peritoneum. Discharge may be the only complaint.
   c. *Stage III* (carrier phase) follows Stage II which lapses into a carrier state where symptoms are minimal but the ability to infect is present for many weeks.
5. Eighty-five per cent of all uncomplicated gonorrhea in the female is asymptomatic.
6. The most common site of infection is the endocervix.
7. Due to changes in sexual behavior, gonorrhea infections of the rectum and throat occur often enough that specific questions about anogenital and orogenital practices should be asked.
8. Pharyngeal infection occurred in 3 to 11.3 per cent of women examined in venereal disease clinics. Of this, 1 to 3 per cent had pharyngeal infection without demonstrable anogenital infection.
9. Nasopharyngeal culture for gonococcus should be obtained when pharyngeal symptoms are present in a patient suspected to have gonorrhea.

DISSEMINATED GONOCOCCAL INFECTION (DGI)

Basic Principles

1. Occurs in 1 to 3 per cent of patients harboring gonococci and 79 per cent of the patients who develop DGI are women.
2. Dissemination occurs during menstruation or pregnancy in 71 per cent.
3. It is more common in the second and third trimester of pregnancy.
4. Arthritis is seen in 90 per cent of cases, dermatitis in 50 per cent, and endocarditis develops in 2 per cent of cases.
5. DGI is characterized by an initial "bacteremic stage" with polyarthritis, skin lesions, and positive blood cultures.
6. In 28 to 40 per cent of women with gonococcal arthritis, pregnancy had been a precipitating factor.

Diagnosis

1. Is confirmed by the presence of intracellular diplococci and by culture of the organism.
2. Cultures should always be taken from the cervix and anus. If there are any pharyngeal symptoms or if there is a history of orogenital sex, nasopharyngeal cultures should also be obtained.

3. The following technique should be followed for taking a cervical culture:

a. Remove cervical mucus plug with a cotton ball held in ring forceps.

b. Insert the cotton-tipped swab into the endocervical canal and move from side to side.

c. Allow 30 seconds for absorption of the organisms to the swab.

4. Neisseria gonorrhea grows best on chocolate-agar-based Thayer-Martin medium in a 5 to 10 per cent CO_2 atmosphere. This agar has been modified recently by the addition of colistin, vancomycin, and nystatin to diminish the overgrowth of the commensal organisms.

Management

1. 4.8 million units of aqueous procaine penicillin G (APPG) I.M., divided into 2 doses. One gram of probenecid should be given orally ½ hour before the injection.

2. When parenteral administration is impossible, 3.5 g. of oral penicillin with 1 g. of probenecid is given orally.

3. If allergic to penicillin:

a. Spectinomycin 2 g. for males and 5 g. for females, given I.M.

b. Tetracycline 1.5 grams orally, followed by 0.5 grams q.i.d. for 4 days.

4. Penicillin is the only drug which is effective for simultaneously incubating syphilis. When regimens other than penicillin are used, follow-up serology for syphilis is mandatory.

Treatment of Complications

1. Pelvic inflammatory disease is treated with 10 to 15 million units of penicillin per day I.V., supplemented by other antibiotics effective against gram-negative organisms.

2. Patients with disseminated gonococcal infection (DGI) should be hospitalized and given 6 to 12 million units penicillin I.V. followed by prolonged therapy for 10 to 14 days with ampicillin, 2 g. daily, once acute symptoms have subsided.

3. Neonatal conjunctival gonorrhea is treated with 150,000 to 600,000 units per day I.M. or I.V., supplemented with topical irrigations of the eye with aqueous solution of penicillin 10,000 U/ml.

CHANCROID (SOFT CHANCRE)

Definition

Is primarily a venereal infection caused by gram-negative bacillus *Hemophilus ducreyi* (Ducrey's bacillus).

Basic Principles

1. The incubation period is 2 to 14 days.

2. The ulceration is irregular and ragged in outline. The edges are undermined and the base is granulomatous and purulent. There is little or no surrounding induration but there is erythema and edema, especially if the lesion is in the labia majora.

3. Pain is a common feature, thus differing from most of the other venereal diseases.

4. The inguinal lymph nodes enlarge and may suppurate.

Diagnosis

1. Is made by the clinical picture of tender, necrotic ulceration and regional, tender, usually unilateral lymphadenopathy.

2. Diagnosis is confirmed by the recovery of *H. ducreyi* from lesions or bubo aspirates.

3. Gram or Wright stain may be used to microscopically identify the short gram-negative rod in characteristic parallel chains.

Management

1. Sulfisoxazole 4 g. initially, followed by 1 g. which may be given 4 times a day for 10 days or longer (up to 3 weeks).

2. Sulfamethoxazole (Gantanol) may be used in doses of 2 g. initially, followed by 1 g. twice a day for 10 days or longer (up to 3 weeks).

3. Tetracycline is also effective in a dose of 500 mg. 4 times a day for 2 weeks.

4. Resistant cases should be treated with kanamycin, 0.5 g., given I.M. twice a day for 2 weeks.

GRANULOMA INGUINALE

Definition

Granuloma inguinale is a chronic granulomatous and ulcerative lesion which is caused by *Klebsiella donovani* and is probably venereal in origin.

Basic Principles

1. It has a venereal spread and the primary lesion is usually on the external genitalia but may be seen on the vagina, cervix, or groin.

2. It is found in tropical and subtropical regions and is more common among the black race.

3. Following a variable incubation period, one or more papular lesions occur, generally in the region of the labia minora.

4. The lesion is of the cutaneous and subcutaneous tissues. It is primarily a nodule which ulcerates and joins with other papules and ulcers to form a large raw area with rolled edges.

5. The disease progresses by fibrous healing so scarring and ulceration are present together. Lymphatic blockage and vulvar elephantiasis can occur.

6. There is little tendency towards lymphadenopathy.

Diagnosis

1. Is by recognition of Donovan bodies, small oval organisms contained in macrophages in the granulation tissue.

2. Biopsy should never be neglected.

3. Microscopically there is an intense infiltration of leukocytes, plasmocytes, and mononuclear cells.

Management

1. Administration of tetracycline, 500 mg. 4 times a day for 3 weeks.

2. For patients who do not respond to tetracycline therapy, intramuscular gentamicin in a dose of 40 mg. twice a day for 2 weeks should be given.

LYMPHOGRANULOMA VENEREUM

Definition

Is a venereal disease acquired by direct sexual contact and caused by a virus that is related to the virus of psittacosis.

Basic Principles

1. Caused by a large virus.

2. Is more common among the black race.

3. The incubation period is 5 to 21 days.

4. Initially there is a small vesicle or ulcer on the labia with inguinal adenitis. This progresses to large tumor-like masses which suppurate and discharge through many sinuses (esthiomene), extending into the perineum and rectum. This may cause elephantiasis of the vulva and stricture of the rectum.

5. The pathology involves primarily the inguinogenital and anorectal regions.

6. Signs and symptoms of systemic involvement may occur during lymphatic spread; these include malaise, anorexia, fever, chills, headache, abdominal and joint pain, toxic rashes or erythema, weight loss, pneumonitis, tachycardia, and rarely meningism or splenomegaly.

7. Proctitis may accompany the fever and weight loss. It is manifested by mucosanguineous discharge, tenesmus, constipation, diarrhea, and/or rectal pains.

Diagnosis

1. Is by Frei's intradermal test. The

test is negative until several weeks after infection and once positive remains so for life.

2. A person who has had the disease is sensitive to an antigen prepared from the virus. Control material is prepared too. The reaction is positive in 48 to 72 hours.

3. Multiple biopsy with this and any other granulomatous disease should be performed to exclude an associated carcinoma, for several studies have indicated the frequency with which this may be associated with either granuloma inguinale or lymphogranuloma venereum.

Management

1. Tetracycline, 500 mg. 4 times a day for 3 weeks is given.

2. Sulfisoxazole, 4 g. initially followed by 1 g. 4 times a day is given for 10 days or longer (up to 3 weeks).

3. Sulfamethoxazole may be used in doses of 2 g. initially, followed by 1 g. twice a day for 10 days or longer (up to 3 weeks).

4. Surgery may have to be undertaken for correction of polypoid tumors or strictures that do not respond to dilatation.

TRICHOMONIASIS

Definition

1. Trichomoniasis may be expressed as an infection of the vagina, the vulva, and less commonly, the urethra, and rarely the endocervix.

2. The causative organism is the protozoan *Trichomonas vaginalis*; it is globular or pear-shaped, is from 10 μ to 30 μ in length (somewhat larger than a polymorphonuclear leukocyte) and has four flagella at the anterior end. There is an eccentrically placed nucleus with attached axostyle.

Basic Principles

1. It is estimated that 2.5 million cases occur annually in the United States. The usual mode of transmission is by sexual contact.

2. Almost all of the female sex partners of infected men are infected.

3. In some patients there are no symptoms or the female may complain of a discharge which comes on during or immediately after menses and is relieved by douching.

4. Characteristically, infestation of the vagina results in symptoms of pruritis and leukorrhea. The discharge is often foul-smelling and may be accompanied by dysuria and dyspareunia.

5. Speculum examination reveals a frothy, bubbly, greenish-yellow vaginal discharge, slight to profuse in amount.

6. There is an associated vaginal and cervical mucosal hyperemia. Not infrequently, hemorrhagic stippling of the posterior vaginal fornix and cervix occurs, resulting in the "strawberry cervix."

7. *p*H ranges from 5 to 7.

8. Vulvar edema, hyperemia, and vulvar excoriations may occur.

9. The upper part of the vagina is most severely infected.

10. The infection appears to be chronic and relapses may occur.

Diagnosis

1. Microscopic examination of a fresh, wet preparation of vaginal discharge in normal saline for evidence of actively motile flagellate protozoa. Motility is necessary for identification on microscopic examination.

2. When the wet mount is negative, the trichomonads, if present, are easily distinguished from leukocytes after Giemsa staining.

3. Cultures of trichomonads are helpful in patients with small numbers of organisms which are not revealed by wet smear. Since the rate of multiplication of the organisms is low, cultures must be

observed for 10 to 12 days before they can be regarded as negative.

4. Recently studies indicate a sensitivity for the wet mount of 76 per cent and for the culture of 91 per cent.

Management

1. Metronidazole, 250 mg. tablet orally 3 times a day for 10 days.

a. When repeat courses are required, 4 to 6 weeks should elapse between courses, and total as well as differential leukocyte counts should be made before, during, and after treatment.

b. Because of metronidazole's reported toxicity in animals, every effort must be made to limit its use to those patients in whom it is clearly indicated.

c. Alcohol should not be consumed during treatment because the patient may experience abdominal pain, flushing, and tremors.

d. The sex partner should be treated simultaneously in order to prevent exogenous reinfection.

2. Vagisec solution (1:100 strength) may be used locally.

3. Clotrimazole, 100 mg. vaginal suppository once daily for 7 days has been found effective.

CANDIDIASIS (MONILIAL VAGINITIS)

Definition

Is the name given to an infection, either acute or subacute, caused by the yeastlike fungus *Candida albicans* or by other species of *Candida*.

Basic Principles

1. Monilia is encountered in all parts of the world and may be seen in all age groups.

2. *C. albicans* is a normal inhabitant of the intestinal tract and results in autoinoculation.

3. Its overgrowth may be predisposed by pregnancy, oral contraceptives, antitrichomonal agents, antibiotics, immunosuppressive drugs, and diabetes mellitus.

4. Symptoms are those of pruritis vulvae and leukorrhea.

5. Speculum examination typically reveals a thick, white, patchy or cheesy vaginal discharge, with the vagina and vulva varying from normal appearance to a state of acute inflammation.

6. *p*H ranges from 4 to 5.

Diagnosis

1. Microscopic examination of a wet saline preparation of the vaginal discharge for evidence of pseudomycelia, the filamentous form of *C. albicans* to which potassium hydroxide has been added.

2. Culture techniques: Nickerson's medium, Monitube, Sabourand medium and speciated on cornmeal agar.

3. It is difficult to determine the significance of a positive culture because of the frequency of candidal colonization in normal individuals.

Treatment

1. 100,000 units nystatin vaginal tablets deposited high up in the vagina by means of an applicator twice a day for 2 weeks.

2. In the gravid patient, a dose of one or two nystatin vaginal tablets daily for 3 to 6 weeks before term probably prevents thrush in the newborn.

3. Miconazole cream should be applied to the vulvae and perineum twice daily for 1 to 2 weeks.

4. Clotrimazole dispensed as 100 mg. vaginal suppositories may be used daily for 7 days.

5. Aqueous gentian violet 1-per-cent to 5-per-cent applied locally has been effective.

6. To prevent seeding of the perineum by fecal matter containing the orga-

nisms, nystatin, 500,000 units orally 3 times a day for 1 week to 10 days or longer may be administered while continuing vaginal treatment.

7. The sex partner should be examined and treated, if symptomatic.

HEMOPHILUS VAGINALIS

Definition

Corynebacterium vaginale (Hemophilus vaginalis) vaginitis is caused by *Hemophilus vaginalis*, now classified as *Corynebacterium vaginale*.

Basic Principles

1. Over 90 per cent of the vaginitides previously classified as nonspecific are caused by *Corynebacterium vaginale (C. vaginale)*.
2. Is probably transmitted sexually.
3. In females with normal ovarian function, who have a gray, malodorous vaginal discharge that is relatively thin and has a *p*H of 5.0 to 5.5, are likely to have *C. vaginale* vaginitis, provided that no trichomonads are demonstrable.
4. The usual complaint is a disagreeable odor.
5. The discharge is often gray and homogeneous.
6. It is not a tissue pathogen and does not cause irritation or soreness. It is simply a surface parasite that proliferates in the vagina to become the predominant organism.

Diagnosis

1. Microscopic examination after Gram's staining reveals a predominance of vaginal epithelial cells with an almost complete absense of polymorphonuclear leukocytes.
2. The organisms present as a pleomorphic gram-negative body which adheres to cell surfaces (clue phenomenon). Sensitivity of Gram's staining has been reported to be greater than 90 per cent.
3. Facilities for culturing *C. vaginale* are not routinely available.
4. When Hemophilus vaginal infection is present, 10 per cent KOH causes a burst of a fishy odor. This is an extremely reliable finding and when one is new at recognizing "clue cells," the finding of this odor should prompt the search for clue cells because they will be present in nearly all cases.
5. Herman Gardner says that if a patient has a malodorous discharge, a *p*H of 5.0 to 5.5, and there are no trichomonads on the wet smear, the patient invariably has *H. vaginalis* infection.

Treatment

1. Ampicillin, 500 mg. orally 4 times a day for 7 to 10 days.
2. Cephalexin monohydrate, 500 mg. every 6 hours for 6 days, or cephradine, 250 mg. every 6 hours for 6 days.
3. Triple sulfa vaginal tablets or cream are also effective.
4. Male sex partners should be examined.
5. Appropriate tests for gonorrhea and syphilis should precede this treatment regimen so as not to make concomitant infection.

MYCOPLASMAS

Definition

1. *Mycoplasma hominis* and T mycoplasma (T for tiny) are the smallest of free-living organisms capable of reproducing themselves without assistance from other forms of life.
2. They are extremely pleomorphic. They appear as granules, ring forms, filaments, coccoids, and other bizarre forms. They possess a limiting cellular membrane rather than a rigid cell wall.

Basic Principles

1. Mycoplasmas were formerly of most concern to veterinarians.

2. Mycoplasma pneumoniae has been implicated in human disease.

3. There are eight recognized species of mycoplasma found in humans.

4. *M. hominis* and T hominis strain frequent genital sites from which they may be cultured by appropriate methods.

5. *M. hominis* and mycoplasma T are the principal mycoplasmas which have been isolated from the human genitourinary tract and have been associated with nongonococcal urethritis, acute salpingitis, abortion, and postpartum fever.

Diagnosis

1. Techniques for identification have improved.

2. The samples are obtained from cervical and urethral swabs and urine.

3. *M. hominis* forms colonies about 100 to 150 μm. in diameter which are just visible to the unaided eye.

4. A colony of *M. hominis* under the microscope has a dense granular center and a foamy peripheral zone ("fried egg" colony).

5. T mycoplasma in contrast form tiny granular colonies with no peripheral growth and with an average diameter of 25 μm.

6. The possible role of mycoplasma in unexplained infertility and recurrent abortion remains to be clarified.

Management

All of the mycoplasma strains are sensitive to tetracycline and resistant to penicillin and other antimicrobial agents that act on the cell wall.

HERPES SIMPLEX VULVOVAGINITIS AND CERVICITIS

Definition

1. Herpesviruses are composed of a single molecule of double strand DNA, one of the simpler forms.

2. Two major serotypes of herpesvirus have been identified and designated Type 1 and Type 2.

a. *Herpesvirus Type 1* (HSV-1), oral herpes, is most often involved in labial, upper respiratory, and central nervous system (CNS) infections.

b. *Herpesvirus Type 2* (HSV-2), herpes genitalis, affects the lower genital tract and causes perinatal infection of the newborn.

Basic Principles

1. Herpesviruses are probably the most widely disseminated human pathogens.

2. The incidence of herpes genitalis is far higher than is generally suspected. It may be the predominant cause of vesicoulcerative disease of the genitalia.

3. Patients observed with recurrent lesions outnumber those with primary lesions in the approximate ratio of two to one.

4. The incidence of active recurrent or secondary disease has far exceeded the combined incidence of all major venereal diseases.

5. The majority of patients with the primary disease are teenage girls and unmarried women.

6. The mean age of those with primary disease has been 26½ years and those with recurrent disease, 36½ years.

7. Once the infection is acquired, generally by sexual contact, the symptoms of the primary attack usually appear in 3 to 7 days.

8. The primary lesions are often extensive, involving all the vulvar tissues, the genitocrural folds, and the peri-anal skin as well as the vaginal and ectocervical mucosa.

9. The primary lesions often appear as widespread indurated papules with vesiculations and ulcerations on the most dependent surfaces. A red areola is invariably present. The lesions often coalesce, forming bullae and large ulcera-

tions, which may involve most of the vulvar and peri-anal skin.

10. Primary lesions last from 3 to 6 weeks. Complete healing without scar result unless there is a secondary infection.

11. The persistence of the herpetic stage of a lesion is dependent upon the degree of moisture at the affected site and the degree of trauma to which the lesion is subjected.

12. Lesions within the labia minora (vestibule) will ulcerate within 24 to 48 hours, whereas those on dryer areas are less subject to maceration.

13. Inguinal lymphadenopathy is almost always present and the majority of patients have a low-grade fever for several days.

Diagnosis

1. The culture is done on human fibroblasts. The material is collected by rubbing the lesions with a cotton-tipped applicator soaked in tissue culture medium. The material is then transferred immediately to tissue culture supplemented with protein. The cytopathic effect is evident after 24 to 48 hours in tissue culture.

2. The material should be stained by the Papanicolaou technique. A saline-soaked cotton-tipped swab is wiped on the lesion and smeared on a dry slide which is immediately fixed in a standard fixative. Staining will demonstrate characteristic nuclear changes with or without intranuclear inclusions. These techniques have given a low yield of positive isolations.

Management

1. Symptomatic relief with wet dressings and Sitz baths (1 part Burrow's solution to 20 parts of water).

2. Ice bag applied to the lesion over a towel may give relief from pain.

3. Antibiotic ointment (bacitracin) to prevent secondary infection.

4. Urinary antiseptics and analgesics such as phenazopyridine hydrochloride (Pyridium) 200 mg. 3 times a day, may give relief from dysuria.

5. Percodan may be required for pain.

6. Hospitalization may be required for patients with extensive vulvovaginal lesions, pelvic lymphadenopathy, and fever.

7. Idoxuridine (Stoxil) applied locally may give relief from the acute symptoms.

8. Inoculation with smallpox vaccine has been used for the prevention of recurrent herpes but is not recommended.

9. Photodynamic inactivation gives symptomatic relief rapidly in 75 per cent of recurrent infections and almost all primary infections.

a. The technique is to apply neutral red dye 1-per-cent or proflurine 0.1-percent directly to the lesion.

b. The physician then exposes the area to light (using a 100- to 150-watt incandescent bulb) for 10 to 15 minutes.

c. The bulb is held about 6 inches from the lesion.

d. Exposure to the light is repeated in 6 to 8 hours and again in 24 hours.

10. The potential effect of producing defective oncogenic viruses in laboratory animals has been demonstrated. There is little evidence to indicate this side effect in humans.

11. The suspected association of cervical cancer and untreated genital herpesvirus 2 must be considered.

CONDYLOMA ACUMINATA (VENEREAL WARTS)

Definition

1. They are the visible manifestations of a viral venereal disease (venereal warts). Condyloma acuminata are the common form of vulvae papilloma but are granulomatous rather than true neoplasms.

2. The infecting agent of genital warts has been identified with the electron microscope as a papillomavirus.

Basic Principles

1. The lesion is usually pedunculated, and there is no induration around the base of the lesion.
2. No ulceration is seen as a rule, but when secondary infection is present, all the patterns of infection with polymorphs, plasma cells, and vascular proliferation may be seen below the epithelial layer.
3. The patient frequently gives a history of a sexual partner having a similar growth, but not always.
4. In most areas the growth becomes luxuriant. Discharge, secondary infection, and bleeding are common.
5. Genital warts seldom grow outside the genital-anal areas. They may spread into the rectum.
6. Monilia infection is seen more often with genital warts than without.
7. Poor personal hygiene seems to play some role in the female.
8. Pregnancy appears to act as a marked stimulus. Some grow so large that a Cesarean section is necessary.
9. Occasionally genital warts disappear spontaneously.

Diagnosis

1. Biopsy should be carried out. Concomitant vulvar cancer may be present.
2. Occasionally the diagnosis can be made by cytology.

Management

1. Podophyllin 25-per-cent is effective when applied to the condyloma acuminata.
   a. The surrounding skin must be carefully protected.
   b. Podophyllin should not be used in pregnancy.
2. Halogenated acetic acid (Nevitol) is effective when applied locally.
3. Triple sulfa cream locally has been reported to be effective.
4. Cryosurgery and hot cautery have been quite successful in eradicating condyloma acuminata.
5. Large condylomata may require surgery and in some instances even vulvectomy.
6. Cancer chemotherapy drugs (thiotepa, methotrexate, 5-fluorouracil cream and bleomycin) have not given a predictably good response.
7. Autogenous vaccines have been reported to be effective.

30. Acute and Chronic Pelvic Inflammatory Disease and Pelvic Tuberculosis

Hugh R. K. Barber, M.D.

DEFINITION

1. Pelvic inflammatory disease is a generalized term describing acute, subacute, recurrent, or chronic infections in the cervix, uterus, tubes, and ovaries, with or without involvement of adjacent supportive tissues as well as the peritoneum and intestines.

2. These infections may be bacterial, fungal, parasitic, or viral in origin.

3. Though commonly used as a diagnosis for any pelvic complaint, the term pelvic inflammatory disease should be replaced by specific descriptive terms as to the type of involvement and causative agent of the infection, if known.

NATURE AND MODE OF INFECTION

There are four causes and types of salpingitis:

1. Gonorrhea. Is an ascending infection which progresses up along the endometrial surface from the cervix to the tubes and peritoneum. Acute attack usually happens at the end of menstruation.

2. Puerperal and Postabortal Infection

a. Is nearly always hemolytic streptococcus, either alone or associated with staphylococcus or *E. coli*.

b. Occurs during the early stage of the uterine infection during the second or third week after labor.

c. Path of infection differs from gonorrhea insofar as it spreads by the lymphatics of the broad ligament and mesosalpinx to those of the tubal wall. It is truly a parametritis.

3. Direct Extension from Acute Pelvic Appendicitis. Infects the serous coat of the tube not the lumen.

4. Tuberculosis. Majority of cases are secondary to a tuberculosis infection of other organs.

BASIC MECHANISMS

1. Pelvic inflammatory disease is usually a problem of young and low-parity females.

2. Pelvic infection has always been a formidable problem in obstetrics and gynecology. With the present rapid rate of increase of venereal disease, this problem has become more formidable and widespread despite current advances in antibiotic therapy.

4. The most frequent cause of acute salpingitis is the gonococcus (*Neisseria gonorrhoeae*), the gram-negative intracellular diplococcus, which invades the pelvic adnexa by direct extension from the lower generative tract.

4. It is difficult to assess the true role of the gonococcus in the disease process because the patient may be asymptomatic initially.

5. With repeated contacts and reinfection or exacerbation, the disease process spreads throughout the reproductive system, crippling it in most cases.

6. In the adult, the method of transmission of the disease is usually sexual contact. In female children, direct nonsexual contamination may occur.

7. The incubation period is from 3 to 8 days and the organism primarily infects the urethra, Skene's ducts, the Bartholin glands, and the cervical glands. Recently there has been an increased incidence of pharyngitis and anal contamination.

8. The fallopian tubes and peritoneum may become involved later by direct extension, especially following the menstrual period.

9. Extension of the disease may take place through the blood stream and involve joints, the heart, meninges, and skin.

10. When acute salpingitis is diagnosed and treated in its early stages, the prognosis is excellent.

11. The patient as well as the consort should be reported to the Department of Health.

12. The organisms most commonly involved in pelvic infections are:

a. *Bacteria. N. gonorrhoeae, Streptococcus* sp., *staphylococcus, Escherichia, Proteus* sp., *Bacteroides, Aerobacter aerogenes, Pseudomonas aeruginosa, Mycobacterium tuberculosis.*

b. *Virus.* Myovirus (mumps).

c. *Parasite. Schistosoma haematobium, S. mansoni.*

d. *Fungus.* Actinomyces bovis, Blastomyces dermatitidis.

ACUTE SALPINGITIS

Basic Principles

1. Pain. Sudden, severe, in the hypogastrium.

2. Temperature. Raised to 102 to 103°F at onset. Is irregular and intermittent. May have chills.

3. Tachycardia is present.

4. Vomiting is not usual.

5. May occasionally have vaginal bleeding.

6. Foul-smelling discharge occurs and may pass tissue via the vagina.

7. In milder cases, the disease process usually subsides in from 4 to 7 days on going to bed.

8. Relapses on getting up too soon are very liable to occur.

9. At first there is extensive endosalpingitis with marked edema, hyperemia, and a heavy purulent discharge.

10. As the process extends, all layers of the tube are involved and pus escaping from the fimbriated end of the tube may result in frank pelvic peritonitis. If the tube is closed at its fimbriated end it may be grossly distended with pus and form a pyosalpinx.

11. Tubo-ovarian abscess is a frequent complication.

12. Drainage of pus out of the tube may become loculated by loops of bowel or mesentery, producing a pelvic abscess.

Orders

1. Bedrest
2. CBC
3. SMA-12
4. Urinalysis
5. Sedimentation rate
6. Measure intake and output
7. Chest radiograph
8. Flat plate of abdomen
9. Intravenous pyelogram and sonogram—optional
10. Smears from urethra, cervix, and anus for aerobic and anaerobic incubation and sensitivity studies
11. Blood cultures
12. Regular diet
13. Infusions as needed. May facilitate the antibiotic regimen.
14. Percodan q.3h. p.r.n. for pain
15. Mineral oil } 15 ml. of each per os at bedtime
16. Milk of magnesia } 15 ml. of each per os at bedtime

17. Dulcolax rectal suppositories as needed
18. To each 1,000 ml. I.V. fluid add 10 to 20 million units of penicillin.
19. If patient is sensitive to penicillin, administer sodium cephalothin, 2 to 4 g. as stat I.V. push, then 2 g. every 4 to 6 hours, totaling 12 to 24 g. per 24 hours.
20. Kanamycin sulfate, 1 g. daily added to penicillin or sodium cephalothin therapy
21. Chloramphenicol has been a valuable drug in doses of 4 to 6 g. per 24 hours. It can only be used as a last-resort drug because of its reported complications.
22. Change antibiotic therapy as indicated after cultures are reported.
23. Nasogastric tube, if indicated
24. Nasal oxygen, if indicated
25. Central venous pressure monitoring as indicated

Management

1. As outlined under orders
2. Cultures of cervix, urethra, and anus
3. Cul-de-sac aspirates
4. Fluids and antibiotics as outlined above
5. Semi-Fowler's position
6. Re-evaluate every 12 hours

CHRONIC SALPINGITIS WITH PELVIC INFLAMMATION

Basic Mechanisms

1. The acute inflammation process will subside into subacute or chronic stages either spontaneously or following treatment although there is marked tendency to repeated re-exacerbations.
2. Is often the result of pelvic inflammation which was inadequately treated and then complicated by the superimposed secondary invasion of other strains of bacteria. When this occurs the patient may be acutely ill.
3. The patient may have remarkably few symptoms.
   a. The chief disability is fatigue or pain following exertion. While the patient is resting there may be no symptoms.
   b. The symptoms usually associated with chronic salpingitis are: pain, menorrhagia, leukorrhea, dyspareunia, and sterility.
4. Abscess formation and pelvic peritonitis may complicate chronic salpingitis and then the clinical picture is similar to that seen in acute pelvic inflammatory disease.

Orders

As outlined for acute salpingitis.

Pelvic Abscess

1. If presenting in the posterior fornix, carry out wide colpotomy drainage.
2. Perform gentle digital exploration of cul-de-sac area to break down pockets of exudate.
3. Keep patient in the semi-Fowler's position.
4. Place adequate and large drains in the lateral pelvis and flanks, if possible.
5. Continue regimen as long as response is adequate.
6. If the condition deteriorates it may be necessary to do an exploratory laparotomy. The technique is covered below.
7. The mortality from ruptured tubo-ovarian abscess prior to 1950 was reported to be between 80 and 100 per cent. It has now been reduced to 6 per cent.

Ruptured Pelvic Abscess

1. Orders, fluids, and antibiotic therapy as outlined above
2. Aspirate pus by culdocentesis to serve as a guide to laparotomy.
3. Cultures for anaerobic and aerobic organisms
4. Remove only infected organs un-

less the infection is so widespread that more extensive surgery is necessary.

5. Explore above and below the liver and spleen to rule out pockets of exudate.

6. Run the small and large bowel to break up sacculations of pus.

7. Aspirate all obvious exudate.

8. Thoroughly wash the pelvis and abdomen with saline.

9. Secure hemostasis.

10. Use drains through vaginal cuff as well as through the right and left lower quadrants. The drains should be large.

11. Close abdomen with retention sutures.

12. Drain above and below the fascia.

13. Sepsis and septic shock are discussed in Chap. 17.

PELVIC TUBERCULOSIS

Basic Principles

1. The causative organism is the acid-fast tubercle bacillus.

2. Majority of the cases are secondary to a tuberculosis infection of other organs.

3. It may be transmitted through the bloodstream from a primary lesion in the lungs, kidney, or peritoneum. Rarely, it is transmitted by the husband who has tuberculosis of the genitourinary tract.

4. About 8 per cent of women dying of pulmonary tuberculosis are found postmortem to have tuberculosis of the genital tract.

5. The diagnosis is often made while investigating infertility problems.

a. The physician inadvertently discovers tubercular lesions in the endometrium by biopsy or curettage.

b. It is the cause of about 5 per cent or more of women seeking help in sterility clinics.

c. When tubercular lesions are found in the endometrium, it can be assumed that the patient has tuberculosis of the fallopian tubes.

6. Frequency of tuberculosis involvement of the various organs in genital tuberculosis is: tubes 90 to 100 per cent, uterus 50 to 60 per cent, ovaries 20 to 30 per cent, cervix 5 to 15 per cent, and vagina 1 per cent.

7. Frequency of presenting manifestations in female genital tuberculosis are: sterility 45 to 55 per cent, pelvic pain 50 per cent, poor general condition 26 per cent, menstrual disturbances 20 per cent, and vaginal discharge 4 per cent.

8. The patient is usually a young woman and the commonest complaints are primary infertility or abdominal pain and menstrual disturbances.

9. Genital tuberculosis has a reputation for appearing unexpectedly; but any woman with a complaint suggestive of pelvic inflammation, and especially if she is infertile, should be regarded with suspicion.

Physical Examination

1. Palpation of the abdomen may reveal a doughy sensation.

2. Ascites, either general or sacculated, may produce distention of the abdomen.

3. Irregular masses may be felt, caused by matting together of intestines, omentum, and pelvic organs.

4. On pelvic examination the tubes may not be palpable. May palpate a unilateral mass with the uterus displaced and tender. The mass is usually completely fixed and tender. The consistency of the mass is not uniform and both firm and fluctuant areas can be palpated.

Diagnosis

1. Symptoms as outlined above.

2. Histological evidence from endometrial curettings is the most easily obtained evidence.

a. When seen in the endometrium it is assumed that the tubes are also infected.

b. A negative report may indicate

that the infected area was missed, the biopsy was not taken at or during menstruation, and that the infection may not yet have spread from the tubes.

3. Bacteriological evidence should always be looked for and curettings sent for Ziehl-Neelsen staining, cultures, and guinea pig inoculation. Growth is slow and at least 6 weeks must be allowed.

4. Biopsy should be made of any ulcerated area in the cervix, vagina, or vulva.

5. If all findings are negative but clinical suspicion remains, a laparotomy or laparoscopy and biopsy of any infected area should be carried out.

6. Once evidence of genital infection is obtained, a search should be made for signs of active tuberculosis elsewhere, particularly in the respiratory and urinary tracts.

Aids in Diagnosis

1. X-ray. Chest radiograph

2. Tuberculin Test. Intracutaneous injection of first-strength purified protein derivative (PPD) on the flexor surface of the forearm. If after 48 hours the transverse diameter of edema and redness measures 10 mm. or more, the result is considered positive.

3. Hysterosalpingography. (Always Use a Water-Soluble Contrast Medium and Never Lipiodol or Other Oily Liquid)

a. The tubal lumen appearances are: rigid "pipe-stem," straight shadow, "fluffy" outline due to thickened mucosa, tube may be closed but often tuberculous tubes are open, signs of adhesions.

b. This test may be dangerous in the presence of active or secondary infection.

Management

1. Must first rule out extragenital tuberculosis.

2. Minimal genital tuberculosis is treated with isoniazid, 300 mg. daily, and ethambutol, 20 mg./Kg. or approximately 1,200 mg. daily.

3. At 6 and 12 months endometrial curettings or biopsies are examined bacteriologically. If negative, a hysterosalpingogram is done.

4. If curettings become positive or tubo-ovarian masses appear during treatment, rifampin, 600 mg. daily is added for 3 months, and the patient is subjected to laparotomy.

5. If no complications arise, isoniazid and ethambutol are continued for at least 2 years.

Management of Advanced Genital Tuberculosis

1. The regimen includes isoniazid, 300 mg. a day, ethambutol, 20 mg./Kg. or approximately 1,200 mg. a day.

2. Patients are re-examined every 4 weeks.

3. For the first 2 months most adnexal masses get smaller.

4. If tubo-ovarian masses are still present after 3 to 4 months of isoniazid and ethambutol therapy, laparotomy is indicated.

5. One week prior to laparotomy, streptomycin, 1 g./day I.M. is given and continued for 2 weeks after surgery.

6. Depending on whether or not residual tuberculosis foci are left in the abdomen, streptomycin administration may be continued twice weekly for a total of three months.

7. Isoniazid and ethambutol are continued postoperatively as they were before the operation.

8. Rifampin, 600 mg. daily, can be used in place of streptomycin.

Indications For Surgery

1. Antituberculosis drugs should be started immediately and administered for 3 to 4 months, following which removal of the tuberculous lesions is made easier.

2. Persistence or increase in size of

adnexal masses after a course of antituberculosis drugs as outlined above

3. Recurrence of endometrial tuberculosis after 1 year of antimicrobial therapy
4. Persistence of pelvic symptoms after long antituberculosis drug therapy
5. In patients over 40 years of age who will not continue long-term therapy or return for follow-up
6. Fistulas which fail to heal

Important Points In Management

1. Preoperative course of antituberculosis drugs is indicated.
2. Antituberculosis drugs should be given postoperatively for 18 months or longer.
3. Preoperative use of antituberculosis therapy makes the surgical procedure technically easier and reduces the risk of operative and postoperative complications.
4. Cure of genital tuberculosis is achieved more quickly with surgery than antituberculosis drugs alone.

ACUTE PELVIC PARAMETRITIS OF NONVENEREAL ORIGIN

Basic Principles

1. Parametritis is an inflammation of the parametrial tissue with cellular infiltration of the broad, cardinal, and uterosacral ligaments. Is described as being of ligneous consistency.
2. Infection travels directly by lymphatics and veins to the loose areolar tissue in the pelvis at the bases of the broad ligament and the sides of the uterus.
3. Factors predisposing to the development of parametritis are: surgical, including conization, cauterization, cervical biopsies, tubal insufflation, hysterosalpingography, dilatation, uterine sounding, and abortion.
4. Traumatic factors include coital trauma, postabortal or delivery laceration of the cervix, douche under high pressure, foreign body, and intrauterine device.
5. Patients become acutely ill and develop sustained fever (103°F) and rapid pulse. If there is associated thrombophlebitis, chills and a spiking temperature will also be noted.
6. Rectovaginal examination reveals thickening and tenderness in both fornices, and eventually a hard cellular infiltration of the uterosacral ligaments and parametria.
7. The WBC and sedimentation rate are elevated.

Management

1. Bedrest.
2. Antibiotic therapy. Type will depend on the organism cultured. Preliminary broad-spectrum antibiotic therapy should be started.
3. Activity and intercourse are contraindicated for at least one month.
4. Antibiotics should be continued for 2 to 4 weeks.
5. Surgery is indicated to manage abscess formation.

31. Fluid and Electrolyte Problems

Hugh R. K. Barber, M.D.

FLUIDS AND ELECTROLYTES

DEFINITIONS

1. **Basic Type Body Fluids.** The plasma, interstitial, and intracellular fluids consist of water, electrolytes, and protein.

2. **Electrolyte.** A substance that is capable of conducting an electric current when it is placed in a solution.

3. **Ions.** Electrolytes dissociated into electrically charged substances.

4. **Ionized Solution**

a. The ions that migrate to the negative electrode (cathode) of the cell have a positive charge and are called cations—i.e., Na^+, K^+, Ca^{++}, Mg^{++}.

b. The ions that migrate to the positive electrode (anode) of the cell have a negative charge and are called anions—i.e., Cl^-, HPO_4^{--}, SO_4^-, HCO_3^- (without equivalent base).

ACIDOSIS AND ALKYLOSIS

1. The hydrogen ion concentration determines whether a solution is acid or alkaline.

2. An increase in hydrogen ion concentration leads to an acid solution, whereas a decrease in hydrogen ion concentration leads to an alkaline solution.

3. There must always be an equal number of positively charged ions (cations) and negatively charged ions (anions) in a solution.

4. The hydrogen ion concentration (H^+), the ion that determines the acidity, will bear a direct relationship to the total anions present and a reciprocal relationship to the other cations present.

5. It is common usage (but not chemically correct) to associate base in terms of cations other than hydrogen.

6. Sodium (Na^+), potassium (K^+), magnesium (Mg^{++}), and calcium (Ca^{++}) are called bases.

a. They are called bases inasmuch as they replace, and are equivalent in electrical charge to, hydrogen ions in maintaining an equal balance of positive and negative ions.

b. Their presence in the body reduces the hydrogen ion (H^+) concentration.

7. Chloride (Cl^-), Phosophates (PO_4^{--}), Sulfates (SO_4^{--}), and much of the protein (proteinates) increase the hydrogen ion concentration and act as acids.

8. Although the hydrogen ion concentration per se in a liter of plasma is small, and the balance between cations and anions greatly influences the hydrogen ion concentration, in the final analysis it is the hydrogen ion concentration that determines acidity or alkalinity.

pH (POTENTIAL OF HYDROGEN)

The term *p*H (potential of hydrogen) is a simple way of representing hydrogen ion concentration.

1. $pH = -\log (H^+)$ or $pH = \log \frac{1}{H^+}$.

2. *p*H represents the negative logarithm of the hydrogen ion concentration.

3. As the hydrogen ion increases, the

pH decreases, and the solution contains more acid.

4. Conversely, as the hydrogen ion concentration falls, the pH rises, and the solution contains more alkali.

5. Normal plasma pH is 7.40, with a range of 7.38 to 7.42.

6. In strict chemical terms, the plasma with a pH of 7.4 is on the alkaline side.

Henderson-Hasselbalch Equation

1. $pH = pK + \log \frac{\text{salt}}{\text{acid}}$

2. It is possible to calculate any of the three unknown variables (pH, $NaHCO_3$, or H_2CO_3) if two are known by direct measurement.

3. At the normal pH of plasma (pH = 7.4) the relation of sodium bicarbonate (salt) to carbonic acid (acid) is $\frac{20}{1}$.

4. In metabolic imbalances of acidosis or alkalosis it is the numerator or salt value that is altered.

5. In respiratory imbalances of acidosis or alkalosis it is the denominator or acid value that is altered.

6. Diagrammatically shown:

a. Metabolic Acidosis

$$pH\downarrow = pK + \log \frac{\text{salt}\downarrow}{\text{acid}} \quad (pH\downarrow CO_2\downarrow)$$

b. Metabolic Alkalosis

$$pH\uparrow = pK + \log \frac{\text{salt}\uparrow}{\text{acid}} \quad (pH\uparrow CO_2\uparrow)$$

c. Respiratory Acidosis

$$pH\downarrow = pK + \log \frac{\text{salt}}{\text{acid}\uparrow} \quad (pH\downarrow CO_2\uparrow)$$

d. Respiratory Alkalosis

$$pH\uparrow = pK + \log \frac{\text{salt}}{\text{acid}\downarrow} \quad (pH\uparrow CO_2\downarrow)$$

7. If the $\frac{\text{salt}}{\text{acid}}$ ratio stays at $\frac{20}{1}$, the pH will remain at 7.4.

8. The pH does not depend on the total sodium bicarbonate or the total carbonic acid, but rather on the relative ratio of salt to acid.

9. Elevation of the sodium bicarbonate fraction without an increase in carbonic acid $\frac{NaHCO_3\uparrow}{HHCO_3}$ will result in an elevated pH and a metabolic alkalosis.

10. If the carbonic acid is elevated at the same time $\frac{(NaHCO_3\uparrow)}{HHCO_3\uparrow}$ as the sodium bicarbonate, and the ratio of $\frac{20}{1}$ is maintained, no change in pH will occur, and a compensated state will exist.

11. By the same token, a decrease in the sodium bicarbonate fraction without a decrease in carbonic acid $\frac{NaHCO_3\downarrow}{HHCO_3}$ will result in a decrease of pH.

12. If carbonic acid content is decreased at the same time as the sodium bicarbonate fraction $\frac{NaHCO_3\downarrow}{HHCO_3\downarrow}$ so that the $\frac{20}{1}$ is maintained, no change in pH will occur.

a. *Illustrated by Use of Formula for Metabolic Alkalosis*

$pH = 6.1 + \log \frac{27}{1.3} = 7.4$ Normal

$pH = 6.1 + \log \frac{36}{1.3} = 7.6$ Uncompensated

$pH = 6.1 + \log \frac{36}{1.8} = 7.4$ Compensated

Equivalent and Milliequivalent

1. It is the power to combine, and not the weight of an ion, that is important in body fluids.

2. The term equivalent, and, more specifically, the milliequivalent (mEq.) has been designated to represent the horsepower of a given electrolyte.

3. An equivalent, as the name implies, means equal to something. The hydrogen

ion (H^+), with a valence* of one has been used as the basis for comparison.

4. An equivalent is that weight of an element which has a combining or reacting value equal to one gram atom of hydrogen ion in change.

a. Milliequivalent is 1/1,000 of an equivalent.

5. $\text{Equivalent} = \frac{\text{atomic weight}}{\text{valence}}$

$\text{Equivalent (sodium)} = \frac{23}{1} = 23 \text{ g.}$

Milliequivalent (sodium) = 1/1,000 of an equivalent = 0.023 g. = 23 mg.

6. With divalent ions, such as calcium with a valence of two:

$\text{Equivalent (calcium)} = \frac{40}{2} = 20 \text{ g.}$

Milliequivalent (calcium) = 1/1,000 of an equivalent = 0.020 g. = 20 mg.

MOL

1. A mol is equal to the molecular weight of a substance.
2. It is independent of valence.
3. A millimol (mM.) is 1/1,000 of a mol.
4. Univalent ions (Na^+, Cl^-) have equal values for milliequivalent and millimol.
5. With divalent ions, millimol is twice the milliequivalent weight.
6. Examples

a. 1 milliequivalent of potasium (K^+) = 39 mg.

b. 1 millimol of potassium (K^+) = 39 mg.

c. 1 milliequivalent of calcium (Ca^{++}) = 20 mg.

d. 1 millimol of calcium (Ca^{++}) = 40 mg.

*Valence of an atom depends on how many atoms of hydrogen (H^+) it can combine with or displace. The monovalent atoms (Na^+, Cl^-) displace one atom of hydrogen, while the divalent atoms (Ca^{++}) displace two atoms of hydrogen.

OSMOL AND MILLIOSMOL

1. The unit of osmotic pressure is termed the osmol.
2. Like the milliequivalent, the milliosmol (mOsm.) is the final unit of measure.
3. Each substance exerts an osmotic effect.
4. Substances that dissociate give rise to dissociated ions, each producing an independent effect.
5. Valence is *not* considered in calculating milliosmols.
6. An equivalent of an univalent substance exerts a pressure of one osmol.
7. Divalent substances such as calcium (Ca^{++}) require two equivalents to produce a pressure of one osmol.

$$1 \text{ mOsm. calcium/liter} = \frac{10 \times 10}{40} = \frac{100}{40} = 2.5 \text{ mOsm.}$$

$$1 \text{ mEq. calcium/liter} = \frac{10 \times 10 \times 2}{40} = \frac{200}{40} = 5 \text{ mEq.}$$

8. A gram of sodium chloride produces a much greater osmotic pressure than a gram of glucose because of the larger number of particles in an ionized solution of the former.
9. One millimol of NaCl (58.5 mg.) in solution in one liter of water has a milliosmolar (mOsm.) effect of two milliosmols, one each for sodium (Na^+) and chloride (Cl^-). The following is an example:

a. 23 mg. Na per liter = 1 milliosmol per liter

35.5 mg. Cl per liter = 1 milliosmol per liter

58.5 mg. NaCl per liter = 2 milliosmols per liter

b. 39 mg. K per liter = 1 milliosmol per liter

35.5 mg. Cl per liter = 1 milliosmol per liter

74.5 mg. KCl per liter = 2 milliosmols per liter

c. 180 mg. of glucose per liter = 1 milliosmol per liter

d. 60 mg. of urea per liter = 1 milliosmol per liter

e. Milliosmolar concentration of 0.9-per-cent NaCl is

$$9 \text{ gm. NaCl per liter} = \frac{9000}{58.5}$$

= 154 mEq. Na^+
154 mEq. Cl^-
308 millosmoles

f. Milliosmolar concentration 5-per-cent glucose in water.
50 g. glucose per liter =

$$\frac{50000}{180} = 278 \text{ milliosmols}$$

10. Sugar and urea do not dissociate and only produce an osmotic effect equal to their molecular weight and concentration.

11. Therefore, in disease states, greatly increased concentrations of glucose and urea can raise the osmolarity of the extracellular water with its physiologic consequences.

12. One milliosmol/liter =

$$\frac{\text{mg. of substance or ion per liter}}{\text{atomic weight of substance or ion}}$$

$$\text{One mOsm./L.} = \frac{\text{mg. per 100 ml.} \times 10}{\text{atomic weight}}$$

DAILY BASELINE REQUIREMENT, EXTRARENAL LOSSES, DEFICITS OR EXCESSES

Basic Principles

1. Fluid and Electrolyte Replacement. The problem of fluid and electrolyte replacement resolves itself into three parts:

a. What are the normal daily baseline requirements?

b. What are the extrarenal losses?

c. What are the deficits or excesses that are present at the beginning of treatment?

2. Fluid Replacement

Daily baseline requirements represent the fluid and electrolyte needs for the day of an average patient who is being maintained on parenteral therapy and who has no abnormal losses, and has not had an excess or deficit present at the start of therapy.

Water Requirements

1. Insensible loss of 700 to 1,000 ml.
2. Urinary output of 800 to 1,500 ml.
3. Total water requirement of 1,500 ml. to 2,500 ml. This is replaced as 5-per-cent glucose and water.
4. Calculated on findings that the average adult requires 35 ml. of water per Kg. of body weight and the obese elderly female only requires 25 ml. per Kg. of body weight.

Electrolyte Requirements

1. Maximal need for sodium chloride is 77 mEq. Na^+ and 77 mEq. of Cl^-. It is supplied by administering 500 ml. of 0.9-per-cent sodium chloride.
2. Approximately 30 to 40 mEq. KCl (2 to 3 g. of KCl) supplies the daily baseline requirement. A urinary output of at least 1,000 ml. in 24 hours must be present before potassium can be added safely.

Calories

1. It is difficult to supply adequate calories with intravenous fluids. In short term replacement therapy it is not necessary.
2. By giving 100 g. of glucose (2,000 ml. 5-per-cent glucose and water) a day, the nitrogen loss of proteins is cut by 50 per cent. 100 g. of glucose can supply only about 400 calories per day.
3. The body can only utilize about 0.5 to 0.7 g. of glucose per Kg. of body weight per hour. An infusion of 5-per-cent glucose and water should not be run faster than 600 ml. per hour, if dehydration is to be prevented.

Vitamins

1. The average postoperative obstetrical and gynecological patient does not need intravenous vitamin supplements.
2. Vitamin B and C are water soluble and when given by the intravenous route are excreted in the urine in high concentrations.

Amino Acids

1. There are pratically no indications for the use of amino acids in the average postoperative obstetrical or gynecological patient. In the immediate postoperative period the enzyme systems are not working at maximum efficiency, and, as a result, the amino acid preparations are excreted at a rapid rate.
2. The reactions associated with protein hydrolysates make their use undesirable, unless they are absolutely needed.

Extrarenal Losses

Are those losses that are going on under observation; are replaced in kind, in amount, and at a rate equal to that at which they are lost; and are divided into external and internal losses.

1. External

a. Vomitus

b. Tube suction

c. Stomach—has a high concentration of chlorides

d. Small bowel—has a high concentration of bicarbonate

2. Surface Losses From Wounds

a. Groin dissection wounds, burns, exenterations, and abdominal perineal resections

b. The losses may be of sufficient magnitude to produce a severe electrolyte problem, especially in the elderly patient

c. Excessive sweating

d. Hemorrhage—must be replaced at the rate it is lost

3. Internal

a. Ileus

b. Peritonitis—resembles a third degree burn

c. Raw pelvic surface—as seen after radical hysterectomy, pelvic exenteration, or an abdominal perineal resection

Excesses and Deficits

1. Excess

a. Expanded extracellular space—may be seen in cirrhotics, cardiacs, and nephrotics

2. Deficit—Dehydration

a. *Rapid*—less than 48 hours in duration, as seen in acute obstruction or ileus. It involves mainly the extracellular space.

b. *Slow*—over a longer period than 48 hours; as seen in pregnancy, ileus, or large bowel obstruction.

It involves the intracellular, as well as the extracellular space.

Management

Replacement of Fluids and Electrolytes After Rapid Dehydration

1. Apply the empiric formula of H. T. Randall to determine fluid requirement.

$$\left(1 - \frac{\text{Normal hematocrit}}{\text{Found hematocrit}}\right) \times 20\% \text{ body weight in Kilograms.}$$

2. Hematocrit is obtained and is designated as the found hematocrit.
3. The normal hematocrit for women is usually 40.
4. The weight in Kg. is obtained by dividing the weight in pounds by 2.2.
5. The weight in Kg. is multiplied by 20% and equals the liters in the extracellular space.

i.e., 20% × 60 Kg. = 12 liters.

6. Assume that a 60 Kg. female is admitted with a diagnosis of acute obstruction and a history of vomiting for 12 hours.

a. Hematocrit on admission is 60 (found hematocrit).

7. By *application of the formula*:

a. $1 - \frac{\text{Normal hematocrit}}{\text{Found hematocrit}} \times 20\%$ body weight in Kg.

$1 - 40/60 \times 20\%$ of 60

$1 - \frac{2}{3} \times 12$ L. $\quad (\frac{3}{3} - \frac{2}{3} = \frac{1}{3})$

$\frac{1}{3}$ of $12 = 4$ L. deficit

b. Inasmuch as the deficit is 4 L. and the patient normally has a 12 L. extracellular space, there are only 8 L. present.

c. 4 liters must be replaced

8. The electrolyte content of the replaced fluid is determined as follows:

a. A serum chloride is obtained.

b. Assume it is returned as 90 mEq./L. and the laboratory normal is 100 mEq./L.

c. The amount of electrolytes to be replaced is worked out as follows:

(1) The value should be:

12 L $\times$ 100 mEq. Cl = 1,200 mEq. Cl^-

(2) The actual value is:

8 L. $\times$ 90 mEq. Cl = 720 mEq. Cl^-

(3) Therefore the deficit is:

480 mEq. of Cl^-

d. In each 1,000 cc. bottle of 0.9-per-cent saline there are 154 mEq. Na^+ and 154 mEq. Cl^-.

e. To find the amount of saline to give, divide: 480/154 = 3.1 L.

f. Of the 4-liter deficit in the extracellular space, 3.1 L. must be replaced as saline or saline and glucose.

g. This leaves 900 ml. that must be replaced as glucose and water.

h. The daily requirement consists of:

(1) Daily baseline requirement:

1,000 ml. 5-per-cent g/w

500 ml. 5-per-cent g/s

1,000 ml. 5-per-cent g/w

40 mEq. KCl—If urinary output is over 1,000 cc.

(2) Extrarenal losses.

(3) Deficit.

HELPFUL HINTS IN MANAGEMENT OF FLUID AND ELECTROLYTE PROBLEMS

Fluid and Electrolyte Imbalance

1. A high sodium level is almost invariably associated with dehydration.

2. Normal adults maintained exclusively on intravenous fluids lose 200 to 300 g. a day.

3. The maximum amount of water that the kidney can excrete is about 15 ml. per minute—or 900 ml. per hour.

4. 500 ml. of citrated whole blood transfused to an adult will raise the hemoglobin about one g. or 7 per cent.

5. Ten per cent of the total body weight can be lost before clinical signs of dehydration start to become obvious.

6. At first, salicylate poisoning gives rise to a state of respiratory alkalosis; if untreated, it leads to a metabolic acidosis.

7. The patient who complains of restlessness, fatigue, dizziness, chest pain, numbness, tingling, and syncope, particularly when under stress, may be suffering from a hyperventilation syndrome.

8. The administration of excessive amounts of intravenous sodium may give rise to hoarseness.

9. The normal urinary flow is 50 to 100 ml. per hour. In treating dehydration a urinary output of about 40 ml. per hour indicates that the dehydration is being corrected.

10. A low serum potassium level means a low cellular, as well as a low extracellular level, whereas a high serum level does not necessarily mean that a high cellular level is present.

11. To each 1,000 ml. of replacement fluid for gastric or small bowel losses, add 20 mEq. of potassium chloride.

12. Every seriously ill surgical patient who is being maintained on intravenous fluids should be weighed daily, and an accurate intake and output record kept.

13. An intravenous solution of 5-percent glucose and saline is hypertonic and should be given at a rate no faster than 300 ml. per hour if dehydration resulting from excess diuresis is to be prevented.

14. Inasmuch as the body is only able to metabolize about half a gram of glucose per Kg. of body weight per hour (0.5 g. × Kg. per hour), it is important to administer an intravenous 5-per-cent glucose and water solution at a rate no faster than 600 ml. per hour, if dehydration is to be prevented.

15. It is important to administer plasma in cases of peritonitis, and also to guard against calcium deficiency, which may occur in these cases.

16. There are times in which the electrolyte imbalance is not appreciated and incorrect therapy is given.

Examples:

a. The use of antibiotics for dehydration fever.

b. The use of the Miller-Abbott for intestinal distention that is secondary to a low serum potassium.

c. Cardiovascular disease or heart failure is often diagnosed when a salt depletion syndrome is actually present.

17. Never give sodium lactate* in the presence of:

a. Liver disease
b. Shock
c. Anoxia
d. Cardiac decompensation
e. Respiratory alkalosis

18. All electrolyte problems are caused by:

a. Disturbance of volume
b. Disturbance of osmotic pressure
c. Disturbance of *p*H

19. The average adult intake of sodium is about 100 mEq. per day and almost all of it is excreted in 1,000 ml. to 1,500 ml. of urine.

20. An early ileus may be detected by noting a decrease in the output with an increase in urine specific gravity.

21. Early in septic shock arterial blood gases frequently reveal a mild respiratory alkalosis.

22. Central venous pressure (CVP) monitoring measures only the function of the right side of the heart.

23. Studies have shown the superiority of pulmonary artery pressure (PAP) and pulmonary wedge pressure (PWP) monitoring by means of a Swan-Ganz catheter over the CVP as an index of left ventricular competence.

24. Pulmonary artery pressure (PAP) and left atrial wedge pressure. Any rise in either pressure is a sign of early pulmonary insufficiency.

25. Following the successful control of septic shock, the patient may develop acute respiratory distress syndrome (shock lung, wet lung of World War II).

26. Therapy of the acute respiratory distress syndrome (shock lung, wet lung of World War II) should include volume-cycled ventilation with "PEEP" (positive end expiratory pressure) as well as frequent higher-dose albumin and lasix. Careful digitalization, if not already accomplished, should be considered to improve enotropic status.

27. Patients in labor who receive general anaesthesia should be given antacids preoperatively.

28. A low p_{O_2} and p_{CO_2} are nearly constant findings in acute pulmonary embolism and if there is a normal p_{O_2} it is possible to rule out pulmonary embolism shock.

29. Patients with massive pulmonary embolism shock will benefit from immediate and total heparinization.

30. The lifesaving capabilities of intravenous hyperalimentation have been confirmed in many clinical studies—in-

*Ringer's injection rather than lactated Ringer's injection has been widely employed in these situations.

testinal (fistulas), renal, and hepatic disease; severe burns and trauma; cancer; congenital malformations; prematurity.

ILEUS

Definition

Obstruction of the intestines.

Types of Ileus

1. Adynamic—inhibition of bowel motility, which may be produced by many causes—i.e., peritonitis.

2. Dynamic—related to mechanical obstruction.

Ileus versus mechanical obstruction: Ileus is probably one of the most frequent complications seen in the postoperative period following gynecological surgery or Cesarean section. It may vary in severity from mild distention to a full-blown picture of paralytic ileus, with its accompanying electrolyte, water, and acid-base imbalance. It is extremely important to make certain that the problem is one of paralytic ileus and *not* one of mechanical small bowel obstruction. Although the fluid and electrolyte replacement may be the same, the definitive approach to the underlying problem is different.

Basic Principles

Ileus is most often preceded by a diminution in urine volume. Fluids and electrolytes collect in the intestines. The extracellular fluid is therefore decreased, and this in turn leads to a decrease in glomerular filtration, with a drop in the urinary output.

1. Vomiting and distention occur on the second or third day after an operation or following a traumatic delivery.
2. Vomitus is first mucus, then bile, and later altered blood.
3. Constipation is the rule.
4. Abdomen rapidly distends with gas.
5. Peristalsis is absent.
6. Bowel sounds are absent.
7. Pain is usually absent, but if present, is never colicky.
8. Patient becomes dehydrated.
9. Pulse becomes rapid.
10. Respiratory rate, temperature, and leukocyte count rise.
11. Urinary output drops.
12. Patient gets toxic.
13. Flat plate of abdomen shows:
    a. Gas-distended loop and multiple fluid levels in the small bowel.
    b. A little gas may be present in cecum and pelvic colon.
14. Must be differentiated from a mechanical obstruction. Four cardinal symptoms of mechanical intestinal obstruction:
    a. Colicky Abdominal Pain—intermittent, comes on suddenly, reaches a peak and subsides. Auscultation at time of pain reveals loud, metallic, high-pitched peristaltic rushes. Most important difference from ileus.
    b. Vomiting—frequent and copious
    c. Distention
    d. Obstipation

Changes Caused by Ileus

A full-blown ileus gives rise to changes in the bowel, kidney, and lung function. This is demonstrated as follows:

1. Intestines

a. Fluids and electrolytes pour into the intestines.

b. The extracellular fluid is decreased in direct proportion to that lost to the intestines.

c. Hematocrit, hemoglobin, and plasma protein concentration reflect this shift by showing an increase in concentration in the intravascular compartment of the extracellular space. (Hct. increases, Hgb. increases, protein increases.)

d. The loss of fluids to the intestine leads to dehydration, which decreases glomerular filtration and may be followed by vasomotor instability.

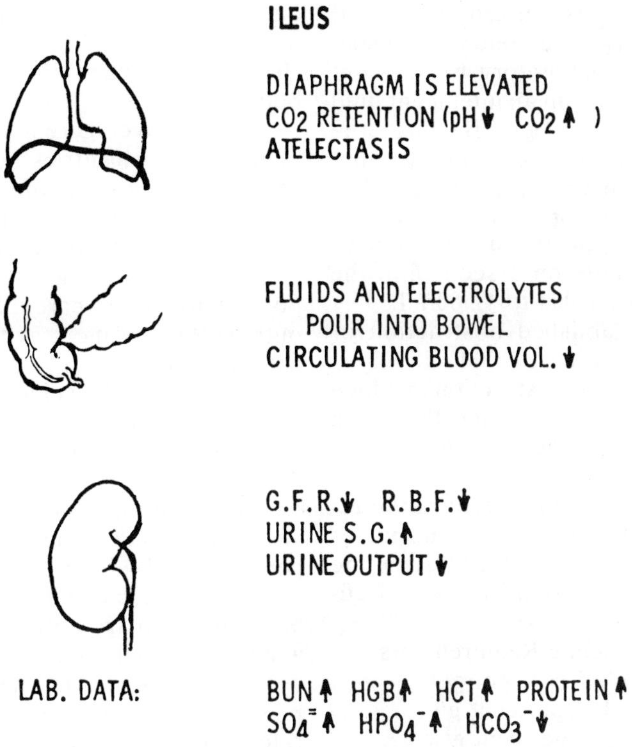

Fig. 31-1. Changes caused by ileus.

2. Kidneys

a. Glomerular filtration rate (GFR) is decreased secondary to the diminished extracellular fluid and to the abdominal distention.

b. Urinary output is decreased. It may occur before the problem of ileus is appreciated. This indicates the importance of following the daily urine output as well as the specific gravity of urine.

c. Specific gravity of the urine is increased.

d. The decreased glomerular filtration leads to an elevation of the urea nitrogen, sulfates, and phosphates. This will increase and aggravate the metabolic acidosis that is present.

3. Lungs

a. The diaphragm is elevated secondary to the abdominal distention.

b. Carbon dioxide retention occurs secondary to the elevated diaphragm and causes a respiratory acidosis.

c. Atelectasis may occur.

Management

1. The replacement of fluids and electrolytes that have been lost by vomiting, or that collect in the intestines during the development of an ileus, is usually an easy matter. The use of the empiric formula

$$\left(1 - \frac{\text{Normal hematocrit}}{\text{Found hematocrit}}\right) \times 20\%$$

body weight in kilograms suggested by Randall provides a useful guide in evaluating the deficit that must be replaced. In addition, the daily baseline requirements and extrarenal losses must also be supplied. Although a decreased red cell mass, such as follows Cesarean section, causes the formula to lose some of its value, it still serves a useful purpose if the daily weight, urine volume, and specific gravity and laboratory findings are evaluated in setting up an intelligent fluid and electrolyte regimen. Because the daily baseline losses are recorded, only the deficit remains to be corrected. The deficit can be estimated as follows:

a. By the time the obstruction or ileus is identifiable on a scout film the deficit is at least 1,000 to 1,500 ml.

b. Well-established obstruction or ileus—deficit is at least 3,000 ml.

c. In an ileus or obstruction in which the pulse rate is elevated and there is a drop in the blood pressure—deficit may be 4,000 to 6,000 ml.

2. Outline for fluid and electrolyte replacement (following plan set up under appendix dealing with Daily Baseline Requirement, Extrarenal Losses, Deficits or Excesses).

a. Daily Baseline Requirements

1,000 ml. 5-per-cent g/w
500 ml. 5-per-cent g/s
1,000 ml. 5-per-cent g/w

plus 40 mEq. KCl, if urinary output is 1,000 ml. or over in 24 hours.

b. Extrarenal Losses—represent the losses from vomiting or tube aspiration. These losses are replaced in kind, according to the level in the gastrointestinal tract from which they are lost and in an amount equal to that lost. (See under deficit.) 20 mEq. KCl is added for each 1,000 ml. of replacement, but only if the urinary output is 1,000 ml. in 24 hours.

c. Deficit

This is replaced by supplying fluid and electrolytes similar to those found in the small intestine. (See chapter on Fluid and Electrolyte Imbalance.) The amount can be calculated from the formula

$$\left(1 - \frac{\text{Normal hematocrit}}{\text{Found hematocrit}}\right) \times 20\%$$

body weight in kilograms or can be judged from the response of the patient to replacement as well as the urinary output, its reaction, and specific gravity.

d. Total fluids replaced in 24 hours should *not* exceed 10 per cent of the body weight.

e. The average early case of ileus occurring in obstetrics and gynecology can be handled by giving the daily baseline requirements, replacing vomitus or intestinal aspirate as described.

f. In treating these cases, it is important to follow carefully the urinary output, the specific gravity, and the reaction of the urine.

g. A metabolic acidosis with accompanying hypotension that cannot be explained points to an intra-abdominal catastrophe.

h. A fixed specific gravity near 1.010 and a low urinary output points to impending renal failure.

i. A specific gravity of 1.028 to 1.030 and a low urinary output indicates that a state of dehydration exists.

j. Acid urine in the presence of plasma alkalosis (elevated CO_2 and chlorides below normal) indicates that more potassium is needed.

k. Alkaline urine with normal plasma potassium and adequate potassium replacement indicates that more saline is needed. This is based on the assumption that there is no urinary tract infection present and that the specimen tested is a fresh specimen. A urinary tract infection caused by a urea-spliting organism gives rise to alkaline urine.*

CHRONIC SHOCK

Definition

Chronic shock is a metabolic imbalance characterized by reduced blood volume as well as protein deficiency.

*The presence of a urinary tract infection can be determined by culture or by an analysis of the ammonia content of alkaline urine. Ammonia is not normally excreted by the kidney when there is alkaline urine. Ammonia present in alkaline urine indicates the presence of a urea-splitting organism.

Basic Principles

1. Hemoglobin and hematocrit may be normal despite the markedly decreased blood volume. There are two important reasons for this:

a. The volume may vary independently from the concentration of substances within a given volume, or the decrease in volume may parallel the decrease in the concentration of substances.

b. There may be a compensatory vasoconstriction working, which reduces the area containing the volume as well as the concentration of substances in that volume.

2. Clinical states in which chronic shock is seen:

a. Bleeding submucous fibroids

b. Intermittent and prolonged bleeding in placenta previa

c. Poor nutrition

d. Carcinoma

3. Review of normal values of red cell mass, plasma volume, and total blood volume:

a. *Normal Blood Volume*—represents 7 to 8.5 per cent of body weight in Kg.

60 Kg. × 7% = 4.2 L. or 4,200 ml.

b. *Normal Red Cell Mass*—represents 3 to 4 per cent of body weight in Kg.

60 Kg. × 3% = 1.8 L. or 1,800 ml.

c. *Plasma Volume*—roughly 4.5 per cent of body weight in Kg.

60 Kg. × 4.5% = 2.7 L. or 2,700 ml.

Application to Clinical Problem

The ideal blood volume, red cell mass, and plasma volume are calculated from these figures after corrections are made for obesity, age, sex, and weight loss. The values obtained are compared with the actual values reported by the laboratory. By this approach an abnormality in the blood volume can be found and corrected.

Examples

1. Age and Sex

a. The average female under 50 years of age has a red cell mass of 32.6 ml ± 4 ml. per Kg. of body weight. Beyond the age of 50 the red cell mass is 28.6 ± 3 ml. per Kg. of body weight.

2. Weight

a. *Obesity*. The obese patient has a lower blood volume than would be expected for her weight. The amount of obese weight over ideal weight increases the blood volume by one-fourth of that expected on a weight basis. This is shown as follows:

(1) If the ideal weight is 120 and the patient weighs 140, the obese weight is 20 pounds.

(2) ¼ × 20 (obese weight) = 5 pounds.

(3) The ideal weight in calculating the blood volume is 120 pounds plus 5 pounds = 125 pounds. It is this weight that is used to calculate the blood volume.

3. Weight Loss

a. If the weight loss has occurred over a period of less than 2 months, the original weight is used.

b. If the weight loss has occurred over a period of 2 to 6 months, the present weight plus one-half of the weight loss is used.

c. If the weight loss has occurred over a period of 6 months to a year, the present weight plus one-fourth of the weight loss is used.

d. If the weight loss has occurred over a 1-year period, the present weight is used.

e. Application.

(1) A female who has lost weight over a 6-month period

(2) The original weight was 160 pounds, and her present weight is 140 pounds. The weight loss is 20 pounds.

(3) 20 pounds (weight loss) × ½ = 10 pounds.

(4) 140 pounds plus 10 pounds = 150 pounds.

(5) This is the weight that should be used in calculating the blood volume.

4. Explanation

Blood volume contracts continually to keep pace with the weight that is being lost.

The weight loss is not obese weight but is loss from the ideal weight.

5. Application

a. The ideal blood volume, plasma volume, and red cell mass for a 53-year-old female who has not lost weight nor is obese for height, can be determined as follows:

(1) 60 Kg. × 28.6 ml./Kg. = 1,716 ml. red cell mass

(2) 60 Kg. × 4.5% body weight = 2,700 ml. plasma volume

(3) Total blood volume 4,416 ml.

(4) If the actual calculations are reported from the laboratory as:

(a) 1,200 ml. red cell mass

(b) 2,300 ml. plasma volume

Then:

	Red Cell Mass	*Plasma Volume*	*Total Blood Volume*
Ideal values	1,716 ml.	2,700 ml.	4,416 ml.
Actual values	1,200 ml.	2,300 ml.	3,500 ml.
Deficit	516 ml.	400 ml.	916 ml.

6. Conclusions

Inasmuch as each 500 ml. of whole blood contains about 225 ml. of red cell mass, it would require about two and one-half transfusions of 500 ml. each to restore the red cell mass to normal values as determined by the above calculations. It is important to restore the values to normal before major surgery is undertaken.

Alternate Approach

1. The hospital may not have the facilities for carrying out blood volume determinations. In a patient suspected of having a contracted blood volume, it is possible to evaluate her response to transfusions by the use of serial hematocrits.

2. If the clinical history and physical examination suggest that the blood volume is decreased, a transfusion can be given and the result evaluated in 24 hours by the hematocrit. A hematocrit change in the range of 0.5 to 2 per cent indicates that more blood is needed, whereas a hematocrit change of 3 to 6 per cent indicates that the blood volume has been restored to normal. It is important to make certain that the patient is in a state of normal hydration.

3. Graphically, this is shown as follows:

Total Blood Volume	*Red Cell Mass*	*Hematocrit*	*Per Cent of Change*
4,000 ml.	2,000 ml.	35	—
500 ml.*	225 ml.		
4,500 ml.	2,225 ml.	36.2	1.2%
500 ml.*	225 ml.		
5,000 ml.	2,450 ml.	39.8	3.6%
500 ml.*	225 ml.		
5,000 ml.	2,675 ml.	44.0	4.2%

*Transfusion

Explanation

It has been shown that the vascular compartment contracts and adjusts to a smaller volume. However, the vascular compartment resists overexpansion after transfusions have restored the blood volume to normal. Further transfusions will cause the red cell mass to expand, and at the same time the plasma portion will be dispersed from the vascular compartment. This supplies an explanation for the hematocrit changes found after giving a transfusion. In the above illustration the blood volume was restored to normal after the second transfusion, and the next transfusion did not change the total blood volume. The red cell mass expanded at the expense of the plasma portion, which is dispersed from the vascular compartment. The hematocrit takes about 18 to 24 hours to stabilize after a transfusion has been given.

Protein Replacement

Transfusions are not a good way to replace protein deficiency. Because each 100 ml. of blood contains only 7 g. of protein, a transfusion of 500 ml. supplies only 35 g. of protein. A patient whose blood protein determination is found to be 5 g. per 100 ml. is deficient 2 g. per 100 ml. of extracellular fluid. The extracellular fluid in a patient who weighs 70 Kg. is 14 L. (20% × 70 Kg. body weight = 14 L. or 14,000 ml. extracellular fluid). In such a patient, the deficit of extracellular protein then would be 14,000/100 = 140 × 2 or 280 g. of protein. Since each transfusion of 500 ml. of blood supplies only 35 g. of protein, in order to replace the protein deficit in the extracellular fluid alone, it would be necessay to give 8 transfusions.

PERITONITIS

Definition

An inflammation of the peritoneum; a condition marked by exudation of serum, fibrin, cells, and pus in the peritoneum.

Basic Principles

1. Peritonitis may occur from many causes, such as a ruptured tubo-ovarian abscess, ruptured viscus, ruptured ovarian cyst, or bacterial contamination.

2. The electrolyte, water, and acid-base problems that arise during the development of peritonitis parallel closely the problems encountered in the treatment of burn cases. The patient with peritonitis usually pours plasma, proteins, water, and electrolytes into the affected area. This gives rise to a depletion of the blood volume, with its unstable vasomotor response, shock, and diminution of glomerular filtration.

3. Although antibiotics may control or alter the signs and symptoms and check the septicemia that so often accompanies peritonitis, an alteration in fluid and electrolyte imbalance still occurs.

Diagnosis

1. Initial stages depend upon the mode of infection.

2. Temperature is elevated.

3. A most important sign of pelvic peritonitis following operation is a pulse that is more rapid than would be expected from the amount of temperature elevation.

4. Once peritonitis is established, the picture is characteristic.

5. Pain spreads with the spread of infection.

6. Vomiting is usual.

7. Constipation is more common than diarrhea.

8. The patient lies motionless and supine, most often with legs drawn up.

9. Expression is anxious and face is drawn.

10. Abdominal muscles over the inflamed site are tightly contracted.

11. In diffuse peritonitis, the whole abdomen is rigid, wooden, and motionless; there is no movement of the abdomen with respiration.

12. Paralytic ileus.

a. Result of direct paralysis of Auerbach's plexus.

Management

1. Because peritonitis resembles a 15- to 30-per-cent third-degree body burn, the basic principles suggested by Evans for fluid and plasma protein replacement in burn cases can be adapted to the patient who has peritonitis. Evans administered 1 ml. of colloid (plasma) and 1 ml. of crystalloid (isotonic saline) per kilogram per cent of body burn, or more

specifically in these cases, as per per cent peritonitis. In applying this concept to replacement therapy in a 60 kilogram female with pelvic peritonitis, we have:

a. 60 Kg. × 15% (pelvic peritonitis) = 900 ml. colloid. 60 Kg. × 15% (pelvic peritonitis) = 900 ml. isotonic saline.

This represents extrarenal loss, and if it has been present for a few days prior to therapy, it may also represent deficit.

2. Fluid Regimen

a. *Daily Baseline Requirements*

1,000 ml. 5-per-cent g/w
500 ml. 5-per-cent g/s
1,000 ml. 5-per-cent g/w

Need for potassium will be based on serum findings as well as the urinary findings.

b. *Extrarenal Losses*

Represent the abnormal losses that are going on under observation. Kilogram body weight × per cent of peritonitis = amount of colloid. Kilogram body weight × per cent of peritonitis = amount of crystalloid.

c. *Excesses and Deficit*

Calculated as indicated if the process has been going on for more than 24 hours.

d. Calcium gluconate as needed.

e. Continue regimen until peritonitis is controlled.

f. As the peritonitis resolves, fluids and electrolytes will be absorbed back into the extracellular space.

g. The clinician must be prepared to supply an extracellular space during the time that fluid and plasma proteins are lost to the site of peritonitis and be prepared to withhold fluids during the time that the third space is resolving.

h. In addition to fluids and electrolyte replacement, the patient should be given the benefit of antibiotics, oxygen, surgery, or any supportive therapy deemed necessary at this time.

Treatment

Four Essentials of Therapy

1. Nothing by mouth
2. Levin, Cantor, or Miller-Abbott tube connected to continuous suction
   a. Measure intake and output and record.
3. Maintain fluid and electrolyte balance.
4. Antibiotic regimen (early and in adequate dosage) Gentamicin up to 1.6 mg./Kg. I.M./I.V. 3 times a day Ampicillin 2 g. I.M./I.V. 4 times a day
   a. If anaerobes are present, add clindamycin 300 mg. I.M. 3 times a day.
   b. In the critically ill patient there is justification for administering ampicillin and Chloromycetin 1 g. in the volutrol every 6 hours for 2 days and then drop the dose to 500 mg. q.6h.

32. Acidosis and Alkalosis

Hugh R. K. Barber, M.D.

BASIC PRINCIPLES

1. Acidosis and alkalosis are not diseases in themselves, but chemical states that are seen in a wide variety of diseases.

2. Clinically, the terms acidosis and alkalosis represent a shift from normal of the hydrogen ion concentration of the plasma, and therefore of the cells.

3. Acidosis and alkalosis may be further subdivided into either metabolic or respiratory. Both may originate from either internal errors in metabolism or externally introduced substances or physical circumstances such as medication, anesthesia, or pneumothorax.

4. There are four basic types of *p*H change: metabolic acidosis, metabolic alkalosis, respiratory acidosis, and respiratory alkalosis.

5. The diagnosis of an acute change is dependent on history and clinical observation of the patient. Its type may be revealed by chemical analysis of the plasma, particularly by plasma *p*H.

6. As compensations take place, alterations in the major electrolytes of the plasma, the *p*H and sometimes electrolytes of the urine, changes in the electrocardiogram, and the presence of abnormal substances in the urine assist substantially in making the diagnosis.

7. The *p*H of the blood or plasma represents one of the most important laboratory determinations since it measures directly the hydrogen ion concentration and the direction as well as the degree of change from normal.

8. CO_2 content, chloride determination, sodium, potassium, and other anions contribute further information to assist in diagnosis.

9. There are buffers in the plasma. In addition, the hemoglobin of the red cells buffers the change in *p*H of the plasma. It does so by the chloride shift as follows:

a. The HCO_3 of the plasma and red blood cells decreases.

b. The chloride content of the red blood cells increases.

c. The chloride content of the plasma decreases.

d. The total fixed cation content of the red blood cells does not change.

e. The water content and volume of the red blood cells decrease.

f. These changes occur in the reverse direction in the capillaries of the tissues.

10. The extravascular buffering that is associated with the movement of K^+ into and out of the ECF with changes in *p*H is probably of the most importance clinically.

METABOLIC ALKALOSIS ($pH\uparrow$ $CO_2\uparrow$)

Etiology

1. The plasma bicarbonate must be primarily elevated. This may be brought about by:

a. Ingestion or infusion of $NaHCO_3$

b. Inappropriate retention of bicarbonate by the kidney, which often occurs in potassium deficit

c. Vomiting in a person who produces HCl in stomach secretions and therefore loses HCl and chlorides

BASIC PRINCIPLES

1. Metabolic alkalosis is a state of decreased hydrogen ion concentration (pH ↑ $NaHCO_3$ ↑) owing to causes other than hyperventilation.

2. It occurs when there is either an increase in base from exogenous sources, a loss of anion (other than HCO_3) in excess of base, or a loss of potassium ion.

3. Addition of excess alkali usually results from the ingestion of large amounts of sodium bicarbonate by patients suffering from peptic ulcer or gastric neuroses. It may be iatrogenic from excessive administration of sodium bicarbonate or lactate.

4. In surgery the commonest cause of metabolic alkalosis is the loss of chloride by vomiting or gastric suction.

a. In the stomach the chloride ion exceeds sodium by a ratio of 3:2 in the normal resting state, and may rise as high as 4:1, with chloride concentrations of up to 150 mEq. per liter.

b. As much as 2,500 ml. gastric juice may be lost in 24 hours, although the average gastric suction in unobstructed cases is usually around 1,000 ml.

c. Even larger volumes may be lost when small bowel content is regurgitated into the stomach.

5. With the excess intake of bicarbonate, 67 per cent of the bicarbonate remains in the extracellular fluid (ECF). Most of the remainder is buffered by H^+ moving out of cells in exchange for Na^+.

a. A small amount of bicarbonate is converted to H_2CO_3 by the production of lactic acid. The H_2CO_3 is then dissociated to CO_2 and H_2O, and the CO_2 blown off by the lung.

b. K^+ probably moves into cells in metabolic alkalosis.

6. Potassium deficiency is now widely recognized as a complication of surgical illness and its management.

a. Potassium cannot be completely conserved by the kidneys and normal dietary intake of 60 to 90 mEq. must be supplied to surgical patients who are unable to ingest potassium-containing food.

b. In addition, potassium losses increase with the alarm response, and frequently large amounts are lost extrarenally from the gastrointestinal tract and through wounds.

c. Alkalosis from other causes results in a shift of potassium intracellularly and also in an increased renal loss, so that plasma levels fall. The plasma level, however, is not a reliable index of the total potassium loss.

d. As potassium is lost, there develops an alkalosis which is characterized by an elevated CO_2, a moderately decreased chloride, a low-normal to low serum potassium level, and a relatively normal sodium. The urine in this condition is acid. The alkalosis does not respond to the administration of NaCl or NH_4Cl but only to potassium administration.

7. Mixed hypochloremic and hypokalemic alkalosis eventuates in many patients, particularly those who are on parenteral fluids without potassium for more than 3 or 4 days, and especially if they are subjected to upper gastrointestinal tract drainage.

a. Often a patient on gastric drainage will start off with chloride loss, mild alkalosis, and with sodium chloride replacement, an alkaline urine.

b. After 2 to 4 days of this, the alkalosis will increase despite adequate sodium chloride replacement, and the urine will become acid.

c. Only the additional administration of potassium will correct the alkalosis.

8. The alkalotic hypokalemic patient is hypersensitive to digitalis and great caution must be exercised in its use.

MAJOR PLASMA ELECTROLYTE IMBALANCES AND URINARY CHANGES OCCURRING IN METABOLIC ALKALOSIS

Basic Principles

1. Metabolic alkalosis is a state of decreased hydrogen ion concentration (pH ↑ $NaHCO_3$ ↑) owing to causes other than hyperventilation.

2. It occurs when there is an increase in base (i.e., Na^+) from exogenous sources, when there is loss of anion (i.e., Cl^-) in excess of base, or in potassium-deficient state.

Compensation

1. Dilution. Extracellular fluid space is increased due to the alkali load.

2. All alkali above 27 mEq./L. of $NaHCO_3$ is excreted by the kidneys.

3. Potassium leaves extracellular fluid and goes into the cells or is excreted by the kidney.

4. If potassium is not replaced, an increased amount of alkali is reabsorbed by the tubules. A metabolic alkalosis with acid urine results.

5. Acid urine results are secondary to the alteration in the $\frac{KHCO_3}{HHCO_3}$ buffer system in the cell. The numerator ($KHCO_3$) is decreased, but the denominator ($HHCO_3$) is not changed. The hydrogen ion concentration in the cell increases and the kidney is stimulated to absorb bicarbonate in larger amounts. $\frac{KHCO_3\downarrow}{HHCO_3}$ = more acid intracellular environment.

6. Respiratory compensations do not occur. If they did, the $HHCO_3$ fraction of the equation would increase, and bicarbonate reabsorption would be elevated. The renal compensations would be ineffectual.

Management

1. Correct underlying disease state causing the imbalance.

2. Rehydrate.

3. Replace gastric losses in equal volume to that vomited or aspirated as:

a. ⅔ in the form of 5-per-cent glucose and saline

b. ⅓ in the form of 5-per-cent glucose and water

***Tab. 32-1.* Metabolic Alkalosis (pH ↑ CO_2 ↑)**

Mechanism	*State*	*Major Plasma and Urinary Changes*
Total base in excess of total anion (except HCO_3^-)	Excess of alkali	Na± ↑ K± ↓ HCO_3 ↑ Cl ↓
	Iatrogenic heartburn	Urine is alkaline.
	Excessive I.V. $NaHCO_3$	
Chlorides are lost in excess of base	Vomiting	Na± ↓ K ↓ HCO_3 ↑ Cl ↓
	Tube aspiration	Urine is alkaline.
Potassium deficiency	Inadequate intake	Na± ↓ K± ↓ HCO_3 ↑ Cl ↓
	Stress	Urine is acid.
	Diarrhea	
	Diuretics	
	Adrenal hormone therapy	Na± ↓ K ↓ HCO_3 ↑ Cl^- ↓
Mixed state	Combination of above	Urine is acid.

4. Add 20 mEq. KCl for each 1,000 ml. of aspirated gastric contents replaced.

5. Only the addition of KCl will correct a persistent plasma metabolic alkalosis in the presence of an acid urine.

6. Add daily baseline requirements.

7. Add only potassium after an output of at least 1,000 ml. in 24 hours is assured (40 ml. per hour).

8. With the mixed type of alkalosis, both sodium and potassium chloride are required, and the urine will again become alkaline when sufficient potassium is being administered if chloride loss continues.

METABOLIC ACIDOSIS (pH ↓ CO_2 ↓)

Etiology

1. Loss of bicarbonate may occur through buffering of strong acids, i.e., diabetic acidosis. Lactic acid may be produced in excess, or strong acids may not be excreted if kidney disease is present. Ketosis and the production of strong acids may occur in starvation.

2. Loss of bicarbonate may occur directly as the result of any body fluid which contains HCO_3^- in a concentration that is higher than plasma, i.e., diarrhea, vomiting of duodenal contents, small bowel fistulas, long-tube suction, pancreatic and biliary fistulas, etc.

3. In certain renal diseases there may be excessive and inappropriate loss of bicarbonate. Retention of fixed acids occur in chronic renal disease.

Basic Principles

1. Metabolic acidosis (pH ↓ CO_2 ↓) is a state of increased hydrogen ion concentration of plasma and cells due to causes other than the retention of CO_2.

2. Metabolic acidosis occurs when there is either an increase in total anion (except HCO_3^-) without equivalent base, or a loss of total base (i.e., Na^+) in excess of anion (i.e., Cl^-).

3. Metabolic acidosis may occur as a result of one or more of the following clinical circumstances:

a. Increase of normal inorganic sulfate and phosphate as the result of failure of renal excretion of these ions in acute or chronic renal failure

b. The appearance of large amounts of organic acid radicals normally present in small or trace amounts, i.e., keto acids in diabetic acidosis or lactic and pyruvic acids in shock and hypoxia

c. It may occur after the administration of certain drugs such as NH_4Cl and/or Diamox.

d. Sodium may be lost in excess of chloride in diarrhea, small bowel fistulas, long-tube suction, and pancreatic or biliary fistulas.

4. In severe acidosis, a little over half of acid is buffered in some other manner than by red cells and plasma.

a. Hydrogen ions leave the ECF in exchange for both Na^+ and K^+.

b. The exchange for K^+ represents about 15 per cent of the total buffering, and the exchange for Na^+ about 36 per cent. This exchange is mainly across cell membranes.

5. The patient is often lethargic, may actually be comatose, and respirations are increased in depth and rate.

MAJOR PLASMA ELECTROLYTE IMBALANCES AND URINARY CHANGES OCCURRING IN METABOLIC ACIDOSIS

Basic Principles in Summary

1. Occurs when the hydrogen ion concentration $\frac{HCO_3^-}{HHCO_3}$ is elevated from causes other than retention of CO_2 (pH ↓ CO_2 ↓).

2. Occurs in situations in which a loss of total base in excess of anion or in

Tab. 32-2. **Metabolic Acidosis ($pH\downarrow$ $CO_2\downarrow$)**

Mechanism	*State*	*Major Plasma and Urinary Changes*
Total anion is increased in relation to total base	$SO_4^{=}HPO_4^{=}$ elevated Shock, renal insufficiency Septic abortion Incompatible blood transfusion Premature separation of placenta	Na$\downarrow$ K$\pm\uparrow$ Ca$\pm\downarrow$ $HCO_3^{\mp}\downarrow$ Cl$\downarrow$ $HPO_4\uparrow$ Urine is acid.
	Keto acids elevated Diabetic acidosis Starvation	Na$\downarrow$ K$\pm\uparrow$ $HCO_3^-\downarrow$ Keto acid$\uparrow$ Urine is acid.
	Lactic and pyruvic acids elevated Adrenal insufficiency Postpartum vasomotor collapse, hypoxia	Na$\downarrow$ K$\pm\uparrow$ $HCO_3^-\downarrow$ Cl$\pm\downarrow$ Lactic acid$\uparrow$ Pyruvic acid$\uparrow$ Urine is acid.
	Chlorides elevated NH_4Cl, Diamox, Ureterosigmoid, transplants	$HCO_3^-\downarrow$ Cl$\uparrow$ Urine is acid.
Excess loss of base over anion, especially chlorides	Exercise loss of base over chlorides Small bowel losses Diarrhea Small bowel fistula Long-tube suction	$HCO_3^-\downarrow$ Cl$\uparrow$ Urine is acid.

which there is an increase of total anion (except HCO_3^-) without equivalent increase of base.

Compensations for Metabolic Acidosis

1. Dilution. There is a shift of water, sodium, and potassium to the extracellular compartment.

2. Relation Between Intracellular and Extracellular Space. Chlorides to intracellular space; Na^+, K^+ to extracellular space

3. Buffer System. Handles about 50 per cent of acid base; $BHCO_3$ + (H) (Acid) $\rightarrow$ B Acid + $HHCO_3$

4. Kidney Compensations

a. Titratable acid (substitute H^+ for Na^+).

$$H_2CO_3 + B_2HPO_4 \rightarrow \underset{\text{(to urine)}}{BH_2PO_4} + \underset{\text{(to plasma)}}{BHCO_3}$$

b. Substitute NH_4^+ for Na^+.

$$NH_4HCO_3 + BCl \rightarrow \underset{\text{(to urine)}}{NH_4Cl} + \underset{\text{(to plasma)}}{BHCO_3}$$

Management

1. Correct the underlying disease state.
2. Rehydrate.
3. Restore electrolyte balance.

4. Keep CO_2 above 15 mEq./L.
5. Potassium as needed after urinary output is at least 1,000 ml. in 24 hours.
6. Add daily baseline requirements.
7. Calculate and give infusions over 24-hour period.

RESPIRATORY ALKALOSIS

Etiology

1. Something must happen to cause the individual to excrete CO_2 at a rate greater than it is produced. This lowers p_{CO_2}.
2. The respiratory center may be stimulated abnormally and directly as:
   a. In encephalitis or meningitis
   b. Hypoxia
   c. Secondary to anxiety or hysteria
   d. Following ingestion of drugs such as aspirin
   e. High fever
   f. From ammonium toxicity in patients with liver disease

Basic Principles

1. Respiratory alkalosis is a state in which p_{CO_2} is reduced by hyperventilation, with a rise in pH as the result of a reduction of the $HHCO_3$ fraction of the bicarbonate buffer system.
2. Tetany may be present transiently.
3. In the presence of a high pH with low p_{CO_2}, the dissociation of oxygen from oxyhemoglobin is impaired, and relative tissue anoxia results. The venous blood tends to be redder than normal.
4. In respiratory alkalosis, the plasma bicarbonate is lowered by other mechanisms in addition to renal compensation. In the early phase of the imbalance they are more effective than renal compensation. The bicarbonate can be lowered by the chloride shift. It can also be lowered further by about the same amount by an increased production of lactic acid. Another means of medication is by exchange of Na^+ and K^+ in ECF for intracellular H^+. The exchange for Na^+ is about four times the exchange for K^+. The two combined represents one-fifth of the total buffering in an animal without kidneys.

MAJOR PLASMA ELECTROLYTE IMBALANCES AND URINARY CHANGES OCCURRING IN RESPIRATORY ALKALOSIS

Basic Principles in Summary

This is a state of decreased hydrogen ion (H^+) concentration $\frac{BHCO_3}{HHCO_3\downarrow}$ secondary to hyperventilation.

Compensation

1. Acute episode of respiratory alkalosis is compensated by renal mechanism.
2. Excess respiratory loss of $CO_2 \frac{(NaHCO_3)}{(HHCO_3\downarrow)}$ results in a decrease in the hydrogen ion concentration.
3. Kidney attempts to restore ratio by excreting bicarbonate.
4. Excretes bicarbonate with water resulting in dehydration.
5. Chlorides shift from the cells to the extracellular space.
6. There is also a derangement in the deposition of glycogen, as well as the utilization of glucose, with an accumulation of lactic acid and ketones in the extracellular fluid.
   a. Lactic acid and ketones are buffered with the result that thee bicarbonate value is decreased ($BHCO_3$ + H Acid $\rightarrow$ B Acid + $HHCO_3$).
   b. $HHCO_3$ is converted to H_2O and CO_2.
   c. CO_2 is released from the lungs.
7. Low potassium values, which may ocur in respiratory alkalosis, result in an increased absorption of bicarbonate by the kidney tubules, with the formation of an acid urine.

Tab. 32-3. **Respiratory Alkalosis (pH ↑ CO_2 ↓)**

Mechanism	*State*	*Major Plasma and Urinary Changes*
CO_2 is blown off in excess quantities by hyperventilation	Hysteria Fever Early salicylate poisoning Ammonium toxicity Respirators High altitudes Eclampsia Panting in labor Early septic shock	Na↓ K↓ HCO_3↓ Cl± ↑ HPO_4↓ Lactic acid ↑ Ketones ↑ Early urine is alkaline and later, after compensations occur, the urine is acid.

8. Late phase of respiratory alkalosis closely resembles metabolic acidosis.

Management

1. Correct the underlying disease state.
2. Give 10-per-cent CO_2, ideally by nasal catheter.
3. Prevent and/or correct dehydration.
4. Do not give bicarbonate in the acute phase. The kidney is excreting it in an attempt to return the ratio of $\frac{NaHCO_3}{HHCO_3}$ back to $\frac{20}{1}$.
5. Sodium lactate should not be given, because the lactic acid value is already elevated and any interference with the metabolism of the lactate ion will merely increase the amount already present.
6. If metabolic acidosis and dehydration result, sodium bicarbonate and water must be given.

RESPIRATORY ACIDOSIS

Etiology

The concentration of H_2CO_3 increases because of the retention of CO_2 that is caused by some impairment in pulmonary function. This may be caused by:

1. Poor exchange of CO_2 across an alveolar membrane when it is thickened
2. Inadequate ventilation
3. Increased CO_2 concentration in the inspired air

Basic Principles

1. Respiratory acidosis develops when there is interference with the respiratory exchange of CO_2 and thus an increase in the $HHCO_3$ fraction of $\frac{BHCO_3}{HHCO_3}$ of the bicarbonate buffer system. As $HHCO_3$ rises, H rises and pH falls.
2. Respiratory acidosis in the acute form is often seen in surgical patients, particularly under anesthesia during surgery, and in the immediate postanesthetic period.
3. Pneumothorax, atelectasis, and pneumonia are fairly common as acute postoperative complications and may produce an acute respiratory acidosis.
4. If the respiratory acidosis persists, compensations take place as in chronic respiratory acidosis.
5. The increase in pCO_2 in respiratory acidosis is buffered by a rise in bicarbonate due to factors other than renal compensation.

a. About 33 per cent of the rise of these mechanisms is accounted for by the chloride shift.

b. Approximately 15 per cent is brought about by the exchange of ECF

Tab. 32-4. **Respiratory Acidosis (*p*H ↓ CO_2 ↑)**

Mechanism	*State*	*Major Plasma Change*
Secondary to inability to blow off CO_2	Narcotic Barbiturate Pneumonia Atelectasis Emphysema Anesthesia Large abdomen in pregnancy Postoperative abdominal distention	HCO_3↑ Cl↓ Urine is acid.

$[H^+]$ for intracellular K^+. This tends to raise the ECF $[K^+]$ but if the renal function is normal, the K^+ will be excreted.

c. A small amount of increase in $[HCO_3^-]_p$ is brought about by a reduction in the organic acid content of plasma.

d. There is a further rise in $[HCO_3^-]_p$ that is thought to be caused by cellular mechanisms, but the exact nature of the mechanism is not known.

MAJOR PLASMA ELECTROLYTE IMBALANCES AND URINARY CHANGES OCCURRING IN RESPIRATORY ACIDOSIS

Basic Principles

This is a state of increased hydrogen ion concentration $(H^+) \frac{(NaHCO_3)}{(HHCO_3\uparrow)}$ secondary to some interference in the ability to blow off CO_2.

Compensation

1. Co_2 retention is in the form of carbonic acid ($HHCO_3$) which changes the ratio of

$$\frac{NHCO_3}{HHCO_3} = \frac{20}{1} \text{ to } \frac{NaHCO_3}{HHCO_3\uparrow} = \frac{20}{1\uparrow}$$

2. Electroloyte shifts occur, sodium shifts to the extracellular space.
3. Main compensation is renal.

a. Increased renal tubular reabsorption of bicarbonate and base.

b. Restores the ratio of $\frac{20}{1}$, a compensated state.

Management

1. Correct the underlying disease state.
2. Give oxygen. If the problem has been longstanding, oxygen may cause cessation of breathing, because the respiratory center now depends on anoxia for its stimulation.
3. Bronchodilators
4. Cold steam
5. Expectorants
6. Antibiotics
7. Tracheostomy

33. Cystocele, Urethrocele, Rectocele, and Enterocele

Hugh R. K. Barber, M.D.

Urethrocele and cystocele should be discussed together. Although they may occur independently of each other, commonly they are present together.

URETHROCELE

Definition

Urethrocele is a protusion downward of the urethra from its attachment just beneath the symphysis pubis.

Basic Principles

1. Results from the inability of the musculofibrous to give the urethra normal support.
2. There is a descent of the urethra from its position under the pubic arch.
3. It may be a cause of stress incontinence and may exist by itself or in company with a cystocele.
4. Childbirth injuries to the urogenital trigone and the pubovesicocervical fascia are chiefly responsible for this condition.
5. When it occurs in a nulliparous woman, a metabolic and/or neurologic disease should be ruled out.
6. Aside from the bulging there may be no inconvenience except for the stress incontinence previously described.
7. A urethrocele must be differentiated from a urethral diverticulum.

Management

1. The urethrocele may be repaired at the time of cystocele repair and will be discussed later.
2. The stress incontinence should be corrected by a suitable operation after careful urological evaluation. This is described under the correction for stress incontinence.

CYSTOCELE

Definition

Cystocele is a herniation of the bladder, causing the anterior vaginal wall to bulge downwards.

Basic Principles

1. It is usually the result of childbirth. The baby's head may stretch the pubococcygeal fibers of the levator ani muscles, permitting gradual sagging of the vaginal walls.
2. Probably the most important factor in the development of a cystocele is incompetency of the pubovesicocervical fascia.
4. One of the most common complaints is that there is a ball bulging between her legs.
5. With a large cystocele frequent cystitis may occur as well as retention of urine. Some women report that they must shove the mass back to void.
6. A large cystocele may stretch the trigone and give urgency and frequency without evidence of any infection.
7. A cystocele seldom gives stress incontinence.
8. An asyptomatic cystocele and/or urethrocele does not require correction.

Indications for Surgery

1. Large cystocele that causes discomfort on sitting or walking.
2. Inability to void without pushing up the anterior vaginal wall manually
3. Marked stretching of the trigone resulting in urinary frequency and urgency
4. Overflow incontinence and/or rarely stress incontinence
5. Difficulty with intercourse
6. Bleeding and ulceration secondary to trauma from the bleeding mass
7. Repeated bladder infections secondary to retention of urine

Management

1. A pessary may be used to support the bladder while treating infections in the bladder, thus reducing the amount of residual urine and increasing the probability of successful eradication of the infection.
2. Often a pessary supporting the bladder results in incontinence.
3. The pessary is rarely successful in controlling the overall clinical problems related to the cystocele but may be helpful in the treatment of urinary infections preoperatively.
4. The definitive treatment of cystocele and urethrocele is surgical.
5. Since both cystocele and rectocele occur so frequently together, the operations for both conditions are often combined.
6. The most important and essential step in the cure of these two conditions is restoring support to the urethra and/or bladder by proper use of the pubovesicocervical fascia.
7. Care must be exercised not to advance the bladder excessively or the urethrovesical angle may be increased with resulting stress incontinence.
8. If there is stress incontinence, which is rare, restoration of the urethrovesical angle must be carried out with meticulous care. A slight tug on a Foley catheter placed in the bladder helps identify the urethrovesical angle permitting precise placement of sutures.
9. A careful urologic and medical workup is indicated and then the following preoperative orders are routinely carried out:
   a. Sulfa vaginal cream twice a day for 2 days
   b. Estrogen vaginal cream for 2 days if the mucosa is very atrophic
   c. Soap suds enema until clear
   d. Crossmatch 1,000 ml. blood
   e. N.P.O. for 8 hours before the operation
   f. Nembutal 100 mg. or Seconal 100 mg. for sleep
   g. Demerol 50 mg. or Seconal 100 mg. plus atropine 0.4 mg. on call to O.R.
   h. Infusion of 1,000 ml. 5-per-cent glucose with heparin 1,000 ml. to be started the evening before surgery, to run during the operation, and for 2 or 3 days postoperatively.

Postoperative Orders

See "Stress Incontinence."

RECTOCELE AND ENTEROCELE

Definition

Rectocele. Protrusion of the rectum into the vagina.

Enterocele. High, posterior vaginal herniation of the small bowel, peritoneum, and fascia bulging forward at the apex of the vagina. It usually dissects down between the rectum and the vagina. Unlike a rectocele it is a true hernia.

Basic Principles

1. If the prolapse is at the level of the middle-third of the vagina, the rectovaginal septum is often involved and the rectum prolapses with the vaginal wall. This is a true rectocele.

2. If the lowest part of the vagina prolapses, the perineal body is involved rather than the rectum, resulting in a relaxed vaginal outlet.

3. If the upper part of the posterior vaginal wall prolapses, the pouch of Douglas is elongated and small bowel or omentum may descend, pushing peritoneum in front of it. This is called an enterocele. Enterocele is usually associated with uterine prolapse and is sometimes called vault prolapse or hernia of the pouch of Douglas.

4. The causes are generally the same as those listed for uterine prolapse and cystocele.

5. Anterior and posterior herniations usually occur concomitantly.

6. Hemorrhoids are frequently associated with the relaxed condition and may contribute to the general perineal discomfort.

7. The rectocele may give rise to very definitive symptoms that require relief.

Indications for Surgery

1. Protruding mass may be annoying, particularly when the patient is walking.

2. Patient may be troubled by a collection of feces in the rectocele pouch, and pressure may be required on the mass through the vagina in order to effect an evacuation of the bowels.

3. Interference with sexual intercourse. The complaint may be legitimate but may sincerely represent sexual incompatibility.

Management

1. A pessary is rarely helpful.

2. Perineal exercises are of little value.

3. Surgery is the treatment of choice.

4. Repair of a relaxed vaginal outlet and repair of a rectocele are two distinct operative procedures.

5. They are frequently done together, but perineal repair is often done when a rectocele is not present.

6. Rarely, a rectocele may be present and require repair in a woman whose outlet is not relaxed.

Vaginal Approach

The aim is to reduce herniation and build a supportive floor from the adjoining muscles and fascia. The cure rate is about 95 per cent.

1. Rectocele

a. A high dissection of the rectum is done from the posterior vaginal mucosa.

b. Imbricate the rectum using the prerectal tissue.

c. Build a firm support utilizing the levator muscles and fascia.

d. The muscles are ensheathed in fascia, and it is not wise to dissect the fascia from the muscles because the firmest union is obtained by the healing of fascia to fascia.

e. The excess vaginal mucosa is trimmed and then closed with continuous or interrupted sutures. It is wise to include some of the prerectal tissue. This closes dead spaces and adds to the support.

2. Enterocele

a. In addition to the symptoms listed for rectocele, the enterocele may give symptoms of pulling in the upper abdomen. This results from a pull on the mesentery as the small bowel protrudes into the vagina, putting a pull on the mesentery of the bowel.

b. The dissection must free the vagina from the rectum and must be carried as high as needed to identify the peritoneal sac.

c. The peritoneal sac should be opened and the contents pushed back into the pelvis.

d. The repair is the same as any hernia and should include high ligation of the sac with excision of the excess peritoneum, approximation of the fascia, and also approximation of the uterosacral ligaments.

e. Then continue as for the repair of a rectocele.

Abdominal Approach

1. Enterocele

a. Indications are:

(1) Failed previous vaginal repair

(2) Dense vaginal scarring

(3) Anatomically short vaginal canal and desire to preserve the existing depth

(4) When the abdominal cavity has already been opened for exploration and an enterocele is known to exist

b. Obliterate the cul-de-sac. It is important to obliterate the space below the level of the uterosacral ligaments (Moschowitz operation).

c. The uterosacral ligaments must be approximated. Care should be taken to avoid including the ureters in the sutures.

PROLAPSE OF THE UTERUS

Definition

Uterine prolapse is a herniation through the pelvic diaphragm with resultant protrusion into the vagina and even beyond the introitus.

Basic Principles

1. The uterus and vagina are held in the pelvis by the cardinal and uterosacral ligaments and by the pelvic floor musculature, mainly the levator ani muscles. When these ligaments and muscles become ineffective, the uterus and vagina descend (prolapse) through the gap between the muscles.

2. The causes of prolapse are:

a. The stretching of muscle and fibrous tissue which occurs with repeated childbirth.

b. Increased intra-abdominal pressure (as in obese women with chronic coughs) and in women who undertake heavy industrial work

c. A constitutional predisposition to stretching of the ligaments as a response presumably to years in the erect position

d. When a nulliparous woman develops a prolapse, she should have a careful metabolic and neurologic workup.

e. Obstetrical trauma with injury to the fascia, muscles, and ligaments that maintain the uterus in its normal position

Clinical Features

1. Sensation of something hanging out when the patient stands or walks
2. Backache. It may be related to other causes than the prolapse.
3. A bearing-down sensation
4. Frequency of urination
5. Difficulty in voiding or moving her bowels
6. Rarely, stress incontinence
7. The uterus gradually descends in the axis of the vagina taking the vaginal wall with it. It may present at any level, but is usually classified as one of three degrees.
8. The degree of descent of the uterus is sometimes difficult to evaluate, because in most cases the cervix usually becomes hypertrophied and elongated.

a. *First Degree or Slight.* Uterus has descended only a slight distance into the vagina.

b. *Second Degree or Moderate.* The cervix appears outside the vulva. The cervical lips become congested and ulcerated.

c. *Third Degree or Severe.* Is a complete prolapse. Is called a procidentia (procidentia means the parts of the body falling out of place). The uterus protrudes through the introitus.

Management

1. Pessary

a. When surgery is contraindicated or refused by the patient, the pessary may provide partial or complete relief of symptoms.

b. The patient must have careful follow-up to detect any ulcerations or pathology that may develop.

c. Sulfa vaginal and estrogenic hormone creams should be prescribed once a week.

2. Surgery

a. The treatment must be individualized and the surgery tailored to fit the patient and the extent of her prolapse.

b. Factors to be considered are:

(1) The age and general physical condition of the patient

(2) The desirability of preserving menstruation

(3) The desirability of preserving the childbearing function

(4) The degree of descensus

(5) The condition of the cervix and the corpus uteri

(6) The presence and degree of cystocele

(7) The presence and degree of rectocele or enterocele

3. Manchester (Donald or Fothergill) Operation

a. Curettage should be done in conjunction with an anterior and posterior repair. The anterior parametrial pillars are cut and plicated in front of the cervix. The cervix is amputated. Scar tissue forms at the level of plication of the cardinal ligaments and gives firm support. Sturmdorf sutures are used to close the mucosa over the amputated cervix.

b. The success rate is high and there are few complications.

c. The procedure is possible with almost any degree of prolapse, if there is no disease in the uterus.

d. The best results are obtained with first and second degree descensus, particularly if the uterus is not in retroposition.

e. Approximating the uterovascular prevents the development of an enterocele.

4. Vaginal Hysterectomy

a. Many consider this the procedure of choice for uterine prolapse, particularly if any uterine pathology is present.

b. After the uterus is removed the surrounding supportive ligaments must be shortened and approximated. Any enterocele must be corrected and if none is present, the uterosacral ligaments must be approximated to prevent one from occurring postoperatively. An anterior and posterior repair are usually indicated and should be carried out.

c. The cure rate is not as good as those reported for the Manchester operation, but this may be because of the selection of patients with the most severe prolapse for vaginal hysterectomy.

d. The complications most frequently encountered are bleeding during and after surgery, urinary tract injuries, urine retention in the postoperative period, and vaginal vault infections.

e. Complications can be kept to a minimum by adequate exposure, careful dissection, and good hemostasis.

5. Abdominal Suspension Operations

a. A variety of operations have been described in the literature. There are few indications for this approach. The operation is mainly used to hold the uterus from the cul-de-sac after endometriosis and endometriomas have been resected.

b. In young women in whom future pregnancies are expected, a modified Gillram operation is considered the operation of choice.

c. The uterosacrals should always be approximated to prevent the development of an enterocele.

6. LeFort Operation

a. Is a short and simple procedure, designed for frail old women who would not be fit for a more extensive operation.

b. It is not, however, as reliable as the Manchester repair and has been made almost obsolete by modern advances in anesthesia and postoperative care.

c. The patient's symptoms must be due to the prolapse and is confirmed if the symptoms are relieved by a pessary.

d. The patient must complain about the prolapse.

e. The operation is carried out by removing a triangular strip of tissue from each vaginal wall. The edges are sutured together, anterior wall to posterior wall. The vagina is now formed into two parallel small vaginas.

f. The disadvantages are that there is no vagina and some develop stress incontinence.

7. Choice of Operation

a. A vaginal hysterectomy is the procedure of choice for a uterus with pathology.

b. For a young woman who wishes to maintain menstruation and preserve childbearing, a vaginoplasty and abdominal suspension may be indicated. If a vaginal repair is undertaken in this patient, the cervix should not be amputated nor the cardinal ligaments plicated.

c. In women who work in industrial jobs and do heavy lifting, the Manchester operation is best.

Preoperative Orders

1. Routine orders for gynecological surgery
2. A careful genitourinary workup with cystoscopy and pyelography is indicated.

Postoperative Orders

Routine for vaginal procedures (see "Stress Incontinence").

34. Urinary Incontinence

Hugh R. K. Barber, M.D.

STRESS INCONTINENCE

DEFINITION

1. Stress incontinence is the involuntary loss of urine at the time of any sudden increase in intra-abdominal pressure, such as sneezing, coughing, laughing, or lifting with the patient in the upright position.
2. To qualify for this diagnosis, a patient must have an intact functioning neurogenic system and the bladder and urethra must be free of disease.

BASIC PRINCIPLES

1. The exact mechanism of urinary incontinence is still not documented.
2. There are many causes of urinary incontinence, only some of which can be treated by surgery. Accurate diagnosis of the cause of stress incontinence requires some consideration of the problems of bladder physiology.
3. The physiology of micturition is summarized as follows:
   a. The bladder stores urine at a low pressure. The bladder wall relaxes its tone and pressure rises very little until over 400 ml. of urine are contained. The pressure does not exceed 20 cm. of water until the bladder is full (600 ml.).
   b. The urethra can normally resist pressures between 20 and 50 cm. which is much higher than the bladder exerts until it is full. The pressure in the urethra is maintained by the urethral wall as well as the sphincter muscle function, which is served by the entire urethra.
   c. Urine is contained in the bladder as long as the intra-urethral pressure is greater than the intravesical pressure.
4. The nervous control of micturition is not completely understood.
   a. Micturition may be described as an autonomic reflex which can be consciously inhibited or facilitated in trained individuals.
   b. A desire to void reaches consciousness when about 300 ml. of urine are in the bladder.
   c. The stimulus passes via the parasympathetic, and reflex detrusor contractions can be inhibited until about 700 ml. are secreted.
   d. The urethra is strongly contracted.
5. Relaxation of the urethra (which is smooth muscle extending from the detrusor to the end of the urethra) is usually a conscious act at the onset of micturition. It may be psychologically inhibited, as in a patient who is not used to using a bed pan or when someone is present.
6. At the end of micturition the urethra contracts and forces the last drops of urine back into the bladder (the urethra is normally empty).
7. Disturbed bladder function may be due to urgency incontinence, fistula, overflow incontinence, neurologic disease, frequency, nocturnal frequency, dysuria, and hematuria.
8. Most agree that the basic problem in the etiology of stress is inadequate

support of the bladder base, vesical neck, and proximal urethra. If the urethra is properly supported, the proximal two-thirds is intra-abdominal.

9. Some believe that stress incontinence results from dilation of the urethra and the urethrovesical junction with funnelling. About 30 per cent of patients with stress incontinence do not have funnelling.

10. Green reports that the posterior urethrovesical junction and the urethral axis are crucial factors in the etiology of stress incontinence and its successful correction. He reports that the posterior urethrovesical angle in the continent female is usually about 90 to 100°. The vertical urethral axis is equally important. A vertical line drawn posterior to the urethrovesical junction is used as a base of an angle drawn to the urethra. Normally, the angle should be 15 to 30°. Management varies for abnormal anterior and posterior angles or combinations.

11. There is not total acceptance of the role that the posterior urethrovesical angle and the loss of the normal urethral inclination play in producing stress incontinence.

12. Ninety-five per cent of significant stress incontinence occurs in multiparas.

13. It is found more frequently in Caucasian women who have delivered vaginally and is aggravated by the erect position with Valsalva stress.

14. Fifty per cent of nulliparous college women will experience stress incontinence at some time or other.

15. Only about 25 to 30 per cent of symptomatic cystoceles have concomitant stress incontinence. There is no correlation between the degree of cystocele and the frequency of stress incontinence.

16. In the presence of a cystocele, if the herniation occurs anterior to the inter-ureteric ridge, patients usually show evidence of stress incontinence. If the herniation is posterior, most patients do not have stress incontinence. Of course, there may be a combination of these.

17. The concept that a short urethra is a primary cause of urinary stress incontinence has not been confirmed.

18. Marked peri-urethral adhesions with distortion of the normal urethra may interfere with urinary continence. The urethra may be a stiff tube through which urine flows. When this occurs it is necessary to release all adhesions before normal function can be restored.

19. Most gynecologists agree that if vesical funnelling, bladder neck descent, and the like are present, it is because of inadequate support of the bladder neck by components of the levator ani in the erect position, as well as loss of adequacy of the attachments of the urethra to the symphysis pubis. This permits the bladder neck to be the target point in the transmission of force from the dome to the base of the bladder. The chief cause is trauma that may not show up until the postmenopausal years.

20. With the patient in the upright position, straining and coughing should not result in urine loss. Another evaluation test that may be helpful is asking the patient to void and voluntarily stop urine flow.

DIAGNOSIS

History

1. Must differentiate stress incontinence from urgency incontinence, irritable bladder secondary to infection, or neurologic disorder.

2. The psychologic stability of the patient must be evaluated.

Physical Examination

1. Should include a general physical evaluation.

2. It is important to evaluate the tone of the levators, the tone of the vagina, and the sensation of the perineal area.

Tests To Perform During The Examination

1. Q-tip Test. This may show an abnormal urethrovesical junction. A lubricated Q-tip is placed into the urethra to the bladder neck with the patient in lithotomy position.

a. In the normal patient the Q-tip will be 13 to 16 degrees above the horizontal and will remain at this angle when the patient strains.

b. In patients with stress incontinence, straining will increase the upward angulation by 20 degrees or more with the majority producing an angle of 50 to 70 degrees. This demonstrates the detachment of the urethra from the symphysis pubis.

2. The Marshall-Marchetti Test

a. 250 ml. of sterile saline is instilled into the bladder.

b. The vagina is infiltrated with a local anesthetic in the area of the bladder neck.

c. Two Allis clamps are placed so that the bladder neck can be elevated without obstructing the urethra.

d. The patient is then asked to cough and the results are noted.

3. The Bonney Test

Similar to the Marshall-Marchetti test. The neck of the bladder is elevated by placing two fingers at the bladder neck and after elevating the bladder towards the symphysis, the patient is asked to cough and the results are observed.

4. The Hodgkinson Test

The largest contraceptive diaphragm fitting ring that the patient can comfortably accommodate is inserted. The patient is then asked to cough and the results are recorded.

5. Cystometry

a. This means the determination of bladder tone and its response to gradual distention with normal saline at body heat.

b. This will provide a measurement of capacity (the normal bladder can hold about 400 to 700 ml.) and of residual urine after voiding (as with cystocele).

c. About 50 ml. are instilled at a time and the bladder wall given time to accommodate.

d. The manometer indicates detrusor contractions, and if these are frequent, and occur early on, an "irritable bladder" is diagnosed. Cystometry cannot determine the cause.

e. The patient should be questioned as to her sensitivity to cold and warmth.

f. The ability to start and stop the urinary flow on demand is important.

g. Bladder hypertonicity is characterized by a contracted, spastic bladder with limited capacity and increased tone.

h. Bladder hypotonicity, which is characterized by low pressures and an increase above the usual capacity of the bladder, may be caused by neurogenic dysfunction.

i. The majority of patients with stress incontinence have a hypotonic bladder with a low resting pressure of 5 to 10 cm. of water.

(1) A sudden increase in the intravesical pressure of an additional 25 to 35 cm. of pressure is sufficient to cause urinary loss.

(2) With a low resting pressure, the spill pressure is correspondingly low.

(3) Although in the continent patient an addition intravesical pressure of 40 to 60 cm. of water is necessary for voiding, the incompetent patient sometimes spills with a rise of only 15 to 20 cm. of water.

6. Urethrocystography

a. The bladder is filled with a contrast medium, and lateral x-ray pictures are taken at rest, straining, and micturating.

b. In the normal resting radiograph, there is a well-formed urethrovesical angle.

c. In the normal micturating radiograph, there is urethral dilatation, downward displacement of the urethrovesical junction, and flattening of the urethrovesical angle.

d. If the appearance on straining are those of micturition, stress incontinence is diagnosed.

e. Urethrocystography is a difficult and specialized technique, uncomfortable for the patient, and not infallible; but it is the best way of demonstrating urethral mobility in cases where there is no obvious prolapse, or much peri-urethral scarring.

7. Urethroscopy

a. Is very important to rule out pathology. Diverticulae, local disease, tone and length of the urethra, inflammatory changes, neurogenic disease, tumors, fistulae, ectopic ureters, as well as other pathology of the bladder and/or urethra can be diagnosed.

b. To undertake the repair of stress incontinence without preliminary cystourethroscopy will reduce the precentage of cure.

8. Chain Cystograms

a. Once considered an essential part of the workup for stress incontinence. Recently there has been controversy over its value.

b. Green has been most consistent in reporting its value. He describes two basic types of anatomic configurations encountered in patients with stress incontinence as revealed by the lateral standing-straining view of the urethrocystogram. In both Type I and Type II, the posterior urethrovesical (PUV) angle is lost; in Type II there is, in addition, an increase in the angle of inclination of the urethral axis, varying from 45 to 120 degrees, depending on the amount of rotational descent of the urethra.

c. Green's major contribution is that with Type I cystograms, vaginal repair is usually successful (90 per cent). On the other hand, with Type II, only 50 per cent were corrected by vaginal operations, while if a Marshall-Marchetti-Krantz procedure was undertaken as the primary therapy, the success rate was 93 per cent.

d. The exact diagnosis is indispensable in treating both hypotonic and hypertonic bladder. It is re-emphasized that in addition to neurological examination, cystometry, cystoscopy, and urethroscopy are mandatory.

e. Older women may have urinary incontinence due to impaired central nervous system control. This is secondary to advanced arteriosclerosis. Little can be done to help this group.

9. Laboratory Tests

a. Routine urinalysis

b. Midstream culture of the urine should be carried out

c. Clearance tests should be ordered as indicated

d. Intravenous pyelograms should be done routinely preoperatively

MANAGEMENT

Nonsurgical—Medical

1. Tincture of hyoscyamus, 10 drops t.i.d.
2. Pro-Banthine, 15 mg. t.i.d., and 30 mg. at bedtime.
3. May be helpful if there is an additional complication of urgency incontinence.
4. Estrogens may help alleviate the symptoms of stress incontinence associated with postmenopausal atrophy. Excessive use of estrogens, on the other hand, may produce or aggravate the problem of stress incontinence.

Exercises

1. Perineal exercises (Kegel) increase pubococcygeal muscular control as well as urogenital diaphragm control.
2. A good voluntary sphincter mechanism alleviates the distress of stress incontinence by permitting a quick forceful contraction of these muscles, thus reducing the involuntary loss of urine under stress.

3. The voluntary contractions of these muscles should be done for 3 or 4 minutes four times a day.

Pessaries

1. Elevation of the neck of the bladder with a pessary may provide control of the stress incontinence. This is used only when the patient is not a good candidate for surgery.
2. In some instances, the pessary may produce or aggravate the problem.

Urethral Dilatation

May relieve a few cases of stress incontinence. Dilatation of the urethra up to a No. 28 French dilator is adequate treatment. The results are unpredictable and often unsuccessful.

Surgery

1. Basic Principles

a. The only type of incontinence that is helped by surgery is stress incontinence. The others will fail.

b. Urgency incontinence must be ruled out prior to surgery for stress incontinence.

c. Cystocele is rarely associated with stress incontinence. Over-vigorous correction of a cystocele may lead to stress incontinence.

d. All infections of the urinary tract must be controlled prior to surgery.

e. The operation should be tailored to the pathologic findings and the physiologic and anatomic imbalance.

f. The initial result is often good. However, within 5 to 10 years only about 50 to 60 per cent prove to be successful.

g. The failure rate with repeat operations is high and the number judged successful drops considerably.

Types of Operations

1. Vaginal Urethroplasty (Kelly's Operation)

a. Is the commonest operation and usually the first choice.

b. It is sometimes called a buttressing or Kelly operation.

c. Is an attempt to prevent urethral dilatation on straining by tightening the para-urethral tissues; and to raise and support the urethra by suturing the fascia beneath it.

d. The injection of Neo-Synephrine (1 ml. in 60 ml. of saline) diminishes the amount of oozing and permits a better dissection of the planes.

e. The anterior wall is carefully dissected from the urethrovesical area.

f. At the level of the urethrovesical junction, a silk suture picks up the periurethral fascia on either side of the urethra. This suture is repeated above and below.

g. After tying the silk sutures, the bladder fascia (sometimes called pubocervical fascia) is pulled together with catgut to give added support.

h. The repair of the cystocele, if present, is now carried out in the usual manner.

2. Marshall-Marchetti-Krantz Operation

a. If the bladder neck is elevated and fixed in the presence of stress incontinence, the primary approach should be suprapubic or a combination of the suprapubic and vaginal operation.

b. The basic function of the Marshall-Marchetti operation is the elevation of the urethrovesical junction and posterior rotation of the bladder.

c. Marked vaginal and urethral scarring is a contraindication to the Marshall-Marchetti-Krantz operation, unless it is combined with release of these from below.

d. The urethrovesical junction is made to adhere firmly to the anterior vaginal wall by suturing the vaginal tissue to the back of the symphysis pubis in the Marshall-Marchetti-Krantz operation. The description of the main steps of the operation are outlined below.

e. The urethrovesical junction is exposed in the space of Retzius. Adhesions are divided and all bleeding points picked up. The urethra must be dissected to within 1 cm. of the external meatus.

f. A Foley catheter in the bladder helps to identify the urethrovesical junction. Silk sutures pick up vaginal tissue on either side and suture it to the pubic periosteum.

g. Additional sutures may be added between the bladder muscle and rectus muscles.

h. Hematuria is common and continuous catheterization is required for 7 days.

i. Periostitis occurs in about 3 per cent of the patients.

j. If an angle that is too acute is produced, the patient may have difficulty in emptying her bladder.

k. The object of this operation is to provide elevation and support for the urethrovesical junction and the proximal urethra.

l. There is a 90-per-cent immediate success rate and 85-per-cent long-term success rate reported.

3. Modification of the Marshall-Marchetti-Krantz Operation

a. *Lapides' Operation*

The urethra itself is sutured to the symphysis and periosteum. The object is to correct the accordion-like shortening of the urethra on straining, which is thought to be a factor in the causation of stress incontinence. It is more traumatic to the urethra.

b. *Burch Operation*

(1) Is an additional suprapubic approach for urinary stress incontinence. Basically, this operation anchors the vagina lateral to the urethra to Coopers ligament on each side. The main advantages are a low surgical morbidity, diminished chance of fistula, decreased postoperative pain, virtual absence of hematuria, and a minimal chance of osteitis pubis.

(2) The disadvantages are that voiding in the postoperative period is slow and incomplete. However, as time passes, the patients begin to void normally.

c. *Ball's Operation*

(1) Advocates a combined repair from below and above. He maintained that freeing the urethra and repairing it from below would prevent failure of the suprapubic suspension. He also preferred suspending the neck of the bladder to the rectus muscle rather than the periosteum of the symphysis pubis, maintaining that this eliminated periostitis, chronic suprapubic pain, and osteomyelitis.

(2) The operation consists of an anterior plication of the urethrovesical junction with the posterior urethroplasty, so as to create good anterior and posterior urethrovesical angles. To do this, the urethra must be well mobilized and all bleeding controlled.

(3) The theoretical basis of Ball's operation rests on the ability of the intact urethra to contract by itself, if free to do so, and on the equal distribution to urethra and bladder of raised intra-abdominal pressure.

4. The Pereyra and Inco procedures to correct stress incontinence have given disappointing results. The initial results were good but long follow-up has been reported to have a 50 per cent failure rate with a high complication rate.

URINARY INCONTINENCE NOT CURABLE BY SPHINCTER PLICATION

Sling Operations

1. Have been popular for many years but the number treated by a sling operation has decreased since the introduction of the Marshall-Marchetti-Krantz operation.

2. The Goebell-Frangenheim-Stoeckel

operation has been reported as the first one of the sling operations described. It has been modified several times.

a. It involves a combined vaginal and abdominal approach.

b. One or two teams attach strips of rectus fascia through the space of Retzius on each side of urethra, thus encircling it. This permits elevation of the urethral base.

c. The tension should be adjusted so that the bladder neck lies behind the upper half of the symphysis pubis.

3. Aldridge's operation and Moir's operation are modifications of the original sling operation.

Millin's Operation

1. Is a sling operation done entirely through an abdominal incision.
2. The abdomen is opened through a lower transverse incision down to the fascia. Fascial strips are cut and these are left attached laterally.
3. The urethra is freed from the vaginal wall by the same approach as used in the Marshall-Marchetti-Krantz operation.
4. The slings are led through the recti and under the urethra and sutured in front of the urethra.
5. If the sling is too tight, voiding is difficult and a urethrovesical fistula may develop. If it is too loose, the operation will be ineffective.

The indications for these operations are a failed Marshall-Marchetti-Krantz operation and a short anterior vagina which cannot be elevated behind the symphysis pubis.

URGENCY INCONTINENCE

It is important to rule out urgency incontinence in evaluating patients with stress incontinence. Two out of three patients with stress incontinence have at least minimal urgency incontinence.

Basic Principles

1. The patient with urgency incontinence is unable to inhibit detrusor contraction and must void urine immediately. She has the sensation of wanting to void but loses her urine before reaching the bathroom.
2. The commonest cause is irritability due to cystitis, but all forms of bladder pathology must be considered, including tuberculosis, calculus, and carcinoma. Urethritis and even vaginal discharge from cervicitis are also causes. It is to be re-emphasized that urgency and stress incontinence may occur simultaneously.
3. It may be either neurogenic in origin (seen in conjunction with spina bifida, multiple sclerosis, diabetes) or to local disease of the bladder, such as interstitial cystitis, cystitis, and trigonitis.
4. If the patient has a cystocele, this may place the trigone on stretch and produce postural frequency.
5. A difficult problem is presented by the patient with urgency or urgency incontinence, usually combined with frequency, in whom no organic lesion is discovered.
6. Such patients are strictly the responsibility of the urologist, but in practice many of them present to the gynecologist.
7. The cause may also be psychological or environmental. Precipitating factors include marital problems, widowhood, accidents or illnesses to close relatives, together with postoperative retention and cystitis.

Management

When there is a diagnosis of urgency incontinence and no organic reason has been discovered:

1. The underlying dysfunction may be one of poor cortical processing of the stimuli resulting from bladder distention. This may be helped by a regimen of "bladder drill."

2. The bladder drill starts with filling the bladder to capacity at the time of cystoscopy. Instead of draining it at the completion, fluid is left in, and on recovering consciousness the patient voids what is usually a very much larger volume of fluid than she has done for a long period.

3. The psychological influence of the anticipated improvement following the bladder drill may have a good effect on the patient.

4. The patient is kept in the hospital and a regimen of voiding "by the clock," regardless of whether or not she desires to micturate, is initiated.

5. Starting one-half-hourly, the time of emptying is increased by one-half hour increments daily to 3 or 4 hours. Even if 2 hours is the longest that can be achieved, this is usually a great improvement over the previous situation.

6. The success of this regimen is often helped by prescribing a mild tranquilizer or sedative, especially at bedtime.

7. Propantheline bromide (Pro-Banthine) 15 mg. t.i.d. plus 30 mg. at bedtime, or atropine, belladonna, or Urispas may diminish the desire to void too frequently (rule out glaucoma before using these drugs).

8. Dilatation of the urethra until it admits a No. 28 French catheter may be helpful. The rationale is unclear, unless it be that some factor causing irritation in the proximal urethra is relieved by stretching.

9. Bladder infection is one of the main causes of urgency incontinence, and a basic part of therapy is to eliminate it if it exists.

10. It cannot be too strongly emphasized that full genitourinary tract investigation must be performed before embarking on the type of regimen outlined above.

11. If this is not done, from time to time patients with serious and treatable pathology of the urinary tract, such as tuberculosis, may be denied specific therapy.

35. Benign Tumors of the Ovary

Hugh R. K. Barber, M.D.

BASIC PRINCIPLES

1. Eighty-five per cent of all ovarian tumors are benign. The overall incidence approximates 7 per cent for all females.
2. Classification of benign ovarian tumors:

Cystic

1. Non-neoplastic
   - a. Follicle
   - b. Lutein
   - c. Stein-Leventhal (polycystic ovary)
   - d. Germinal inclusion
   - e. Endometrial
   - f. Tubo-ovarian inflammatory

2. Neoplastic
   - a. Epithelial
     - (1) Serous
     - (2) Mucinous
     - (3) Endometrioid
   - b. Germ cell
     - (1) Benign cystic teratoma (dermoid)

3. Solid
   - a. Fibroma
   - b. Brenner
   - c. Other associated rare lesions

DIAGNOSTIC SYMPTOMS AND SIGNS

1. Often none are present.
2. In many instances, the first symptom noted is a palpable mass or abdominal enlargement.
3. Vague heaviness, pressure, and dull aching may occur.
4. As a rule, there is no destructive influence exerted on menstrual function.
5. Because of lack of any specific symptom, uncomplicated tumors are often large by the time the doctor is consulted.
6. The symptoms are usually related to the complications that occur.

PHYSICAL SIGNS

1. Small tumors remain in the pelvis and will only be detected on bimanual examination.
2. Larger tumors fill the pelvis and usually lie between the uterus and the sacrum. If the patient is not too fat, the uterus can be distinguished on palpation as separate from the tumor.
3. A tumor occupying the abdomen causes a midline swelling and is usually tense.
4. Little can be done at this stage to classify the tumor or exclude malignancy. Very large tumors are likely to be benign; a primary malignant tumor would probably have killed the patient before reaching such a size.
5. If the patient is very thin, irregularities may be palpated, and sometimes two tumors may be suspected.
6. Some tumors of moderate size have a long pedicle composed of the attenuated broad ligament and fallopian tube, which allows the tumor to be displaced from side to side or to occupy a high abdominal position.
7. Adhesions, inflammation, displacement of pelvic organs may all exist along with a tumor and confuse the examiner.

DIFFERENTIAL DIAGNOSIS

1. Full bladder
2. Ascites
3. Pregnancy
4. Myomata
5. Pelvic inflammatory disease
6. Diverticulitis
7. Appendiceal abscess
8. Distended cecum
9. Pancreatic cyst
10. Mesenteric cyst
11. Broad ligament cyst
12. Pelvic kidney
13. Retroperitoneal tumors

COMPLICATIONS

1. Torsion of pedicle
2. Rupture of cyst
3. Suppuration of cyst
4. Hemorrhage
5. Malignant change

NON-NEOPLASTIC (PHYSIOLOGIC) CYSTS

FOLLICLE CYSTS

Basic Principles

1. Persistence of enlarged follicle may lead to temporary enlargment of the ovary.
2. May result when a follicle does not rupture at the time of ovulation.
3. Usually small but may attain a size of 6 cm.
4. Are unilateral.
5. If the patient is observed for one or two menstrual cycles, the cyst will usually disappear.
6. The patient is usually asymptomatic but may complain of fullness or pain in one adnexal area.

Management

1. Observation and re-examination after two periods.
2. Surgical intervention is only indicated if a complication arises.

CORPUS LUTEUM CYSTS

The cyst develops from abnormally excessive secretion and accumulation of fluid associated with the involution process.

Basic Principles

1. Usually larger than a follicle cyst and may increase to 8 cm. in size.
2. Most of these cysts are due to a vascular or lymphatic disturbance.
3. The symptoms are similar to those seen with a follicle cyst.
4. May be asymptomatic or mimic a tubal pregnancy. May be associated with amenorrhea, pain, and a mass.
5. Ruptured hemorrhagic cyst may produce typical signs of intraperitoneal bleeding.
6. Halban's syndrome is characterized by a persistent corpus luteum cyst, amenorrhea followed by irregular uterine bleeding, unilateral pelvic pain, and a small, tender, moveable adnexal mass. It is obvious that in most cases the disease is diagnosed after ectopic pregnancy has been ruled out.

Management

1. Laparoscopy, culdoscopy, colpotomy, or occasionally exploratory laparotomy, are needed for diagnosis and therapy, if there is no accident in the cyst or the diagnosis is unclear.
2. In this age group it is possible to follow the patient through one or two periods to see if there is regression of the mass.

THECA-LUTEIN CYSTS

Basic Principles

1. In corpus luteum cysts ovulation has preceded its development; in the in-

stance of theca-lutein cyst or cysts, the abnormality occurs in the absence of ovulation.

2. They may be unilateral and solitary but more often are multiple and bilateral.

3. They are the result of disturbances in the normal hypothalamic-pituitary-gonadal axis, in which an elevated gonadotropin level is observed.

4. Theca-lutein cysts may be iatrogenic.

5. They usually regress without treatment.

6. Theca-lutein cysts may be found in the newborn, with hydatidiform mole, choriocarcinoma, twin pregnancy, erythroblastosis fetalis, and with the use of clomiphene citrate or Pergonal.

Management

1. Is conservative.

2. Surgery is not necessary except in the management of complications.

NON-PHYSIOLOGICAL, NON-NEOPLASTIC OVARIAN CYSTS

Stein-Leventhal Syndrome [S-L]

1. May be referred to as the polycystic ovary syndrome (PCO). Is characterized by amenorrhea or oligomenorrhea, infertility, and usually clinical evidence of excess androgenicity.

2. The ovaries are often bilaterally enlarged, but may be of normal size or only one ovary may be affected.

3. The ovaries are usually enlarged, have a thick gray capsule and numerous subcapsular cysts (oyster or potato ovary). There are varying degrees of theca-cell hyperplasia.

Diagnosis

1. Usually made on clinical grounds.

2. Confirmatory laboratory findings include a moderately elevated serum testosterone (usually not over 200 ng. per 100 ml.), normal urinary 17-hydroxycorticosteroids, normal or slightly elevated urinary 17-ketosteroids (rarely over 25 mg. per 24 h.), elevated serum LH, and normal serum FSH.

3. If the diagnosis is in doubt, visualization of the ovaries by laparoscopy, culdoscopy, or laparotomy may occasionally be necessary.

Differential Diagnosis

1. Adrenal hyperplasia
2. Adrenal tumor
3. Pituitary tumors

Management

1. If pregnancy is not desired, menstruation should be induced by Provera or one of the oral contraceptive agents.

2. If there is evidence of adrenal hyperplasia, cortisone should be given and monitored by following the 17-ketosteroid levels.

3. If pregnancy is desired, these patients will usually ovulate in response to clomiphene. If there is no response to clomiphene and if other factors contributing to infertility have been ruled out, Pergonal and HCG may be used.

4. Surgery offers an opportunity to explore the patient. In some patients who do not respond to medical therapy, a wedge resection of the ovary is indicated. This requires excision of about half of the ovarian tissue and the resection must be carried to the hilus of the ovary.

NEOPLASTIC OVARIAN CYSTS

(BENIGN CYSTIC TERATOMA [DERMOID])

Basic Principles

1. Dermoids are rarely large, often bilateral (25 per cent).

2. Is usually found in the childbearing age but may be present at any age.

3. Grossly, there is a rather thick, opaque, whitish wall, and on opening the cyst one frequently finds hair, bone, and cartilage as well as a large amount of greasy fluid, which rapidly becomes sebaceous on cooling.

4. There are no pathognomic signs. In pregnancy the cyst frequently lies anterior to the uterus, overlying the bladder.

5. The malignancy rate is low and has been reported from 1 to 3 per cent.

6. The complications that occur are torsion, hemorrhage, rupture, and infection.

Management

1. Resection of the cyst and, if this is not possible, excision of the ovary

2. The other ovary should be bisected, inspected, and biopsied.

3. In the over-age-35 patient, the treatment of choice is total hysterectomy and bilateral salpingo-oophorectomy.

NEOPLASTIC EPITHELIAL CYSTS

SIMPLE SEROUS CYSTS

Basic Principles

1. Represents 15 per cent of all benign ovarian tumors.

2. May vary in size from a few centimeters to a huge cyst occupying the entire abdominal cavity. Usually is about 5 to 6 cm.

3. Is most often unilateral.

4. Usually there are no symptoms unless torsion, rupture, or hemorrhage occurs.

Management

1. Resection of the cyst in the younger age group

2. In the over-35-years age group, hysterectomy and bilateral salpingo-oophorectomy is indicated.

SEROUS CYSTADENOMA

Basic Principles

1. A unilocular or multilocular cyst lined by epithelium similar to the fallopian tube

2. They are common and form 20 per cent of all ovarian neoplasms.

3. It is smaller than its mucinous counterpart and grows to a maximum of 10 cm. in diameter.

4. About one-third are bilateral.

Management

Is dependent upon the age of the patient. In young women a unilateral salpingo-oophorectomy is sufficient therapy. However, in the peri- and postmenopausal patient and patients over age 35, a total hysterectomy and bilateral salpingo-oophorectomy is the treatment of choice.

PAPILLARY SEROUS CYSTADENOMA

Basic Principles

1. Comprise 10 per cent of all benign ovarian tumors.

2. It is most common in women in their reproductive years.

3. Bilaterally is seen in 50 per cent of this type of tumor.

4. Grossly, papillary serous cystadenomas are globular and multiloculated.

5. Reveals intracystic and extracystic papillary growths.

6. May show clinically malignant tendencies.

Management

1. After age 35 years, a total hysterectomy and bilateral salpingo-oophorectomy is indicated.

2. A more conservative operation may be carried out during the childbearing years, if the patient is informed that she is at risk to develop a more serious problem.

MUCINOUS CYSTADENOMA

Basic Problems

1. A unilocular or multilocular cyst of the ovary lined by tall columnar epithelium resembling that of the cervix or large intestine
2. May reach a very large size, occupying the whole abdomen.
3. Are the second most common type of ovarian tumor. It accounts for 15 per cent of all ovarian tumors and 25 per cent of all benign ovarian tumors.
4. Are usually unilateral.
5. Malignant changes occur in about 5 per cent of the cases.
6. Torsion is common because of the well-defined pedicles, which are often present.

Management

The same as for serous cystadenoma

FIBROMA

Basic Principles

1. Is composed of fibrous tissue and resembles fibromata found elsewhere.
2. It is common in the elderly.
3. Accounts for about 5 per cent of all ovarian tumors.
4. May represent a thecoma that has undergone fibrous transformation.
5. May be associated with Meig's syndrome. When hydrothorax is present, the right side is involved 75 per cent of the time, the left side 10 per cent of the time, and both sides are involved in only 15 per cent of the cases.

Differential Diagnosis

1. Malignancy with pulmonary metastases
2. Cardiac or renal disease with fluid retention
3. Hepatic cirrhosis
4. Tuberculous peritonitis

Management

1. In the peri- and postmenopausal patient, hysterectomy and bilateral salpingo-oophorectomy is indicated.
2. In younger patients, a conservative operation is acceptable.

BRENNER TUMOR

Basic Principles

1. Is a rather uncommon type of ovarian neoplasm and grossly is identical to a fibroma.
2. Makes up 1 to 2 per cent of all ovarian tumors.
3. Is most common in the sixth decade.
4. Is rarely malignant.
5. Microscopically, the epithelial cells show a "coffee bean" pattern due to the longitudinal grooving of the nuclei.

Management

The same as for fibromas

PREGNANCY LUTEOMA

Basic Principles

1. Is not a true neoplasm even though it may attain a diameter of 15 cm. and have numerous mitoses.
2. It is best interpreted as a focus of reversible, nodular, lutein-cell hyperplasia, since it depends on chorionic gonadotropin stimulation for its structural and functional integrity.

Management

1. Conservative since it is reversible in most instances
2. Surgery is reserved for the complications that may arise such as torsion or hemorrhage.

36. Benign Uterine Tumors

Hugh R. K. Barber, M.D.

ENDOMETRIAL POLYPS

Definition

1. The term "polyp" is a clinical rather than a pathologic one, referring to a growth which is attached by a pedicle or stem, and not indicating in any way its histologic characters.
2. The polyp has a structure like the endometrium itself, consisting simply of a localized heaping up of the latter. Most reveal only estrogen response, i.e., proliferation or hyperplasia.
3. They are usually benign growths that occur after age 35 years and may be single or multiple.

Basic Principles

1. May be small or large enough to fill the uterine cavity.
2. It is impossible to assess their frequency.
3. Most often endometrial polyps are asymptomatic.
4. Some may be associated with menorrhagia, postmenstrual staining, and postmenopausal bleeding.
5. There is cramping pain, usually mild, as the uterus tries to expel the polyp.
6. The polyp may be present at the external os.
7. The histologic types of endometrial polyps are:
   a. Those made up of functional endometrium
   b. Those made up of immature endometrium
   c. Adenomatous polyps
8. Endometrial polyps undergo malignant degeneration, particularly in the postmenopausal period.
9. May have a chronic vaginal discharge.

Diagnosis

1. Suspect from history.
2. Pap smear
3. Hysterogram (fractional and should be carried out with a water-soluble dye)

Management

1. Remove the polyp with a tonsil snare or twist it off with a polyp forceps.
2. A fractional curettage and cervical biopsies should be carried out.
3. The base of the polyp must be carefully curetted.

ENDOMETRIAL HYPERPLASIA

Definition

A term used to describe a uterine condition in which the endometrium remains in the proliferative phase for many weeks or years, which results in hyperactivity and growth of both glandular and stromal elements of the endometrium.

Basic Principles

1. The majority of patients are between 35 and the menopause, but this condition may affect young women and even postpubertal adolescents.
2. Functional (dysfunctional) uterine bleeding presents without a causative uterine lesion (such as tumor, infection, or complication of pregnancy), although frequently there may be associated follicle cysts of the ovary.

3. Functional bleeding is a clinical term, while hyperplasia is a histologic diagnosis.
4. The underlying cause is excessive or unopposed endometrial stimulation by estrogen in the absence of progesterone.
5. It is usually associated with anovulation or extended periods of amenorrhea. It may be secondary to ovarian unresponsiveness, disturbed pituitary gonadotropin secretion, Stein-Leventhal syndrome, adrenocortical hyperplasia, functioning ovarian tumors, and administration of estrogens.

Symptoms

1. Hemorrhage is common, irregular, often continuous for weeks, and liable to be profuse.
2. Amenorrhea for one or two months intervenes between spells of hemorrhage.
3. Anemia may be marked.

Diagnosis

1. History indicating anovulation or prolonged periods of amenorrhea
2. Endometrial biopsy
3. Fractional curettage

Management

1. Postpubertal until Age 30 Years

a. Improve diet and recommend more rest. Anemia, obesity, and underweight for height should be corrected.

b. Rule out endocrine, metabolic, and other pathologic states.

c. Progesterone in oil, 100 mg. I.M.

d. Provera, 10 mg. q.4h. until improved.

e. Combined estrogen-progesterone pill for three cycles.

f. Premarin 20 mg. I.V. in emergency cases; response is seen usually in one hour; if not, repeat the dose q.3 to q.4h. times three doses.

g. Give cyclic progestin therapy after the immediate bleeding problem is over.

2. Over Age 30 to Age 45 Years

a. Rule out pathologic conditions, i.e., fibroids, chronic pelvic inflammatory disease, etc.

b. If present, correct anemia.

c. Fractional curettage is indicated.

d. Rarely is hysterectomy required to control the bleeding.

3. Postmenopausal Patient

a. Rule out pathologic condition, i.e., carcinoma of the endometrium, ovarian tumors, etc.

b. Fractional curettage with cervical biopsies

c. If bleeding recurs, do a repeat fractional curettage.

d. Hysterectomy may become necessary for recurrent bleeding.

e. If the patient is not a good candidate for surgery, she may be treated with large doses of Depo-Provera or Delalutin, which produces hemostasis through the production of endometrial atrophy.

ADENOMATOUS HYPERPLASIA

Definition

Adenomatous hyperplasia, a typical precancerous lesion, may be a focal or general change, with its greatest prevalence in women of perimenopausal age with dysfunctional bleeding.

Basic Principles

1. Histologic examination of curettings shows the glands to be back-to-back; there is pseudostratification of the glandular epithelium and, in the most intense form, a characteristic pallor or eosinophilic stain reaction of these glands with intense proliferation of the glandular epithelium, forming buds and islands within the gland lumen.
2. Carcinoma in situ of the endometrium has been reserved for those lesions of undoubted invasion of the stroma,

high differentiation, and confinement to a local area of endometrium; in the past this lesion was called adenoma malignum.

3. Adenomatous hyperplasia is a precursor lesion and these patients are at high risk for later invasive carcinoma of the endometrium.

4. Young women may have a syndrome of the cystic ovary and oligomenorrhea and may present with adenomatous hyperplasia in their reproductive years.

Management

1. Young Women

a. Fractional curettage is indicated if there is any lawless bleeding.

b. Initiating ovulation and the subsequent progestational effect on the endometrium can reverse the pattern of adenomatous hyperplasia and restore normal cycling of the endometrium.

c. This may be achieved by giving progesterones, Clomid, cortisone, and in some instances by wedge resection of the ovary.

2. Peri- and Postmenopausal Years

a. Fractional curettage and hysterectomy will confer upon the patient a lasting prophylaxis without the requirement for further follow-up.

b. If hysterectomy is not indicated at that moment, a repeat curettage should be done at 4 months following the initial diagnosis.

c. If adenomatous hyperplasia is not present, the patient may be followed with endometrial biopsies at 6-month intervals.

d. If adenomatous hyperplasia is present at the time of the second curettage, a hysterectomy is indicated. In this age group the ovaries should also be removed.

e. Treatment with progesterones is not indicated in this age group.

LEIOMYOMATA (FIBROIDS)

Definition

1. Benign, well-circumscribed tumor of nonstriated muscle with supporting fibrous tissue. Though not encapsulated, it can be shelled out from the uterine muscle.

2. It may arise from immature or undifferentiated cells in the myometrium or possibly from cells in blood vessel walls. It has been definitely shown that the tumor arises from a muscle cell, probably an undifferentiated myoblast.

3. Rarely, they are found in the ovary or the round ligament.

Basic Principles

1. The fibroid is the commonest tumor found in women (present in 15 to 20 per cent), especially after 35 years of age.

2. Location of the fibroid describes the type. They may be conglomerate and multiple and vary in size from tiny (millet seeds) to several centimeters in diameter.

3. Some fibroids develop a long pedicle and present as a polyp.

4. It is seemingly hormone-dependent and will continue to grow with varying degrees of rapidity during the menstrual era, with postmenopausal regression and shrinkage of the tumor.

5. As leiomyoma contain either A or B type G-6-PD, but not both, they are considered to arise from a single cell and are therefore neoplasms.

6. Fibroids bind approximately 24 per cent more estradiol per mg. of cytoplasmic protein than does the normal myometrium.

7. Erythrocytosis associated with uterine fibroma is mediated through direct production of erythroprotein by the tumor.

8. The finding of abnormally large venous spaces in the endometrium overlying fibroids could be an objective source

of associated menorrhagia. The finding is usually associated with glandular atrophy and stromal hyperplasia, not an uncommon finding in anovulation associated with fibroids.

9. Varieties According to Position

a. *Interstitial or Intramural.* Probably all fibroids begin to grow in the substance of the uterine wall. As they grow they continue to be surrounded by a layer of muscle of varying thickness. Most fibroids as they increase in size, pass into one of the following positions: subserous (subperitoneal), submucus, or cervical.

b. *Subserous* develops on the outer surface of the uterus. It may become very large and cause only minimal symptomatology. It may be sessile or pedunculated and may become intraligamentous, retroperitoneal, or parasitic depending upon growth.

c. *Submucus* migrates toward the uterine cavity and projects therein. Is probably the most important myoma since it involves the endometrial cavity and leads to increased bleeding and cramps.

10. Cervical fibroids make up about 5 per cent of all fibroids. They are always solitary tumors and may attain a large size.

11. Secondary changes in myomas include hyaline degeneration (most common), cystic degeneration, infection, calcification, necrosis, fatty degeneration, and sarcomatous degeneration (in 0.5 per cent or less, usually postmenopausal). Carneous degeneration is a particularly interesting degenerative process, which most often is a curious phenomenon of pregnancy, and is probably related to an impaired circulation in the myoma.

Symptoms and Diagnosis

1. In many instances the patient is totally asymptomatic.

2. There is a history of heavy menstrual periods.

3. Pain is not a symptom of myoma unless there is a torsion of a pedunculated lesion.

4. There may be a palpable abdominal tumor.

5. Vaginal examination. Irregularly enlarged uterus and bulky ovaries

6. As the tumor grows there may be pressure symptoms according to the location.

7. If bleeding is sufficient there may be an associated anemia.

8. Fractional curettage is indicated in the presence of lawless bleeding.

Management

Depends upon the following:

1. Associated symptoms
2. Size and location of tumors
3. Age of patient
4. Childbearing status

Conservative Treatment

1. Asymptomatic Tumors. Most fibroids are small and free of symptoms. They are found on routine examination and require no treatment other than periodic follow-up examinations in the absence of any developing symptoms.

2. Symptomatic Tumors

a. Treat conservatively if fibroids are small.

b. Analgesics for dysmenorrhea and minimal pressure symptoms.

c. Perform a fractional curettage for any abnormal bleeding to rule out endometrial polyps, hyperplasia, submucus fibroids, or carcinoma of the endometrium.

Surgery

1. Indications for Surgery

a. Excessive size (generally 16 weeks or more)

b. Exclusive of pregnancy, excessive or rapid growth may be associated with sarcomatous changes

c. Submucus fibroid associated with heavy and recurrent bleeding

d. Pedunculated fibroid may be susceptible to torsion and possible necrosis

e. Pronounced pressure symptoms on the bladder or rectum; obstruction to ureter

f. Cases in which myomas by size or location are believed to contribute to infertility, habitual abortion, or premature labor

2. Type of Surgery

a. Myomectomy is usually reserved for patients in whom the preservation of reproduction is of importance.

b. Patients so treated have a high incidence (5 to 40 per cent) of subsequent myomata necessitating further surgery. If in the interim the patient has one or two full-term deliveries, it is a small price to pay.

c. Slightly higher morbidity than with hysterectomy.

d. Hysterectomy is the usual and preferable procedure, particularly in older women, and when the myomata are large. Ideally, a fractional curettage must be carried out prior to hysterectomy.

e. If at the time of curettage (for heavy and repeated bleeding in women over age 40 years) a diagnosis of submucus fibroid is made, hysterectomy is probably indicated.

Radiotherapy

1. Today there is scant indication for an irradiation menopause. Most gynecologists prefer surgical treatment.

2. Rarely, in the occasional bad-risk patient it is effective. A fractional curettage or endometrial biopsy should be done prior to the radiotherapy.

3. It is contraindicated in the presence of submucus fibroid, pedunculated subserous myoma, degenerated myoma, pelvic infection, or a myoma exceeding 12 weeks size.

Adenomyosis

See Chapter 37.

Plexiform Tumorlets

Plexiform tumorlets found in the endometrium are benign. They are incidental lesions of stromal-cell origin that are noted microscopically and are associated with a high incidence of uterine fibroids.

Hemangiopericytoma

1. Are cellular tumors, rarely malignant, that are found in the uterus as well as other parts of the body.

2. It is a vascular lesion not unlike the glomus tumor and may be distinguished by a tendency toward concentric arrangements of pericytes around capillaries.

3. The malignancy rate is reported as 20 to 25 per cent.

4. Differential diagnosis includes endometrial stromatosis and sarcoma.

37. Adenomyosis

Hugh R. K. Barber, M.D.

DEFINITION

1. Is characterized by benign invasion of the myometrium by the endometrium, which normally lines the uterine cavity superficially.

2. It continues to be an elusive disease of the perimenopausal years.

BASIC PRINCIPLES

1. Adenomyosis results from direct extension of the basal endometrium down into and rarely through the myometrium. Serial sections will reveal this direct continuity.

2. Previous pregnancy seems to play a role in etiology; less than 6 per cent of patients are nulliparous.

3. Although no firm relationship between adenomyosis and a precancerous or malignant condition of the uterus has been established, on a few occasions adenocarcinoma has been reported as arising from adenomyosis in conjunction with a normal-surface endometrium.

4. On occasion the adenomyosis may penetrate through the uterus and involve the rectosigmoid, uterosacral ligaments, and other adjacent organs.

The presence of concomitant pelvic endometriosis is frequent.

DIAGNOSIS

1. The clinical diagnosis is presumptive. It is based on the three following findings:

a. Progressive severe dysmenorrhea, with or without menometrorrhagia

b. Normal to slightly enlarged, globular uterus

c. A patient 35 to 45 years old.

2. The diagnosis is only made definitively if the uterus has been removed and the diagnosis confirmed on histologic examination.

MANAGEMENT

1. The progress of adenomyosis depends on continued ovarian function.

2. If the patient is immediately premenopausal and the symptoms are mild, conservative therapy is indicated.

3. Menopause will completely correct the condition.

4. When the symptoms are severe and getting progressively worse, hysterectomy is indicated. In this age group oophorectomy should also be carried out.

38. Endometriosis

Hugh R. K. Barber, M.D.

DEFINITION

1. Endometriosis is a disorder characterized by the presence of functioning endometrial tissue outside the uterine cavity.

2. Aberrant tissue may be found in many locations including the ovaries, uterosacral and other pelvic ligaments, rectovaginal septum, pelvic peritoneum, umbilicus, laparotomy scars, hernia sac, bowel or bladder, lower genital tract, tubal stumps, and lymph nodes.

BASIC PRINCIPLES

1. The development and extension of endometrial tissue into the myometrium is termed adenomyosis. This disease entity seems histogenetically unrelated to endometriosis and is characterized by an entirely different clinical situation. Furthermore, findings on pelvic examination show none of the characteristics of endometriosis.

2. Endometriosis implies proliferating growth and function (usually bleeding) in an extrauterine site.

3. An endometrioma may be defined as an area of endometriosis, usually in the ovary, which has enlarged sufficiently to be classified as a tumor.

4. When the endometrioma is filled with old blood (resembling tarry or chocolate-colored, syrupy fluid) it is commonly known as a chocolate cyst.

5. While the complaint of infertility should be sufficient to alert the physician to the possibility of endometriosis, the index of suspicion is elevated if the woman has progressively severe dysmenorrhea, dyspareunia, or pain on defecation.

6. Endometriosis has been noted with increasing frequency and is found in about 15 per cent of pelvic operations.

7. It is seen among women of the higher socioeconomic groups. As such, it has been correlated with delayed or deferred motherhood.

8. Endometriosis has been called the "disease of civilization."

9. The median age of patients at the time of diagnosis is approximately 37 years, but approximately 15 per cent of patients are under age 30 years.

10. Histogenesis has been suggested by several theories: the transplantation or tubal regurgitation theory, coelomic metaplasia doctrine, lymphatic spread, hematogenous route, and the composite or unified concept.

MANEUVERS TO AVOID

1. Pelvic examination during the menstrual period or after diagnostic dilatation and curettage

2. At the time of menstruation or just premenstrually, uterotubal insufflation should not be done.

3. Pelvic examination after endometrial biopsy is contraindicated because of the possibility of endometrial spillage inside the peritoneal cavity.

4. Cryosurgery should be avoided in young females because of the high incidence of subsequent cervical stenosis.

DIAGNOSIS

Diagnostic Triad

1. A period-linked symptom that gets progressively worse.
2. An interval of 5 years since the last delivery despite the number of previous deliveries.
3. Tender nodules in the cul-de-sac, uterosacral ligaments, and the ovaries, particularly noticeable during menstruation. A fixed retroversion of the uterus may be present.

Diagnostic Aids

1. Culdoscopy
2. Laparoscopy
3. Barium enema
4. Intravenous pyelogram
5. Cystoscopy
6. Examination under anesthesia

Differential Diagnosis

1. Chronic pelvic inflammatory disease
2. Ovarian tumor or cancer
3. Rupture of an ovarian endometrial cyst may simulate an attack of pelvic peritonitis, appendicitis, ectopic pregnancy, ovarian cyst with twisted pedicle, a ruptured dysfunctional ovarian cyst, or carcinoma of the rectosigmoid.

Management

1. Asymptomatic endometriosis may be safely dealt with by close observation. Mild pain can be controlled by analgesics.
2. For more pronounced symptoms, surgery or hormone treatment still constitutes the only available therapy.

Surgery

1. Endometriosis is probably best treated primarily by surgery and this is mandatory if there is an adnexal mass present.
2. Hormone therapy over a long period of time is expensive, often unsatisfactory, and the result is not predictable.
3. Where the disease is very extensive with adnexal masses and particularly in older women, hysterectomy and bilateral salpingo-oophorectomy is indicated.
4. In young women with less extensive disease than described above, it is possible to preserve an ovary since hysterectomy alone will relieve most if not all the symptoms.
5. In young women desirous of pregnancy, conservative surgery should be carried out, if possible. It should include resection of endometrial cysts, unilateral adnexectomy if required, fulguration of implants, suspension of the uterus, and presacral neurectomy.
6. If there is a recurrence of the endometriosis following conservative surgery that requires a second operation, it should probably include castration. Following castration surgery subsequent hormonal replacement therapy in the premenopausal woman is an accepted practice.

Hormonal Therapy

1. Pregnancy has often been suggested as the optimum prophylactic and therapeutic treatment for endometriosis.
2. Regression of endometriosis following suppressive hormone therapy is probably due to a combination of anovulation and amenorrhea brought about by adenohypophyseal suppression.
3. Hormones that have given subjective or objective relief of signs or symptoms are: estrogens, androgens, progestins, combined estrogen-progesterone pill, hydroxyprogesterone caproate, and medroxyprogesterone.
4. A new testosterone derivative, 2,3 isoxazol ethisterone (Danazol), with weak androgenic and no estrogenic or progestational activities is also reported effective in suppressing endometriosis.

It acts by inhibiting gonadotropins or gonadotropin-releasing factors. More clinical trials are necessary to evaluate its overall value in the management of endometriosis.

5. **Contraindications to Hormone Therapy**

a. Unproved endometriosis especially in presence of adnexal masses

b. Large myomata that may be stimulated to grow during hormone therapy

c. Excessive side effects, either physical or psychological

d. Hepatic disease

e. Previous thrombophlebitis or embolic phenomenon

f. Previous mammary cancer

g. Patients over age 35 years

h. Patients who use cigarettes excessively

6. Prolonged therapy is applicable in:

a. Unmarried patients with maximal symptoms and minimal palpable findings in whom a biopsy diagnosis has been established

b. Patients with persistent or recurrent disease after previous conservative surgery

7. Short-term hormonal therapy is indicated:

a. Prior to conservative surgery

b. Subsequent to conservative therapy in order to inhibit ovulation and prevent reactivation of the disease

Results

1. Only 25 per cent of successful pregnancies are reported after hormone therapy that results in pseudopregnancy.

2. Between 50 and 60 per cent of successful pregnancies are reported after surgery.

3. Surgery not only eliminates endometriosis but also corrects factors relating to tubal distortion or uterine fixation.

Complications

1. Endometriosis, untreated, is rarely a fatal disease and the complications arising from it are few.

2. Occasionally there will be some obstruction of the rectosigmoid at the level of the cul-de-sac.

3. Obstruction of the small bowel is infrequent but may occur. It is usually in the low ileum or at the ileocolic junction. It is most likely due to adhesions between loops of the intestine, which may produce kinking and obstruction.

4. An ovarian endometrial cyst may rupture, become infected, and occasionally is associated with malignant changes.

5. The ureters may be invaded, although most infrequently.

39. Gynecological Cancer

Hugh R. K. Barber, M.D.

Exclusive of the ovary and the fallopian tube, carcinoma in the female reproductive system can be readily detected early by presently available diagnostic techniques. The question is raised and rightfully so, if indeed this is the situation, then why are cancers of the vulva, vagina, cervix, and corpus not diagnosed at an early stage? Why have screening programs failed to accomplish this? The blame must be shared by the patient as well as the doctor. Only a well-informed public and profession can work cooperatively together to search for cancer in its early, most curable stage. Each doctor's office should serve as a screening clinic for detection of gynecological cancer.

BASIC PRINCIPLES

1. Exclusive of choriocarcinoma, there are only two definitive types of therapy that result in cure in a significant number of gynecological cancers, i.e., surgery and radiation.
2. The philosophy has changed from which is a better form of treatment for a given cancer, to what is the better form of treatment for a given patient. Individualization has replaced standardization.
3. Chemotherapy—the treatment of cancer with drugs and with hormones—can be used effectively for disseminated as well as localized cancer. It has not only added to the longevity of the patient with gynecological cancer but has also improved the quality of life.
4. Therapy is no longer rigidly instituted for a state of disease but rather to eradicate a volume of cancer in a patient.

GENERAL MANAGEMENT

1. Although there are individual variations in management of a patient with different forms of gynecological cancer, there is an overall plan for all of these patients.
2. The patient admitted to the hospital for treatment of cancer is subject to a general evaluation of her physical status. A complete history is taken, and specific answers to the following questions are included: duration of present symptoms, history of weight change, previous neoplastic disease at any site, family history of neoplastic disease, whether or not she is a twin, menstrual history, abortions, histories of pregnancies, and previous operations of any kind.
3. In the routine physical examination, a careful pelvic and rectal examination should be carried out on admission and recorded. The speculum examination should not only visualize the cervix but should be manipulated to expose the entire vagina.
4. A patient who has cancer generally suspects the nature of her illness; or, as often happens, she has been told the diagnosis, or that such a diagnosis is to be ruled out. When entering the hospital she is apprehensive, regardless of appearance. A well-organized admission routine can be most reassuring.
5. The admitting doctor or house officer should refrain from general discussion of neoplastic disease, methods of treatment, specific diagnoses of her case, and prognosis. The term tumor or growth should be used in relation to her condition and not the word cancer.

6. On admission, the patient should be put at ease and medication should be prescribed to attain two objectives: tranquilizing drugs that allay apprehension should be given as necessary; to insure sleep, medication should be given at a stated time so that the patient does not have a restless night.

7. If pain is present, the patient is asked what she has been taking and with what effects; the medication is ordered immediately and, if necessary, in increased doses to insure maximal relief.

LABORATORY DATA

1. Papanicolaou smears of the vagina, cervix, and endometrium should be obtained.
2. Complete blood count
3. Urinalysis including cultures and sensitivity
4. SMA-12 (total protein, albumin, calcium, cholesterol, glucose, blood urea nitrogen, uric acid, creatinine, total bilirubin, alkaline phosphatase, LDH, SGOT)
5. SMA-6/60 (chloride, CO_2, potassium, sodium, BUN, glucose) as indicated
6. CEA and AFP as indicated
7. Clotting mechanism is assessed by thrombin time, prothrombin time, and partial thromboplastin time. Bleeding time, platelet count, and clot retraction are optional.
8. Roentgenologic Studies. Chest radiograph, intravenous pyelogram, and in indicated cases a bone survey.
9. Electrocardiogram
10. Proctoscopy and cystoscopy as indicated
11. Sonogram (ultrasonography)
12. Barium enema and GI series are optional.
13. Lymphangiography is optional and is not recommended in the elderly.
14. Computerized axial tomography as indicated
15. Liver scan if deemed necessary.

PREOPERATIVE REGIMEN FOR RADICAL ABDOMINAL SURGERY

1. The general principles in preparation for laparotomy and major pelvic surgery are followed with the addition of the list below for radical pelvic surgery.

2. The preparation for intracavitary radiation does not need to be as extensive but should include certain of the following orders as deemed appropriate for the patient.

3. Upon return of laboratory reports, any abnormal values are rectified by appropriate measures—i.e., blood transfusions for anemia, plasma for hypoproteinemia, indicated parenteral fluids for chloride, potassium or sodium deficiencies, vitamin K for prolonged bleeding and clotting time, and so on.

4. In debilitated patients, preoperative blood volume studies may be carried out and blood replacement ordered as needed and indicated. Ordinarily such studies are not necessary.

a. If the blood volume is thought to be depleted and facilities for blood volume determination are not available, it is possible for a blood volume determination to be made by watching the response of the patient's hematocrit to transfusions.

b. If there is a rise of 2 to 3 per cent after the transfusion of 500 ml. of whole blood, it can be assumed that the blood volume deficit has been overcome.

5. In certain debilitated patients in whom it is felt that there is a chance for cure or significant palliation, hyperalimentation (TPN—total parenteral nutrition) should be administered. This is discussed elsewhere.

6. Counseling of the patient should be intensive, and the husband or another relative should be involved. The type of procedure, the complications, and the period of hospitalization must be presented.

7. The team of social worker, oncology nurse, and inhalation therapist, as

well as others should be involved preoperatively.

Preoperative Bowel Preparation

1. Ideally, the intestinal tract should contain the minimal amount of material, but stringent measures are not necessary. Regular diet may be permitted up to and including the evening meal prior to the day of operation. Nothing by mouth is permitted after midnight.
2. Enemas are ordered daily and until clear the evening before surgery. It is to be emphasized that mechanical cleansing is the most important factor in a bowel prep.
3. 60 ml. of 50-per-cent magnesium sulfate is given twice a day for 2 days prior to surgery.
4. 45 ml. of castor oil are given in the afternoon before surgery. It serves to flatten the small intestine.
5. Neomycin, 1 g. q.lh. × 6 doses, is given in the afternoon and evening before surgery.
6. Sulfathalidine, 2 g. 4 times a day for 1 week, provides an excellent bowel prep.
7. If the patient has had any barium studies, it is important to take a flat plate of the abdomen the evening before surgery to make sure that there is no residual barium.

Additional Preoperative Measures

1. The patient is given a pHisohex shower the night before surgery.
2. A sulfa cream or antibiotic suppositories are inserted into the vagina the day before surgery.
3. No pelvic laparotomy for cancer should be undertaken without adequate blood readily available for transfusion. Thus, typing and crossmatching of several units of blood is a routine order, the number depending upon the anticipated magnitude of the procedure.
4. The vagina is prepared with Betadine in the operating room.
5. If the patient has a carcinoma in situ, it is better not to prepare the vagina because the superficial layer of cells may be denuded.

Management in the Operating Room

1. After induction of anesthesia, the patient is placed in lithotomy position and pelvic examination is performed. With complete relaxation, palpation often permits different impressions than can be obtained with the patient awake, uncomfortable, and exhibiting varying degrees of muscle rigidity.
2. A Foley catheter is inserted into the bladder. Care must be taken to insure that it is not in the vagina or the urethra, but is well placed in the bladder.
3. The indicated operation is then carried out.

POSTOPERATIVE MANAGEMENT AFTER RADICAL SURGERY

1. Immediately following surgery, the vital signs, i.e., blood pressure, pulse, and respirations, are noted at 15-minute intervals until sensoria are fully recovered.
2. Special attention is directed to the pulmonary response and ventilation.
3. Urine output per catheter is recorded at hourly intervals. 40 ml. per hour is considered satisfactory.
   a. In the immediate postoperative period urinary output may be minimal, but after 12 hours the normal rate of excretion generally increases if fluid intake is adequate. An excess secretion of antidiuretic hormone (ADH) may decrease the urinary output.
   b. A good urinary output indicates good tissue perfusion. An output of 1,000 ml. a day is considered adequate.
   c. Absence of urine indicates a mechanical block. Caution must be exercised in administering fluids.
   d. The urine excretion from ileal or colon conduits is especially noted. In

case of ileal conduits, prompt urine flow is anticipated, but not infrequently the first 24-hour output may be less than normal.

e. In the case of colon conduits, urine excretion may be delayed for several hours, or even 1 or 2 days. This is because of the usual excessive edema that may occur at the uretero-colon implantation sites as compared with the uretero-small bowel implantation sites.

f. In the case of wet colostomy there may be little or no urine excretion for 1 or 2 days. These patients must be carefully observed and controlled.

4. The insertion of nasogastric tube is carried out at the discretion of the operator.

5. Oral ingestion of fluids is not permitted until the bowel sounds are completely normal.

a. When oral feedings are started, it is best to give 60 ml. of water each hour as desired by the patient. If the patient is reluctant to take fluids or has any nausea, fluids should be withheld.

b. Generally, fruit juices and milk produce an increased amount of gas accompanied by gas pains that may be severe. They should not be given.

6. The use of prophylactic antibiotics in the postoperative period should be individualized.

7. Fluid and electrolyte intake is discussed elsewhere, Chap. 31.

8. The treatment of ileus, intestinal obstruction, and peritonitis is discussed elsewhere.

9. When large denuded areas have been created, such as result from radical Wertheim hysterectomies with pelvic node dissection, pelvic exenterations, and radical vulvectomies, excessive exudation from these sites may result in significant fluid, electrolyte, and protein loss. This should be corrected by the addition of 250 to 500 ml. of plasma added to the daily baseline fluid and electrolyte replacement.

10. Blood chemistry studies should be obtained at least every other day.

11. The protein level should be maintained at a minimum of 6 g. per 100 ml. and the hemoglobin at least 11 g.

12. The extended radical procedure that includes excision of the hypogastric arteries and veins result in removal of the branches of the autonomic nervous system and interferes with bladder and bowel function.

a. In this instance, the catheter should be kept in place for at least 6 weeks. This keeps the bladder from overdistending, reduces residual urine with its accompanying infection, and maintains the ureters in position where there is no pull on their blood supply.

b. If a lesser procedure is carried out, the catheter can be removed in 2 weeks. The patient should be catheterized for residual urine until the residual is below 150 ml.

40. Cancer of the Lower Genital Tract

Hugh R. K. Barber, M.D.

CANCER OF THE VULVA

Basic Principles

1. Cancer of the vulva accounts for 0.7 per cent of all female cancers at a rate of 1.8 per 100,000 females. It is the fourth most common malignant tumor of the female genital tract, accounting for 3 or 4 per cent of all gynecologic malignancies.

2. It occurs most frequently after the age of 65 years; it makes up 30 per cent of the malignant gynecologic tumors arising in the seventh decade. It is rare under age 45 years and is very rare in pregnancy.

3. There are about 500 deaths annually in the United States from vulvar carcinoma.

4. Cancer of the vulva is usually diagnosed in the localized stage—about 60 per cent of all cases.

5. Surgery is the usual treatment in over 80 per cent of all cases. The 5-year survival rate is 64 per cent.

6. Almost all lesions are squamous cell in origin, although adenocarcinomas of Bartholin's glands, basal cell carcinoma, malignant melanomas, and malignant sweat-gland tumors also occur.

7. The most common symptom of vulvar carcinoma is long-standing pruritus.

a. Chronic inflammatory changes are always present for varying periods, sometimes for several years, before cancer appears as an ulcerating lesion, with raised rolled borders and surrounded by induration of the uninvolved skin and subcutaneous tissues.

b. Rarely, multiple or one other cancerous lesion is present simultaneously in different portions of the vulva. They may appear as kissing lesions, one ulcer on each side, directly opposite from one another.

8. Approximately 50 per cent of the patients with cancer of the vulva have positive lymph node involvement. About 30 per cent have superficial involvement, about 15 per cent have superficial and deep involvement, whereas only about 3 per cent have deep involvement as the only metastases.

9. The most frequent site of the initial lesions is the labia majora, in the mid or anterior portion.

a. The clitoris is also a common site.

b. Encroachment upon the urethra or actual involvement of its occurs in larger lesions.

c. Less frequent primary sites are the region of the fourchette and posterior labial areas.

10. In the differential diagnosis other common conditions to be considered are: lymphogranuloma inguinale, chancre, chancroid and acuminata condylomata.

11. All white lesions of the vulva must be biopsied if short-term medical treatment is unsuccessful.

12. Any suspicious lesion should be biopsied immediately.

Precancerous Lesions

1. Carcinoma in situ now represents 35 per cent of all vulvar cancers. With no characteristic symptoms of lesion, a high index of suspicion and interest in vulvar disease are necessary to detect these lesions.

2. Vulvar carcinoma in situ is frequently multifocal, and multiple biopsies must be taken. Painting the vulva with 1-per-cent toluidine blue and then rinsing with 1-per-cent acetic acid will allow some unsuspected areas to be identified and biopsied, since the neoplastic areas will retain the dye.

3. Paget's disease may be in situ as well as invasive.

a. The final diagnosis for any in situ lesion remains with the histologic examination.

b. Paget's disease may resemble amelanotic melanoma on microscopic examination.

c. When the section is stained with periodic acid-Schiff and the glycogen has been digested, the Paget's cells become PAS positive.

d. The staining techniques assist in differentiating the lesion from the amelanotic melanoma.

4. The treatment for localized carcinoma in situ may be wide local excision or hemivulvectomy.

a. However, widespread in situ cancer may require a simple vulvectomy with or without skin graft.

b. There is increasing evidence to support an attempt at eradication of the in situ with 5-per-cent fluorouracil (5-FU) cream or lotion.

c. If the lesion fails to respond to this, the indicated and appropriate surgery can be carried out.

5. Paget's disease of the vulva is usually considered an in situ lesion. However, it may be associated with a sweat gland carcinoma.

a. Instead of the usual superficial vulvectomy which does not include all of the underlying fat pad, this lesion is best treated by a simple vulvectomy that is carried through all layers, including the fascia over the underlying muscle.

b. The procedure is probably best called a radical local excision of the vulva.

c. If invasive cancer is diagnosed, a superficial and deep node dissection can be carried out at that time or as a secondary procedure.

Staging of Carcinoma of the Vulva

Cases should be classifed as carcinoma of the vulva when the primary site of growth is in the vulva. Tumors present in the vulva as secondary growths from either a genital or extragenital site should be excluded from registration, as should cases of malignant melanoma.

Stage O.	Carcinoma in situ, e.g., Bowen's disease, noninvasive disease, noninvasive Paget's disease.
Stage I.	Tumor confined to the vulva, 2 cm. or less in largest diameter. Nodes are not palpable, or are palpable in either groin, not enlarged, mobile (not clinically suspicious of neoplasm).
Stage II.	Tumor confined to the vulva more than 2 cm. in diameter. Nodes are not palpable, or are palpable in either groin, not enlarged, mobile (not clinically suspicious of neoplasm).
Stage III.	Tumor of any size with adjacent spread to the urethra and any or all of the vagina, the perineum, and the anus, and/or nodes palpable in either or both groins (enlarged, firm, and mobile, not fixed but clinically suspicious of neoplasm).
Stage IV.	Tumor of any size infiltrating the bladder, mucosa, or the rectal mucosa, or both, including the upper part of the urethral mucosa, and/or fixed to the bone or other distant metastases.

Treatment

1. Established invasive malignant disease of the vulva is not suitable for radiation therapy.

a. The blood vessels are end-type of vessels with poor collateral circulation. As a result, endarteritis with necrosis may follow radiation therapy.

b. Many vulvar lesions are very big and therefore not suitable for implantation with radium or new radioactive substances.

2. Invasive cancer must be treated by radical vulvectomy. This means removal of the entire vulva, including the labia majora, labia minora, hymenal remnants, and clitoris.

a. The lateral incision is made at the labiocrural fold; superiorly, the mons pubis is removed; inferiorly, the perineum is incised near the anus; and the medial incisions usually lie just outside the level of the urethral meatus.

b. The procedure must encompass the disease even though the distal one-half of the urethra has to be removed.

c. The superficial nodes bilaterally are excised and a decision must be made about the removal of the deep nodes.

3. Hemovacs are used to facilitate the apposition of flaps and prevent the accumulation of serum. The hemovacs are removed when the daily drainage is less than 50 ml.

4. Postoperative ambulation is begun on the day following surgery and progresses rapidly each day.

5. Postoperative antibiotic therapy is ordered as indicated.

6. Oral feedings are usually started the day after surgery.

7. The catheter is removed on the tenth postoperative day.

8. Sitz baths are started within the first week.

9. Wound breakdown at the margin of the skin flaps continues to be a problem.

a. The wound should be denuded and an enzyme ointment applied to and in the debridement.

b. Most close without requiring a skin graft.

Certain cases of recurrence can be managed by pelvic exenteration.

Results

1. The cure rates range around 60 per cent in most cases.

2. Patients with positive superficial nodes have a 40-per-cent cure rate. In patients with negative nodes the cure rate approaches 80 per cent. Approximately 60 per cent of patients will have negative nodes.

CANCER OF THE VAGINA

Basic Principles

1. Cancer of the vagina is extremely rare. It comprises less than 1 per cent of all genital malignancies.

2. Cancer of the vagina usually occurs after the age of 70 years.

3. There are about 300 deaths from cancer of the vagina each year.

4. Cancer of the vagina is usually diagnosed in the localized (43 per cent) or regional (36 per cent) stage.

5. The ratio of cancer of the cervix to vaginal cancer is roughly 50:1. It is often difficult to tell whether the tumor arises primarily in the vaginal epithelium or extends to it from a primary locus in the cervix. When both are involved together, the cervix is considered the primary locus.

6. Usual treatment is radiation—60 per cent of all cases.

7. The 5-year survival rate is 45 per cent.

8. Persisting bloody vaginal discharge, at first relatively painless, is the initial sign of primary vaginal cancer.

9. Because of its relatively infrequency, primary vaginal cancer is not often considered; if an ordinary solid-blade speculum is used for examination, the instrument may cover the anterior midportion of the vaginal tube, at which point the lesion frequently originates.

10. The most common form of primary vaginal cancer is the squamous cell type. Macroscopically, it presents as a rounded or elongated ulcer with raised rolled edges and central excavated ulcer.

11. Vaginal cancer generally arises in the upper-third of the posterior wall of the vagina and involves the rectovaginal septum early.

12. As the cancer invades and spreads, the cancer usually destroys the cervix and then invades the parametria. Involvement of the vulva is rare, and spread to the lymph nodes is usually late.

13. Occasionally, adenocarcinoma is seen. When it is diagnosed, it is important to determine whether the lesion is primary or is actually a metastasis from an unsuspected primary cancer elsewhere.

14. Cancer of the endometrium is prone to metastasize to the vagina and is almost always found on the anterior wall.

15. Less often, secondary vaginal lesions may have their origins from the ovary, paraurethral glands, or gastrointestinal tract (especially the colon), or from hypernephroma or uterine choriocarcinoma.

16. Since many alleged primary vaginal cancers are really metastases from an unsuspected primary cancer elsewhere, it is important to have a careful workup including biopsies and fractional uterine curettage.

17. Clear-cell adenocarcinoma (Müllerian type) is discussed elsewhere.

Staging of Carcinoma of the Vagina

Excluded from this classification are secondary cancers in the vagina, cervical cancers involving the vagina, and malignant lesions extending into the vagina from the urethra or vulva.

Stage O.	Carcinoma in situ; intraepithelial carcinoma
Stage I.	The carcinoma is limited to the vaginal wall.
Stage II.	The carcinoma has involved the subvaginal tissue but has not extended to the pelvic wall.
Stage III.	The carcinoma has extended to the pelvic wall.
Stage IV.	The carcinoma has extended beyond the true pelvis or has involved the mucosa of the bladder or rectum. Bullous edema as such does not permit a case to be allotted to Stage IV.
Stage IVa.	Spread of the growth to adjacent organs
Stage IVb.	Spread to distant organs

Treatment

Since the 5-year survival rate in primary epithelial cancer of the vagina is approximately 45 per cent with primary radical surgery with or without supplemental radiation, it is important to concentrate on making an early diagnosis.

1. Upper Two-Thirds of the Vagina

a. *Stage O (Carcinoma In Situ).* Simple excision or, in select cases, total hysterectomy and total vaginectomy.

b. *Stage I.* Radical hysterectomy, bilateral pelvic node dissection, and total vaginectomy. Radiation therapy is an alternate and the modality chosen for certain patients.

c. *Stage II.* Radical surgery as listed above. If it is not possible to encompass the cancer, radiation therapy, both external and intravaginal, should be carried out. Exenteration is reserved for recurrent cases of cancer of the vagina.

d. *Stage III.* Primary radiation therapy

e. *Stage IV.* Primary radiation therapy. It may be necessary to divert the fecal and/or urinary stream before therapy.

2. Lower-Third of Vagina

a. *Stage O.* As listed above

b. *Stage I.* Total hysterectomy and total vaginectomy plus radical vulvectomy and bilateral groin node dissection. Radiation therapy may be chosen followed by a groin dissection.

c. *Stage II.* As for Stage I

d. *Stage III.* Primary radiation therapy

e. *Stage IV.* Radiation therapy with or without diversion of the urinary and fecal steams depending on the condition of the patient

CLEAR-CELL ADENOCARCINOMA (MÜLLERIAN TYPE)

It was reported that a study at Massachusetts General Hospital revealed a highly significant association between the treatment of mothers with diethylstilbestrol (DES) during pregnancy and the later development of adenocarcinoma in their daughters.

Basic Principles

1. The natural estrogens have apparently not been associated with this problem.
2. Nonsteroidal estrogens, i.e., diethylstilbestrol, dienesterol (nestrol, Synestrol), hexestrol, and benzestrol, have also been associated with this type of vaginal and cervical cancer.
3. The incidence rate for the development of clear-cell carcinoma of the vagina or cervix is approximately 0.1 per cent in the female fetus whose mother took stilbestrol.
4. About 80 to 90 per cent of these patients develop adenosis of thc vagina or have a congenital anomaly of the cervix and/or vagina. From these observations it was suggested that diethylstilbestrol (DES) acts as a teratogen rather than a carcinogen.
5. All teen-age girls with irregular periods should receive a thorough pelvic examination including palpation and direct visual inspection of the cervix and vagina plus cytologic studies.
6. DES-exposed females should start to have pelvic examinations after their first period and at any age if they have symptoms.
7. Although the cytology studies are often negative because the tumors have a low grade of malignancy and are often covered with either intact mucosa or slough, the studies should still be carried out, and it is suggested that the lesions or fornices be scraped with a spatula.
8. In all cases of clear-cell adenocarcinoma with a history of diethylstilbestrol ingestion by the mother, adenosis has been found.
   a. Adenosis is defined as the persistence of glandular elements in and under squamous epithelium of the vagina.
   b. There is no current evidence that indicates that adenosis is a precursor of clear-cell adenocarcinoma.
9. In studies carried out with the microspectrophotometer, all clear-cell adenocarcinomas had aneuploid DNA distribution; all areas of adenosis had a diploid or tetraploid distribution pattern, which is usually seen in proliferating epithelium.

Diagnostic Signs

1. The anterior fornix often appears shortened and is less elastic than usual.
2. A cervical hood may be present and gives the appearance of a cockscomb.
3. The cervix appears red.
4. There is often a red granular mucosa, small cysts, or a papillary lesion that may be multicentric in appearance.
5. On palpation there is a sandy irregularity.
6. The involved area takes Schiller's or Lugol's stain poorly, if at all.
7. The same findings may exist in patients with adenocarcinoma. Usually the findings are more marked, and often polypoid, nodular, or papillary lesions are present.

Treatment

1. Following representative biopsies, the general program for managing adenosis is close observation and repeated

examinations. Adenosis is benign and there is currently no evidence that it will turn directly to cancer.

2. Although some authors recommend partial or total vaginectomies for vaginal adenosis, treatment is conservative in most institutions. Laser beam therapy is being tried in a few centers.

3. Clear-cell adenocarcinoma of the cervix and fornices is best treated with radical surgery. Early lesions (Stage I vaginal or cervical carcinomas) can and do metastasize to regional pelvic lymph nodes.

4. Radical hysterectomy, pelvic lymph node dissection, and placement of split-thickness graft from the buttock into the area from which the vagina was excised.

a. The ovaries are preserved unless they are diseased.

b. Pelvic exenteration has been employed to encompass disease too extensive to be cured by a less radical surgical procedure.

5. Clear-cell adenocarcinoma can also be treated and cured by radiation.

a. Many radiotherapists are reluctant to deliver large doses of cancerocidal radiation to a young woman.

b. However, radiation therapy is considered by some to be preferable to pelvic exenteration as therapy for the more advanced lesion.

6. The criteria for prognosis depends on the degree of mitotic activity (one or more mitoses per high-power field carries a bad prognosis), involved regional lymph nodes, and the stage of disease.

7. The recent observation of pulmonary and/or supraclavicular lymph node metastases indicates that prolonged follow-up of treated individuals is essential.

CANCER OF THE CERVIX

Cancer of the cervix is a disease of the inner city. About 1.6 per cent of newborn girls, or 1 out of 63, will develop invasive cancer of the cervix uteri at sometime during their lives. In 1978 there were about 20,000 new cases of invasive cancer of the cervix reported and about 7,700 deaths.

Basic Principles

1. The high-risk group includes those starting intercourse in their teens, having multiple sexual partners, or having many children, and women from the low socioeconomic groups.

2. The peak incidence for carcinoma in situ of the cervix is between 30 and 40 years of age, whereas for invasive cancer it is between the ages of 40 and 50 years.

3. In understanding the natural history of cancer of the cervix, it is important to know the cause of death from disease. Uremia, infection, and hemorrhage are the leading cause of death from invasive cancer of the cervix, but some women die from distant metastases.

Diagnosis

1. There are no symptoms characteristic of cancer of the cervix. A high index of suspicion is necessary.

2. Bleeding is probably the most common symptom associated with cancer of the cervix and is usually bright red and "lawless." It may result from contact with the cervix—contact bleeding.

3. The cervix should be examined carefully with rotation of the speculum in order to see all fornices as well as the entire cervix.

4. A cervix involved with a malignant process may show nothing if the disease is localized in the canal or if the lesion is smaller than an ulcerated mass.

5. The spectrum of findings may include red areas, erosions, ulcers, nodularity, an exophytic or endophytic lesion, or nodularity with ulceration.

6. An accurate histologic diagnosis is essential before definitive treatment is instituted.

7. A differential diagnosis should rule out chancres, tuberculosis, granuloma

inguinale, lymphogranuloma venereum, condyloma acuminata, and radium eschars.

8. A point to emphasize is that each of these lesions can be present concurrently with cancer, and this argues strongly for biopsy proof of disease.

9. The Papanicolaou smear is merely a screening method and has its greatest application in the asymptomatic woman.

a. Any lesion visible on the cervix should be biopsied since an obvious lesion may result in a negative Pap smear, despite the invasive nature of the lesion.

b. The combination of Pap smear and biopsy will give a high yield of positive results in those patients in whom "early" cancer is present.

10. Pregnant patients represent a captive group and afford the physician the opportunity of not only doing a Pap smear but also for training the patient in the need for routine physical examination, cytology, and biopsy screening.

11. When positive or suspicious cells are reported on Pap smear examination, it is important to have a systematic approach to establishing a diagnosis.

a. Repeat smears are submitted to another laboratory.

b. A colposcope can be used to outline the lesion and obtain colposcopically directed biopsies.

c. On an outpatient basis, punch biopsies of the Schiller's or toluidine-blue-treated cervix and vagina are taken. Endocervical curettage with a small curette may be performed.

d. Hospital admission for fractional D and C, further biopsies, or conization of the cervix, if deemed necessary.

e. Biopsy revealing invasive cancer avoids the need for conization.

f. Vaginal bleeding should be evaluated systematically.

g. The D and C should be preceded by a careful pelvic examination under anesthesia.

h. The endocervix should be carefully curetted with a small curette and the tissue sent as a separate specimen.

i. Then the depth of the uterine cavity is determined with a sound.

j. The cervix is then dilated and the uterine cavity is explored with a polyp forceps.

k. The endometrial cavity is systematically curetted including the top of the fundus and both cornua. An attempt should be made to identify the site of the tumor.

l. Multiple-punch biopsies are then taken of the cervix.

Staging of Carcinoma of the Cervix Uteri

Stage O.	Carcinoma in situ, intraepithelial carcinoma
Stage I.	The carcinoma is strictly confined to the cervix (extension to the corpus should be disregarded).
Stage Ia.	Microinvasive carcinoma (early stromal invasion).
Stage Ib.	All other cases of Stage I; occult cancer should be marked "occ."
Stage II.	The carcinoma extends beyond the cervix, but has not extended to the pelvic wall. The carcinoma involves the vagina, but not as far as the lower third.
Stage IIa.	No obvious parametrial involvement.
Stage IIb.	Obvious parametrial involvement.
Stage III.	The carcinoma has extended to the pelvic wall. On rectal examination there is no cancer-free space between the tumor and the pelvic wall. The tumor involves the lower-third of the vagina. All cases with a hydronephrosis or nonfunctioning kidney are included.

Stage IIIa.	No extension to the pelvic wall.
Stage IIIb.	Extension to the pelvic wall and/or hydronephrosis or nonfunctioning kidney.
Stage IV.	The carcinoma has extended beyond the true pelvis or has clinically involved the mucosa of the bladder or rectum. A bullous edema as such does not permit a case to be allotted to Stage IV.
Stage IVa.	Spread of the growth to adjacent organs
Stage IVb.	Spread to distant organs

Notes About the Staging

1. Stage Ia (microinvasive carcinoma) represents those cases of epithelial abnormalities in which histologic evidence of early stromal invasion is unambiguous. The diagnosis is based on microscopic examination of tissue removed by biopsy, conization, portio amputation, or removal of the uterus. Cases of early stromal invasion should thus be allotted to Stage Ia.

2. The remainder of Stage I cases should be allotted to Stage Ib. As a rule, these cases can be diagnosed by routine clinical examination.

3. Occult cancer is a histologically invasive cancer that cannot be diagnosed by routine clinical examination. As a rule, it is diagnosed on a cone, the amputated portio, or on the removed uterus. Such cancers should be included in Stage Ib and should be marked "Stage Ib, Occ."

4. *Stage I* cases can thus be indicated in the following ways:

Stage Ia.	Carcinoma in situ with early stromal invasion diagnosed on tissue removed by biopsy, conization, or portio amputation, or on the removed uterus.
Stage Ib.	Clinically invasive carcinoma confined to the cervix
Stage Ib, Occ.	Histologically invasive carcinoma of the cervix which could not be detected at routine clinical examination but which was diagnosed on a large biopsy, a cone, the amputated portio, or the removed uterus.

Treatment

1. Dysplasia when moderate or marked is usually adequately treated by conization or multiple biopsies plus endocervical curettage. This is followed by Pap smears. Cautery and cryotherapy should only be used after a firm histologic diagnosis has been established.

2. Carcinoma in situ should only be treated after accurate clinical and histologic findings are determined.

a. The colposcopically directed biopsies are helpful.

b. In most cases, a cone biopsy or multiple biopsies and an endocervical curettage should be performed.

c. In young women desirous of children, a biopsy may be therapeutic as well as diagnostic.

d. Older women are probably better treated by hysterectomy after an invasive lesion has been ruled out.

e. Cautery or cryotherapy is not recommended in the management of carcinoma in situ.

3. Stage Ia or early stromal invasion in general is treated as invasive cancer. When invasion is indefinite or only 1 mm. in depth, does not cover a wide area, and involves no vascular or lymphatic area, the treatment is the same as that suggested for carcinoma in situ.

4. Stage Ib is usually treated by radical hysterectomy and bilateral pelvic lymphadenectomy. Radiation therapy is chosen for those patients in whom sur-

gical therapy is not to be performed because of age or general health.

5. Stage IIa receives the same treatment as Stage Ib.

6. Stages IIb, IIIa, and IIIb are treated by primary radiation. External therapy is started first, followed by intracavitary radiation.

7. Stage IV is generally treated by primary radiation therapy. This therapy may require preradiation diversion of the fecal and/or urinary stream. Primary pelvic exenteration may be selected for those patients with central disease that extends into the bladder usually with a vesicovaginal fistula and in whom it is possible to completely encompass the disease.

Cancer of the Cervix Complicating Pregnancy

1. Approximately 1 pregnancy in 3,000 is complicated by cervical cancer.

2. The disease is not different from that found in the nonpregnant state.

3. A comparison of cure rates in comparable stages of disease between pregnant and nonpregnant patients shows no difference.

4. Prognosis depends on the extent of the disease.

5. Primary treatment usually chosen is surgery. However, radiation therapy gives equally good results but produces more late side effects in these young patients.

41. Cancer of the Upper Genital Tract

Hugh R. K. Barber, M.D.

CANCER OF THE ENDOMETRIUM

Basic Principles

1. Cancer of the endometrium is a disease of suburbia.

2. About 2.2 per cent of newborn girls or 1 in 45 will develop cancer of the corpus uteri sometime during their lives.

3. Malignant neoplasms of the corpus uteri generally occur in patients a decade older (of peri- and postmenopausal age) than those who develop cancer of the cervix.

a. It does occur in women less than 40 years of age in 5 per cent of cases and has been found as early as age 17 years.

b. More than 70 per cent of the cases occur after age 50, while 20 per cent occur between the ages of 40 and 50.

c. There is an increasing number of patients in the older age group presenting with adenosquamous cancer of the endometrium.

4. Early diagnosis is the key to successful treatment in cancer of the endometrium.

5. The physical habitus of these patients is well known to the gynecologist.

6. They are patients with an abnormal pituitary function and a long history of hyperestrogenism which may have many causes.

7. Reports indicate that there is a higher incidence of cancer of the endometrium occurring at an early age among patients with continuous unopposed estrogen stimulation of the endometrium, i.e., patients with the Stein-Leventhal syndrome, a long history of anovulation and/or amenorrhea.

8. It appears that the postmenopausal prehormone is androstenedione and that the notable postmenopausal estrogen is estrone.

a. Conversion of androstenedione to estrone is increased with age, massive obesity, and liver disease.

b. Increased production of the precursor androstenedione for conversion to estrone is noted in chronic anovulators, in polycystic ovarian disease, in certain functioning ovarian tumors, and in ovarian cortical stromal hyperplasia.

c. The significance of exogenous estrogens in the etiology of endometrial carcinoma is generally suspected but not completely understood.

9. Negative cytology does not have the same accuracy in prognosticating that the development of cancer is highly unlikely, because on cytologic evaluation the preinvasive lesions are not diagnosed with the same accuracy as obtained in cancer of the cervix. Adenomatous hyperplasia should be considered a precursor lesion.

10. The first and most significant symptom is abnormal vaginal bleeding. In any age group it should be suspect for a serious problem and a fractional curettage should be carried out.

11. Pelvic examination may reveal a normal or nearly-normal-sized uterus for the stated age and parity. In most instances, there is some enlargement of the uterus, which may be of softer than normal consistency. The coexistence of fibroids may distort the estimation of uterine size. In more advanced cases, the uterus is definitely enlarged and softer

than normal. Tumor may fungate out of the cervix and fragments may become detached during bimanual examination.

12. The diagnosis of endometrial carcinoma should not be difficult. Although the diagnosis may be made in the office by endometrial biopsy, a careful pelvic examination under anesthesia, and a **careful fractional curettage is mandatory for accurate clinical staging.**

13. Pyometra may be the first manifestation of endometrial cancer because of blockage low in the endometrial cavity. In patients in the peri- and postmenopausal age groups who present such a condition, an underlying carcinoma must be ruled out.

14. Adenocarcinoma of the endometrium is either localized or diffuse over the surface of the endometrium. Cancer arising in the endometrium tends to remain within the uterus for a long period of time.

a. As it grows it invades the myometrium and spreads toward the isthmus and the endocervix.

b. From the myometrium it spreads through the serosa to the peritoneal cavity and from the endocervix spreads to the pelvic nodes.

c. The lymphatics increase in amount as the serosa of the uterus is approached; deep penetration of the myometrium is associated with an increased incidence of positive node involvement.

d. Since the myometrium in the postmenopasual women is much thinner than in the premenopausal patient, a little penetration of the myometrium may bring the cancer into contact with the lymphatics and account for the greater potency of endometrial cancer among the postmenopausal woman.

e. The high-risk group for extrauterine spread are those with involvement of the lower uterus or cervix, histologic Grade III lesions, and deep myometrial invasion.

Clinical Staging of Carcinoma of the Corpus Uteri

Stage O.	Carcinoma in situ. Histologic findings are suspicious of malignancy; cases of Stage O should not be included in any therapeutic statistics.
Stage I.	The carcinoma is confined to the corpus.
Stage Ia.	The length of the uterine cavity is 8 cm. or less.
Stage Ib.	The length of the uterine cavity is more than 8 cm.

Stage I Subgroups. It is desirable that the Stage I cases be subgrouped with regard to the histologic type of the adenocarcinoma as follows:

G1.	Highly differentiated adenomatous carcinoma
G2.	Differentiated adenomatous carcinoma with partly solid areas
G3.	Predominately solid or entirely undifferentiated carcinoma
Stage II.	The carcinoma has involved the corpus and the cervix but has not extended outside the uterus.
Stage III.	The carcinoma has extended outside the uterus but not outside the true pelvis.
Stage IV.	The carcinoma has extended outside the true pelvis or has obviously involved the mucosa of the bladder or rectum. A bullous edema as such does not permit a case to be allotted to Stage IV.
Stage IVa.	Spread of the growth to adjacent organs
Stage IVb.	Spread to distant organs

Management

Stage O

Carcinoma in situ. The management should be tailored to fit the needs of the patient, her age, and desire for future childbearing. In selected young patients with minimal disease, an alternative to hysterectomy may be repeat curettage in 3 to 4 months or a course of progestational agents followed by repeat curettage.

Stage Ia, GI

1. Total hysterectomy and bilateral salpingo-oophorectomy and followed by postoperative vaginal radiation.

2. In patients in whom the histologic grade is G2 or G3, external pelvic radiation should be given preoperatively followed by total hysterectomy, bilateral salpingo-oophorectomy, and vaginal radiation postoperatively.

3. If preoperative external radiation has not been given and the surgical specimen reveals a histologic grade of G2 or G3 (instead of G1) or moderate or extensive myometrial invasion (one-third or more myometrial penetration), postoperative external radiation should be given.

Stage Ib

The same management as for Stage Ia.

Stage II

Preoperative external pelvic radiation is followed in 6 weeks by a modified radical hysterectomy and pelvic node dissection, if possible. Otherwise, a total hysterectomy is chosen.

Stage III

If the lesion involves only the adnexal structures, preoperative x-ray therapy is followed by total hysterectomy and bilateral salpingo-oophorectomy. Postoperatively, vaginal radiation is given. An alternate plan is modified radical hysterectomy.

Stage IV

Primary therapy is external and intracavitary radiation therapy. The patient is evaluated to ascertain whether supplementary progestational agents should be used. If the cancer is limited to the pelvis but involves bladder, rectum, or both, the patient is evaluated for pelvic exenteration. External therapy may be employed before pelvic exenteration is selected. In certain instances, despite the presence of widespread disease, it is necessary to remove the uterus to control hemorrhage.

Alternate Plan of Therapy

1. Recently the protocol has been changed to include hysterectomy as the first step in the management of all stages of cancer of the endometrium.

2. All patients will receive vaginal radiation postoperatively and the external therapy will be tailored to fit the needs of the patient.

3. This plan will allow a comparison between the value of preoperative as opposed to postoperative x-ray treatment.

Procedures for Different Types of Cancer

1. Distant Metastases

a. Primary progestational therapy is indicated. Depo-Provera 400 mg. intramuscularly a day for 7 days and then every 7 to 10 days, or Delalutin 250 mg. following the same schedule. In addition, Megace is given in doses up to 200 mg. by mouth a day.

b. Localized disease without response to progestational therapy is treated with x-ray therapy.

c. In the presence of widespread disease and no response to the treatment suggested above, chemotherapy is indicated.

d. Chemotherapy has not been particularly effective to date. However, combination therapy employing Cytoxan, Adriamycin, and platinum has shown some promise for help.

2. Adenosquamous Cancer

a. The increasing number of mixed adenosquamous cancer detected in the endometrium adds a new dimension.

b. This cancer has both malignant-appearing glandular and squamous components.

c. Venous involvement is observed in one-half of the cases, and blood vascular and transtubal routes may be involved in the dissemination of the neoplasm.

d. The mean age at detection is 65.5 years.

e. The duration of symptoms tends to be short, and abdominal or distal spread is frequently observed.

f. These tumors respond poorly to ionizing radiation. The 5-year survival rate is 19 to 20 per cent.

g. The treatment is total hysterectomy and bilateral salpingo-oophorectomy.

3. Sarcoma of the Uterus

a. Is a very rare disease.

b. The main varieties are leiomyosarcoma—true malignant neoplasms of smooth muscle cells (most common form); endometrial stromal sarcomas, which are composed of rounded and fusiform cells arising from mesoblastic elements of the endometrium itself; mixed mesodermal tumors of the uterus, the counterpart in the adult of sarcoma botryoides of infants and children; and very rare forms such as fibrosarcoma and carcinocarcinomas (mixtures of leiomyosarcoma and endometrial carcinoma).

(1) One form of leiomyosarcoma arises within the myometrium and has a poor prognosis.

(2) The other form arises within a fibroid and has a better prognosis.

c. The diagnosis of malignancy is established by counting the number of mitoses per 10 high power fields (HPF). Tumors with less than 5 mitoses per 10 HPF are benign, those with higher mitotic counts are malignant. The prognosis for leiomyosarcomas with greater than 10 mitoses per 10 HPF is poor and metastases are frequent.

d. There are no characteristic symptoms of sarcoma. Early bleeding does not occur unless polypoid lesions project into the endometrial cavity.

e. On physical examination the uterus is enlarged, suggestive of fibroids.

f. Rapidly enlarging masses in the uterus, especially of soft consistency, suggest sarcoma, but histologic study must be carried out to confirm this.

Treatment

1. Total hysterectomy and bilateral salpingo-oophorectomy is the keystone of therapy.
2. Combination chemotherapy (Cytoxan, actinomycin D, vincristine, and Adriamycin) have shown promise in controlling the sarcoma. Among those patients with a cellular stroma, the addition of a progestational agent has given some benefit.

CANCER OF THE FALLOPIAN TUBE

Basic Principles

1. This is the rarest carcinoma of the female genital tract.
2. The average age at diagnosis is 49 years.
3. The commonest form arises from the mucosa, forming papillary or medullary anaplastic lesions.
4. The metastatic pattern is similar to that for ovarian cancer.
5. The fallopian tube is commonly involved secondarily in advanced cases of endometrial and ovarian cancer.
6. There are usually no or only slight symptoms until the disease is advanced.
7. A profuse, intermittent, watery discharge, often blood-tinged, the so-called hemohydrops tubal profluens, may be present.
8. A positive Pap smear in the presence of a negative curettage should alert the clinician to this diagnosis.
9. On pelvic examination an adnexal mass is present, with the corpus and cervix seemingly normal, but the exact diagnosis is rarely made preoperatively.

10. Staging for cancer of the fallopian tube is similar to that for ovarian cancer.

Treatment

1. On opening the abdomen, fluid or peritoneal washings should be sent for cytologic examination.

2. The treatment is similar to that for ovarian cancer.

EMBRYONAL RHABDOMYOSARCOMA (BOTRYOID TYPE) OF THE VAGINA

Basic Principles

1. This is an uncommon, highly malignant neoplasm, which is encountered in infants and young children and has a very poor prognosis. It may be seen in adults.

2. When seen in the vagina it usually starts as a small, broad-based, polypoid mass, and as it grows it takes on the typical appearance of lobulated masses of vesicular or hemorrhagic polyps which soon fill the vagina and project through the vaginal introitus.

3. Widespread metastases are the rule rather than the exception.

4. The most common metastatic sites are the lungs and the regional nodes.

5. Bloody discharge, vaginal bleeding and/or mass are the most common signs.

6. Formerly, pelvic exenteration with pelvic node dissection was the treatment chosen. However, now an attempt is made to favor a less radical procedure and to treat the patient with combination anticancer chemotherapy.

OVARIAN CANCER

Basic Principles

1. Deaths from ovarian cancer have slowly increased over the last 40 years, and the rate is now 2.5 times that of 1930.

2. 1.4 per cent or 1 of every 70 newborn girls will develop cancer of the ovary at sometime during their lives.

3. In 1978 there were 18,000 new cases reported. The age-specific incidence rates for ovarian cancer show a steady rise up to age 80 where they drop off slightly in the older ages.

4. Cancer of the ovary is the leading cause of death from gynecologic cancer. There are about 11,000 deaths a year from ovarian cancer.

a. It constitutes about 25 per cent of gynecologic cancers but accounts for 44 per cent of all deaths from cancers of the genital tract.

b. Ten out of every 1,000 women in the United States over age 40 years will develop ovarian cancer and only one or two will be cured.

5. Early diagnosis is a matter of chance at present rather than a scientific method.

6. Common epithelial ovarian cancers spread along the surface of the peritoneum and organs involving structures in the upper abdomen.

7. Although it is stated that there are no early symptoms of ovarian cancer, a careful history will reveal vague abdominal symptoms and mild digestive disturbances and may be present for months before the diagnosis is made. In women after age 40, with a history of ovarian dysfunction and bouts of dyspepsia, indigestion, and abdominal pain in whom no definite diagnosis can be made, it is important to rule out ovarian cancer.

8. What is interpreted as a normal-sized ovary in the premenopausal woman represents an ovarian tumor in the postmenopausal woman.

9. It is advisable to do a laparotomy when any pelvic mass has appeared after the menopause; an adnexal mass in a woman of any age that progressively enlarges beyond 5 cm. while under observation; an adnexal mass 10 cm. or more in size; normal-sized ovary in the postmenopausal woman; and a mass which cannot be definitely diagnosed as either a fibroid or carcinoma.

10. Common epithelial ovarian cancers make up about 80 per cent of all

ovarian cancers. Only 8 per cent occur in women under age 35 and most occur in women over age 40 years.

Classification

1. Common primary epithelial tumors of the ovary (benign, borderline, or malignant)
   Serous
   Mucinous
   Endometroid
   Mesonephric
2. Germ cell tumors
   Dysgerminoma
   Extraembryonal teratomas
   Adult teratomas
   Carcinoids
   Struma ovarii
3. Gonadoblastoma
4. Gonadal stromal (sex cord-mesenchymal) tumors
   Female type
     Granulosa cell tumor
   Male type
     Sertoli-Leydig
5. Tumors not specific for the ovary
   Lymphoma
6. Metastatic tumors
   Krukenberg
   Adenocarcinoma of large intestinal origin
   Miscellaneous

Clinical Staging of Carcinoma of the Ovary

Staging is based on findings at clinical examination and surgical exploration. The final histologic findings (and cytologic, when required) after surgery are to be considered in the staging.

Stage I. Growth limited to the ovaries

Stage Ia. Growth limited to one ovary; no ascites
i. No tumor on the external surface; capsule intact
ii. Tumor present on the external surface, or capsule(s) ruptured, or both

Stage Ib. Growth limited to both ovaries; no ascites
i. No tumor on the external surface; capsule intact
ii. Tumor present on the external surface, or capsule(s) ruptured, or both

Stage Ic. Tumor either Stage Ia or Stage Ib, but with ascites* present or with positive peritoneal washings.

Stage II. Growth involving one or both ovaries with pelvic extension

Stage IIa. Extension and/metastases to the uterus and/or tubes

Stage IIb. Extension to other pelvic tissues

Stage IIc. Tumor either Stage IIa or Stage IIb, but with ascites present or with positive peritoneal washings

Stage III. Growth involving one or both ovaries with intraperitoneal metastases outside the pelvis, or postive retroperitoneal nodes, or both. Tumor limited to the true pelvis with histologically proven malignant extension to small bowel or omentum.

Stage IV. Growth involving one or both ovaries with distant metastases. If pleural effusion is present, there must be positive cytology to allot a case to Stage IV. Parenchymal liver metastases equals Stage IV.

*Ascites is peritoneal effusion which, in the opinion of the surgeon, is pathologic, or clearly exceeds normal amounts, or both.

Special Category. Unexplored cases that are thought to be ovarian carcinoma

The Cancer Committee endorses the histologic typing of ovarian tumors as presented in WHO Publication No. 9, 1973, and recommends that all ovarian epithelial tumors be subdivided according to a simplified version of this. The types recommended at the present time are as follows: serous tumors, mucinous tumors, endometrioid tumors, clear-cell (mesonephroid) tumors, undifferentiated tumors, and unclassified tumors.

After separation of cases according to histologic types, the groups shall be staged using above classification.

Treatment of the Common Epithelial Ovarian Cancer

Stage I

1. Aspiration of fluid for cytology
2. Total hysterectomy and bilateral salpingo-oophorectomy
3. Omentectomy
4. Appendectomy
5. Instillation of P^{32} } optional
6. Chemotherapy }

Stages II, III, and IV

1. The same as for Stage I, if possible
2. Chemotherapy for therapy in Stages III and IV

Treatment of Nonepithelial Tumors

1. Germ Cell Tumors

a. *Dysgerminoma*

(1) In the presence of spread beyond the ovary, total hysterectomy, bilateral salpingo-oophorectomy, omentectomy, and biopsy of the para-aortic nodes. Postoperative x-ray therapy and combination chemotherapy should be given as indicated.

(2) In a young woman with a unilateral, encapsulated dysgerminoma, acceptable treatment includes a unilateral salpingo-oophorectomy, biopsy of the other ovary and of the para-aortic nodes, as well as cytologic examination of peritoneal fluid.

b. *Endodermal Sinus, Embryonal Teratoma, and Choriocarcinoma*

(1) Management is generally total hysterectomy and bilateral salpingo-oophorectomy.

(2) No strong argument can be made for the more radical procedure over a conservative management.

(3) The tumors are not radiosensitive.

(4) Combination chemotherapy has shown some encouraging results.

2. Gonadal Stromal Tumors—Granulosa Cell Tumors

a. In women over 35 years, treatment includes total hysterectomy and bilateral salpingo-oophorectomy.

b. In children and adolescents, the tumor is usually unilateral and encapsulated, and therefore unilateral salpingo-oophorectomy is sufficient treatment.

3. Gonadoblastoma

a. Is a rare tumor composed of germ cell and gonadal stromal elements.

b. Most occur in patients who are intersexual with phenotype female habitus, who are amenorrheic and possibly virilized.

c. The malignancy rate is near zero, but the gonads are useless and both ovaries should be removed. The gonads should be removed in the presence of an XY chromosome pattern, even though the gonads are not enlarged.

Advanced Cancer of the Ovaries with Ascites

1. Ascites from carcinoma of the ovaries indicates the most advanced stage. Only palliative treatment is possible. Occasionally a patient may live for years.
2. Ascites of any appreciable degree produces mechanical symptoms, which are promptly relieved by paracentesis; this is indicated whenever symptoms of fullness, dyspepsia, and respiratory im-

pairment are present. If surgical intervention is contemplated, this should be done expeditiously and is preferable to paracentesis.

3. If roentgenograms indicate accumulation of fluid in either or both chest cavities, thoracentesis is indicated.

4. All aspirations of abdominal or chest fluids should be sent to the laboratory for cytologic diagnosis.

5. After maximal drainage of ascites, abdominal and pelvic examinations are performed for evaluation of masses. Often a large ballotable abdominal mass is identified as a possible "omental cake." Under propitious circumstances, laparotomy is then indicated.

6. If large, fixed masses are palpated and surgery is not selected, P^{32} and/or radiation therapy have little to offer for these patients.

7. A single alkylating agent is the treatment of choice. If the patient responds and then relapses, she should be evaluated for combination chemotherapy.

8. When mechanical interference with intestinal tract function occurs owing to neoplastic blockage of the bowel or infiltration of the bowel wall, and causing carcinomatous ileus, a long tube should be given a trial.

9. If the tube fails to relieve the obstructed bowel, the question of surgical intervention to relieve obstruction arises. Such procedures may entail bowel resection or by-pass procedures. Unfortunately, it is generally found that little can be done.

10. In unusual circumstances, when all factors indicate ovarian carcinomatosis, and laparotomy is performed for palliation, it is discovered that the cancer is indeed localized and totally excisable with bowel resection. A few patients operated upon under such circumstances have survived for years free from evidence of active cancer.

42. Breast Diseases

Hugh R. K. Barber, M.D.

CANCER OF THE BREAST

Basic Principles

1. One out of every 13 women, or about 7 per cent, will develop cancer of the breast.
2. There are approximately 91,000 new cases in the United States each year and 34,000 deaths from breast cancer.
3. Among women in the United States who are 25 to 74 years of age, breast cancer is the leading cause of cancer mortality.
4. It is the leading cause of death from all causes in women 39 to 44 years of age. Every 15 minutes one women dies of this disease.
5. Carcinoma is more common on the left than right side, more in the outer than inner quadrant, more in women without children, and more in women who have not suckled.
6. Bilateral in breast—successive in 4 per cent or more of cases.
7. Male to female ratio is 1:100.
8. Familial incidence (five-fold increase)
9. The typical presentation is that of a lump in the breast which in the early stages is isolated, moveable, and painless.
10. As the cancer advances, fixation, retraction of skin or nipple, ulceration, pain, erythema, and nodal axillary masses may appear.
11. Early detection depends on self-examination by women at monthly intervals and semi-annual examination by physicians. The breast self-examination (BSE) should be performed at monthly intervals, one week after the menses.
12. To make an early diagnosis, the physician must have a high degree of suspicion regarding all breast lesions as well as a basic knowledge of the following factors:
    a. The common types of breast lesions and their relative frequency
    b. The age-periods at which these lesions usually occur
    c. The characteristic symptom complexes
    d. The various risk factors that increase a patient's chance for developing breast cancer
13. The most common type of breast lesion and their frequency are: fibrocystic disease 34 per cent, cancer 27 per cent, fibroadenoma 19 per cent, intraductal papilloma 6 per cent, duct ectasia 4 per cent, and other 11 per cent.
14. *Patients at high risk* include: those over 40 years of age, those with a family history of breast cancer, nulliparous women or those with first parity after 34, women with a previous history of cancer in one breast, those with a precancerous mastopathy type of fibrocystic disease, those with adverse hormonal milieu, those with lowered immunological competence, patients with excessive exposure of the breast to ionizing radiation, those exposed to carcinogens, those with endometrial or ovarian cancer, those with a high dietary intake of fat, patients with chronic psychological stress, those living in the western hemisphere, those belonging to the upper socioeconomic group of the white race.
15. *Biopsy* is mandatory in patients with:
    a. True three-dimensional dominant

lumps even if diagnostic aids are negative, excluding cysts which can be safely aspirated under controlled conditions

b. Suspicious lesions found by diagnostic aids, even if there are no clinical findings

c. Serous, serosanguineous, bloody, or watery nipple discharge, even if there are no palpable masses and cytology and breast x-ray studies are negative.

d. Other adverse signs, i.e., eczema of the nipple, unexplained retraction or elevation, suspicious axillary adenopathy, redness of the skin of the breast, underlying induration without signs of infection, unexplained skin dimpling, or a persistent dominant area of unexplained thickening of the breast

16. *X-ray studies* of the breast are advised for all patients over 50 years on a yearly basis, for those with symptomatic breasts that are difficult to diagnose clinically, for those with an abnormal thermogram, for women possessing factors related to increased risk of breast cancer, preoperatively when a breast lump is present, except when the patient is under 25 years, after cyst aspiration, for multinodular breasts, for large pendulous breasts, for areas of thickening without a true mass, for breasts with dense scar formation due to previous biopsies or trauma. The observed median survival time for cancer of the breast is 6 years for all ages; over 10 years under 45; 9.5 years between the ages of 45 and 54; 6.5 years between the ages of 55 and 64; 5.2 years between the ages of 65 and 74; and 3 years at 75 years and over.

Schematic Anatomic Staging Outline (Clinical Observations)

1. Stage I. Breast mass localized, all nodes negative.

2. Stage II. Breast mass localized, axillae positive.

3. Stage III. Breast mass locally extensive, axillae, supraclavicular, and internal mammary nodes positive.

4. Stage IV. Distant metastases.

5. The UICC and the AJCCS has provided a TNM classification for cancer of the breast.

Treatment

1. Radical mastectomy or modified radical mastectomy and axillary node dissection is the preferred treatment. However, the procedure can be tailored to the extent of the disease and the needs of the patient.

2. Recommendations for surgery, radiation, and chemotherapy depend on the type, size, location, and extent of the tumor, age, relation to the menopause, as well as other pertinent factors.

Differential Diagnosis and Characteristic Symptom Complexes

1. Fibrocystic Disease

a. Is commonly bilateral and multiple.

b. Characterized by dull, heavy pain, sense of fullness and tenderness.

c. Changes with menses are common.

d. Tenderness is common

e. Axillary nodes should be normal.

f. There is no venous engorgement.

g. Occurs in women between 20 to 50 years of age.

2. Fibroadenoma

a. Are very mobile, solid, firm, well delineated.

b. It is the classical rubbery, slippable mass.

c. They are multiple and bilateral in about 14 to 25 per cent of patients.

d. A fibroadenoma grows slowly and does not change with menses.

e. Occurs in women between 15 to 40 years of age.

3. Cystosarcoma Phylloides

a. A rare variant of fibroadenoma.

b. May cause massive enlargement of the breast.

c. The skin is seldom involved and the axillae are usually clear.

d. Venous engorgement and skin inflammation may be present.

4. Galactocele

a. Typically occurs following lactation.

b. It is usually found beneath the areola.

c. It is occasionally tender.

d. A milky discharge is sometimes found.

5. Cyst of the Glands of Montgomery

a. This is essentially a sebaceous cyst involving periareolar glands and presents under the areola. It is usually very small.

b. It may be fixed to the skin but not the chest wall.

6. Fat Necrosis

a. Usually results from trauma.

b. Skin dimpling and a firm, indistinct mass are characteristic.

c. It may be very difficult to differentiate from cancer.

d. The lesion is occasionally tender.

7. Mondor's Disease

a. Is caused by superficial thrombosis of veins overlying the breast and may produce skin dimpling.

b. Typically, tenderness is present in early phases.

c. The lesion is self-limited and disappears with time.

8. Intraductal Papilloma

a. Presents with a serous (yellow), serosanguineous (pink), sanguineous (bloody), or watery type of discharge.

b. Usually no lump can be palpated.

9. Mammary Duct Ectasia (Comedo Mastitis)

a. Is usually subareolar.

b. Commonly manifests with nipple discharge.

c. The discharge is usually multicolored and sticky, bilateral and from multiple ducts.

d. The patient may experience a burning, itching, or dull pulling type of pain around the nipple and areola and there may be palpable, tortuous, tubular swelling under the areola.

e. Nipple retraction, skin retraction, and a diffuse mass may be present.

f. There may be edema and axillary adenopathy.

g. If is very difficult to differentiate from cancer.

Treatment

Unless the diagnosis is obvious or there is regression of the lesion within a short period of time, a biopsy is indicated and appropriate therapy selected. If any malignancy is found, tissue should be sent for estrogen receptor assay.

Alternative Types of Treatment

A current controversy over the surgical treatment of breast cancer has tended to divert attention from the importance of early diagnosis through breast self-examination (BSE) and periodic physical examination of the breasts by physicians aided by new diagnostic advances.

There is a definitive trend to do less radical operations for breast cancer. However, even when the breast cancer is found early, at least 20 per cent of the cancers have already spread to adjacent lymph nodes. At present, there is no completely satisfactory method of identifying those tumors which have already undergone limited extension, and those which have spread beyond the confines of customary treatment. While studies continue in many disciplines on these exceedingly important questions, we must understand the nature and description of the various methods of treatment of breast cancer that apply to the tumor itself.

1. Extended Radical Mastectomy or Supraradical Mastectomy. Surgical removal of the internal mammary chain of lymph nodes, the entire involved breast, the underlying chest muscles, and the lymph nodes in the axilla (armpit).

2. Halsted Radical Mastectomy. Surgical en-bloc removal of the entire involved breast, the underlying chest muscles, and the lymph nodes in the axilla.

3. Modified Radical Mastectomy. Surgical removal of the entire involved breast and many lymph nodes in the axilla. The underlying chest muscles are removed in part or are left in place after removal of the nodes in the axilla.

4. Simple Mastectomy (More Recently Called Total Mastecomy). Surgical removal of the entire involved breast. The underlying chest muscles and lymph nodes in the axilla are not removed.

***Note*: All of the above procedures remove the involved breast completely.**

5. Limited Procedures. They have received a variety of names, including lumpectomy, local excision, partial mastectomy, tylectomy (comparable to lumpectomy). In each instance, the tumor is surgically removed with a varying amount of surrounding tissue.

6. Treatment of Choice. For many years surgeons have preferred the Halstead radical mastectomy as the operation of choice for most cancers of the breast. More recently, some surgeons have preferred the modified radical mastectomy for early cancers, or a simple mastectomy for in-situ (extremely early and noninvasive) breast cancer. Subcutaneous mastectomy with subsequent implant has also been recommended for lobular carcinoma in-situ but *not* for invasive cancer.

43. Radiation Therapy in Gynecology

Hugh R. K. Barber, M.D.

A working knowledge of the physics, basic radiation biology, permissible radiation exposure, and the application of radioactive isotopes is important in the evaluation and management of clinical problems in oncology. Because of the great advances made in radiophysics, radiation therapy has become too complex for the average gynecologist. Proficiency in radiotherapeutic techniques demands teamwork between the different specialists and competent radiotherapists and physicists. It is not within the province of this short discussion to create radiotherapists but certain fundamentals are emphasized, so that the gynecologist may be an efficient member of the therapeutic team.

BASIC PRINCIPLES

1. All matter is made up of chemical substances which can be divided into two kinds, elements and compounds.

    a. An element is a distinct kind of matter which cannot be decomposed into two or more simpler kinds of matter.

    b. A compound is formed when two or more elements combine together chemically to produce a more complex type of matter.

2. Atoms are the smallest particles of an element that can exist without losing the chemical properties of the element.

3. Molecules are the smallest particles of a compound that can exist without losing the chemical properties of the compound.

4. The atom is an electrical structure having three basic units, the proton, the neutron, and the electron.

    a. This concept is adequate for an understanding of most phenomena in radiological physics.

    b. The nucleus contains the protons and neutrons while the orbits—circular or elliptical—contain the electrons.

5. The simplest atom is one of the element hydrogen. This consists of a central nucleus comprising one proton around which one electron moves in a shell or orbit.

6. The proton is a heavy particle carrying a positive charge and the electron is a very much lighter particle with a negative charge of exactly equal magnitude (but of opposite sign) to that of the proton.

7. Therefore, almost all of the mass of the atom is in the nucleus, and the positive charge of the nucleus is balanced by the negative charge of the electron to make the atom as a whole electrically neutral.

8. The next simplest atom is that of the element helium. Its nucleus comprises two protons and two neutrons and there are two orbital electrons moving around the nucleus.

9. A neutron is a particle with a mass approximately equal to that of a proton but with no electrical charge.

10. The electron is a much lighter particle than a proton having a mass only 1/1,840 of the mass of a proton, and it has a negative charge of exactly equal magnitude (but of opposite sign) to that of the proton.

11. Positrons have the same mass as an electron but with a positive charge existing only while in motion.

12. The nucleus of the helium atom

therefore has a positive charge of 2 units (due to two protons) and a mass of approximately 4 units. The two positive charges of the nucleus are balanced by the two negatively charged electrons around the nucleus.

13. Every element has a mass number and an atomic number (Z).

a. The atomic number of an element is the number of protons in the nucleus (which is equal to the number of electrons around the nucleus) of an atom of that element.

b. The mass number of an atom is the total number of protons and neutrons in the nucleus. It gives a measure of the mass of the nucleus or its atomic weight.

14. Protons and neutrons are known collectively as nucleons because they are found in the nucleus.

15. The atomic number is written to the left and below (subscript) the symbol for the element. For sulfur it is $_{16}S$. The atomic mass is written above (superscript) and to the right, i.e., S^{32}. It may also be written with the mass number being placed above the atomic number, i.e., $\frac{32}{16}$.

16. An isotope is a chemical element having the same atomic number as another (i.e., same number of nuclear protons) but possessing a different atomic mass (i.e., different number of nuclear neutrons).

17. Isobar is a term applied to two or more substances that have the same atomic weight but different atomic numbers.

18. Radionuclide is an atomic nucleus which will decay spontaneously into some other nuclear species, accompanied by the liberation of energy—a nuclear species that is radioactive.

19. Bremsstrahlung (Brems rays) is a name applied whenever high-speed electrons, regardless of their source, are abruptly slowed down, and their energy is converted to electromagnetic radiation. If the energy is large enough the electromagnet radiation is in the x-ray region.

20. High energy β-particles, passing close to atomic nuclei and undergoing deceleration, also give rise to Brems radiation.

TYPES OF RADIATION EMITTED

1. These radiations, whether natural or artificial radioisotopes, are of three kinds, named after the first three letters of the Greek alphabet: (1) alpha rays (or particles), (2) beta rays (or particles), and (3) gamma rays (energy).

a. Alpha particles are streams of high-speed helium nuclei (two protons and two neutrons packed tightly together) that have been ejected from radioactive substances.

b. Beta rays are streams of fast-moving electrons (particles) ejected from radioactive substances with velocities that may be as high as 0.98 of the velocity of light. In soft tissues, beta rays can travel distances ranging from small fractions of a millimeter up to about one centimeter, producing ionization in their path.

(1) The beta particle comes from a neutron in the nucleus. Neutrons change into a proton and an electron. The electron is then ejected from the nucleus.

(2) Emission of the beta particle from the nucleus (beta decay) does not change the mass number (the total number of particles in the nucleus) but does increase the atomic number by one, i.e., $_{15}P^{32} \rightarrow {}_{16}S^{32} + {}^{-}\beta^{o}$.

c. Gamma rays come from radioactive substances. When they are produced by electrical machines, we call them x-rays. They differ fundamentally from alpha and beta radiations, as they are not particles but waves of the same type as light and radiowaves, but with different properties of their very much shorter wave length.

RADIATION QUANTITIES AND UNITS

1. Units for activity are measured by curie.

2. Units of exposure are measured by rotengen.

3. Units for absorbed dose are measured by rad.

DEFINITIONS

1. Roentgen (r) is a measurement of radiation exposure. Is defined as "that amount of x- or gamma radiation such that the associated corpuscular emission per 0.001293 gram of air, produces in air, ions carrying one electrostatic unit of quantity of electricity of either sign. A milliroentgen is 1/1,000 r.

2. Roentgen-equivalent-man (rem) is defined as that quantity of radiation which produces the same biological effect in man as 1 r.

3. The rad is a unit of absorbed dose. It is defined as an energy absorption of 100 ergs per gram of any material (roughly equivalent to the roentgen).

4. Curie (C) is the quantity of any radioisotope which disintegrates at the rate of 3.7×10^{10} disintegration per second. The subunits of the Curie unit are: millicurie (mCi) = 1/1,000 of C, microcurie (μCi) = 1/1,000 of mCi.

5. mg.Ra (Milligram Radium). Used for radium only (1 mg. radium = 1 mCi radium = 8.2 rhcm).

6. mg.Raeq. (Milligram Radium Equivalent). Used for gamma-emitting radioisotopes which are applied in radiation therapy as substitutes for radium or radon. Defined as the activity which produces the same ionization in air by gamma radiation as 1 mg. of radium (1 mg.Raeq. = 8.25 rhcm).

7. Linear Energy Transfer (LET). Is the energy released (usually in Kev) per micron of medium (tissue) along the tract of any ionizing particle.

CHARACTERISTICS OF RADIATION

Basic Principles

1. Radiation can be defined as the propagation of energy through space or matter. In radiology they can be divided into two main groups, corpuscular and electromagnetic. Radiations produce their effect principally by the process of ionization—the ejection of outer orbital electrons from atoms.

2. Corpuscular radiation consists of moving particles of matter. Electromagnetic radiation consists of a transport of energy through space as a combination of an electric and magnetic field, both of which change in magnitude as a function of time and space.

3. X-ray and gamma rays are examples of these types of energy. Cesium, radium, cobalt, and x-irradiation are examples of this type of energy.

4. X- and gamma rays lose their energy in matter by three primary processes:

a. Photoelectric absorption and

b. Compton scattering, which result in the ejection of an orbital electron, while

c. Pair production involves a change of the photon energy into mass (a positive and negative electron are formed).

5. The radiobiological effects on cells may be inhibition of cell division, chromosome mutation, or gene mutation. The energy of x-ray or gamma rays may cut through a chromosome allowing the severed ends to join together with little change of function. The use of potentiators such as hydroxyurea or actinomycin D inhibit the chromosome from reforming.

Physical Aspects of High LET Particles

1. Protons, helium ions, and heavy ions are heavy-charged particles.

a. The particles pass through matter and travel in nearly a straight line and come to stop after passing through a certain depth of absorber, depending upon their initial energy.

b. The rate of energy loss increases sharply near the end of the range. There the dose reaches a peak, known as the "Bragg peak."

c. The dose falls off very rapidly beyond the Bragg peak.

2. P ions, unlike other heavy charged particles, are unstable and have a very short half-life. They have not been used in gynecological malignancy.

3. Neutrons interact with tissue and release highly ionizing, heavy charged particles; most of the dose is contributed by recoiling protons from hydrogen in tissue. Current research with neutron therapy has promise but has not added any significant survival in the treatment of gynecological cancer.

Gross Effects of Intracavitary Radiation

1. Erythema—1 week
2. Exudation—2 weeks
3. Slough—6 to 8 weeks
4. Scarring—6 months
5. Contraction—1 year

Radiobiological Effects on Skin

For 6,000 r in 6 weeks, 250 KV, HVL 2 mm. Cr, 10 × 10 cm^2 field. With supervoltage, approximately twice the doses are required to produce the same early effects.

1. Early Effects

First week	Faint (first erythema after 6 to 12 hours, fading in 2 to 3 days)
Second week	Sharply defined (second) erythema
Third week	Deepening erythema
Fourth week	Dry desquamation
Fifth week	Beginning moist desquamation
Eighth week	Complete moist desquamation
Twelfth week	Complete healing

2. Late Effects

Three months to years	Atrophy, telangiectasis, depigmentation, subcutaneous fibrosis

ADMINISTRATION OF RADIATION

Points of Reference Used in Calculating Dosages

1. Cervical cancers are not very sensitive tumors and high dosage must be used.

2. The adjacent normal tissue must be protected.

a. The function of the uterus and ovaries must be sacrificed, but it is often desirable to retain the sexual function of the vagina.

b. This is destroyed by shrinkage and fibrosis if too high a dosage is given.

c. In addition, the bladder and rectum must be completely protected.

Tab. 43-1. **Data on Permissible Radiation Exposure**

The exposure in the United States for a 30-year period (reproductive life of average person)	*Rads*
For diagnostic radiology	4.1 R
For radioisotopes around us	1.4 R
For radioisotopes in body	0.8 R
For cosmic radiation	0.4 R
From luminous dial watches	0.4 R
From nuclear testing	0.1 R
Total	7.2 R

***Tab. 43-2.* Radiation Contribution of Roentgenographic Diagnostic Procedures**

Procedure	*Skin Doses*	*Female*
Chest film 14″ × 7″	100 mR	0.07 mR
Chest photofluoroscopic film	1,000 mR	0.70 mR
Pyelogram	1,200 mR	1,300 mR
Pelvimetry	12,000 mR	1,300 mR

***Tab. 43-3.* Point at Which Radiation Exposure Damages Fetus**

Fetal Damage (Month of Gestation)	*R*
First	40 R
Second	90 R
Third	140 R
Fourth	200 R
Fifth	250 R
Sixth	350 R
Eight	500 R
Tenth	600 R

No threshold for gene mutation. Estimates for doubling of the spontaneous mutation rate in man run from 10 R to 140 R.

***Tab. 43-4.* The Development of Regulations for Maximum Permissible Dose to the Whole Body as is Follows:**

1931	1,000 mR per week	50 R per year
1935	500 mR per week	25 R per year
1946	300 mR per week	15 R per year
1958	100 mR per week	5 R per year

Currently 100 mR per week; 15 times as much for hands and feet; 1/10 as much for nonradiation workers.

***Tab. 43-4.* Radioisotopes**

Isotope	*Symbol*	*Half-Life*	*Alpha*	*Beta*	*Gamma*
Radium 226	^{226}Ra	1,620 years	+	+	+
Cesium 13	^{137}Cs	26.6 years	−	+	+
Cobalt 60	^{60}Co	5.4 years	−	+	+
Iridium 192	^{192}Ir	74.4 days	−	+	+
Phosphorus 32	^{32}P	14.3 days	−	+	−
Iodine 125	^{125}I	60.0 days	−	−	+
Radon 222	^{222}Rn	3.8 days	+	+	+
Gold 198	^{198}Au	2.7 days	−	+	+
Yttrium 90	^{90}Y	2.7 days	−	+	−

3. One method of avoiding damage to adjacent structures is to plan the radium dosage with reference to an imaginary point in the pelvis called point A.

   a. This is the basis for the Manchester method.

   b. Point A is 2 cm. from the central canal of the uterus, and 2 cm. above the lateral fornix, and is in the middle of an area arbitrarily called the paracervical triangle.

4. Too large a dosage in this vascular area will cause ischemia and fibrosis with a risk of subsequent stricture of the ureter. This is, however, a very rare complication and the real limiting factor in intracavitary radiation is the sensitive loops of bowel lying in the pelvis.

5. The size of the tumor and the space available in the uterus and vagina vary from patient to patient.

   a. Sometimes the uterine canal cannot be found because of the invasiveness of the tumor; and the degree of lateral distention of the vaginal vault affects the dosage delivered to the pelvic wall.

   b. The treatment of each patient must therefore be adapted to the conditions found on examination under anesthesia.

6. Afterloading technique is now commonly used. This means using a special tandem and colpostat which are first placed in position in the uterus and vagina and then loaded with radium, cobalt, or cesium.

   a. The technique has been developed to allow the radiotherapist to take more time and care in inserting and adjusting the applicators without exposing himself to radiation while doing so.

   b. It also allows more flexibility in dosage: one applicator can be unloaded, or the amount of radium altered, without interrupting treatment.

Preparation for Radiotherapy

1. Anemia must be corrected. It increases the anoxia of cancer and renders it less radiosensitive.

2. Local infection must be corrected. It will be impossible to sterilize a septic fungating growth; and some whole-pelvis radiation might be given as a preliminary to bring about some regression. Antiseptics and antibiotics may be needed.

3. If a pyosalpinx exists it should be removed surgically and radiation delayed for a week. The presence of sepsis both increases tissue anoxia and endangers the patient's life. The very small mortality associated with radiotherapy is due to sepsis.

4. Intravenous pyelogram is most important.

5. Bone scan should be done as indicated.

6. Psychologically the patient should be prepared by a frank discussion of the treatment.

Postoperative Care

1. If there is a temperature elevation of 101°F or more for 12 hours, remove the radium.

2. The patient should remain flat and use only one pillow. She may turn from side to side.

3. Indwelling catheter in bladder with continuous drainage

4. Adequate fluid intake

5. Percodan or codeine and aspirin for discomfort

6. Seconal for sleep

7. Check any bleeding.

8. Low residue diet

9. Exact time for removal of radioactive material should be placed on the order sheet.

Complications from Radiotherapy

1. Early

   a. Variation in size and shape of the fornices and extent of tumor

   b. Dilatation of the cervical canal may sometimes cause a tear into the broad ligament.

   c. Pyrexia

   d. Frequency and dysuria

e. Proctitis, diarrhea, and bleeding

f. Whitish membrane may cover the vagina.

2. Late

a. Vaginal atrophy

b. Fibrosis of the ureter

c. Intestino-vaginal fistula and/or rectal drainage

d. Avascular necrosis and spontaneous fracture have been observed.

e. Surface erythema, ulceration, and subcutaneous fibrosis

EVALUATION OF MACHINES FOR EXTERNAL RADIATION THERAPY

Units of Measurement

1. 1 electron volt = 1 ev
2. 1 thousand electron volt = 1 kiloelectron volt = 1 Kev
3. 1 million electron volt = 1 Mev
4. 1 billion electron volt = 1 Bev

Advantages of Megavoltage

1. Less skin reaction due to their lower surface dose. This is the most important advantage of megavoltage and permits radiation therapy without the bothersome skin reactions.

2. Greater depth doses, especially for small and medium fields. This permits simple set-up—usually opposing megavoltage fields are satisfactory as multiple fields or rotational therapy with kilovoltage.

3. Less dose in bone and less bone "shadowing." Less side scatter.

Disadvantages of Megavoltage

1. Much higher cost for machine and installation

2. Beam shaping more difficult

Megavoltage is essential for up-to-date curative and palliative radiation therapy.

Cobalt 60 vs. Cesium 137

Isotope	*Half-Life*	*Gamma Lines*	*Corresponding Voltage of Electrical Generators*
Cobalt 60	5.24 years	1.7 and 1.33 Mev	2–3 M
Cesium 137	26.6 years	0.67 Mev	1–1.5 Mv

1. Advantages of Cobalt

a. Better skin sparing (surface dose about one-half that of Cesium 137)

b. Better field shaping (source diameter about one-half that of Cesium 137)

c. Higher output

2. Disadvantages of Cobalt

a. Source replacement every 2 to 5 years

b. Room shielding more difficult

c. Cobalt 60 is preferable.

X-ray and Gamma Rays Versus Electrons

1. Advantages of X-Rays and Gamma Rays

a. Better skin sparing

b. Larger beams

2. Disadvantages of X-rays and Gamma Rays

a. Depth sparing more difficult

b. Lower ouput

c. Megavoltage electron-beam therapy is worthwhile only for very large institutions.

RADIATION THERAPY FOR GYNECOLOGICAL CANCERS

Cancer of the Cervix

Radiation therapy is the treatment chosen for stages IIb, III, and IV. It is chosen for those patients in stage Ib who are poor operative risks.

Outline of Standard Pelvic Field for External Radiation

1. Superior Border. A transverse line at the upper end of L5. It is centered on the midline of the vertebral body.

2. Inferior Border. A transverse line at the lower edge of the obturator foramen (or pubic symphysis). It is centered on the midline of the pubic symphysis. In stage IIIa (disease extending to the lower vagina), the lower edge of the pelvic field should be extended to include all disease, with at least 1 cm. margin.

3. Lateral Border. Perpendicular lines on each side, through the center of the acetabulum (not the head of the femur).

Whole Pelvis Irradiation and Intracavitary Radium Therapy

Tab. 43-5. **Irradiation Schedule for Specific Stages of Pelvic Cancer**

Stage	*External RT Whole Pelvic Rads*	*Intracavitary Parametrium Rads (Point A)*	*Max. Mg.–Hrs.*	*Ext. RT Booster Rads*	*Minimum-Dose Pelvic Wall Rads*
Ia	None	3,500–3 wks,–3,500	9,000	None	None
Ib, IIa	4,000 in 4 wks.	3,000–3 wks.–3,000	7,600	None	5,500
IIb	4,000 in 4 wks	3,000–3 wks.–3,000	7,600	1,000 involved side wall	6,500
IIIa	4,000 in 4 wks.	3,000–3 wks.–3,000	7,600	None	5,500
IIIb, IV	4,000 in 4 wks.	3,000–3 wks.–3,000	7,600	1,000 involved side wall	6,500

Starting 2 to 3 weeks after completion of external radiation: if the cervical os is not identifiable, this step is replaced by additional 2,000 rads by multiple fields, followed by intravaginal radiation.

up to 2,000 rads one-half centimeter below the mucous membrane.

Postoperative Radiation

1. Stage Ia G1. Speculum shows penetration of myometrium for more than one-third of its thickness.

a. External pelvic radiation 4,000 rads in 4 weeks plus vaginal radiation by an applicator up to 2,000 rads one-half centimeter below the mucous membrane.

b. If there is no penetration of the myometrium and the cancer is well differentiated, only intravaginal radiation is given.

2. Stages Ia G2, Ia G3, and Ib G1 (or G2 or G3). Uterine cavity greater than 8 cm. and/or poorly differentiated malignancy

a. 4,000 rads in 4 weeks plus intravaginal radiation

3. Stages II, III, and IV. External therapy of 4,000 rads in 4 weeks plus intravaginal radiation

Currently a number of institutions have been carrying out primary surgery and

Cancer of the Endometrium

Fields as outlined for cancer of the cervix.

Preoperative Radiation

1. Stage Ia G1 (uterine cavity less than or equal to 8 cm. and/or well-differentiated malignancy). No preoperative radiation

2. Stage Ia G2 or G3, Ib G1, G2 or G3 (uterine cavity greater than 8 cm. and/or poorly differentiated malignancy). External radiation to pelvis including the upper vagina—4,000 rads

3. Stages II, III, IV. External radiation to pelvis including the upper vagina—4,000 rads

All patients receive vaginal radiation by insertion of radium, cesium, or cobalt tailoring the radiation to the pathology found at surgery.

Care of Patient Receiving External X-ray Therapy

1. Requires close supervision.
2. Ambulatory patients appear to tolerate therapy better than one confined to bed.
3. The diet should contain adequate protein, vitamin B complex, and vitamin C.
4. Heat, sunlight, and irritating chemicals applied to the skin over the area of treatment are hazardous and may produce an accelerated or exaggerated skin reaction.
5. CBC should be checked each week.
6. The care of the patient should be shared by the radiation therapist and the referring physician.

44. Chemotherapy

Hugh R. K. Barber, M.D.

BASIC PRINCIPLES

1. In contrast to surgery and radiation therapy, chemotherapy (the treatment of cancer with drugs and hormones) can be used effectively for disseminated as well as localized cancer.

2. Within the last decade, it has become clear that although chemotherapy had long been considered largely a palliative procedure, capable of extending but not saving lives, certain kinds of cancer can now be cured by chemical treatment.

3. A major goal of current cancer chemotherapy is to achieve cures by prompt and vigorous treatment of such cancers. By "cure" is meant that the life expectancy of the treated patient is the same as "normal" life expectancy; specifically, the same as that of a matched cohort in the general population.

4. It has long been known experimentally that chemotherapy is more effective when tumor masses are small than when the tumor cell burden is high.

5. The concept of the first-order kinetic cell kill by drugs (fixed-percentage kill rather than fixed-number kill per effective dose) means that, with a small tumor burden, total cell kill can be achieved with a reasonable number of repetitive doses which, with a large tumor cell burden, would still leave residual cells which would eventually develop "resistance" and start to grow again.

6. Immunotherapy is postulated to kill tumor cells by zero-order kinetics (fixed number of tumor cells).

7. In humans, the effect of chemotherapy on the host is based on cell-kill hypothesis. In an attempt to represent cell kill, volume reduction is approximated because most clinical lesions can be measured only in two dimensions. As an example, oncologists refer to the greater-than-50-per-cent objective response. This criterion implies at least a halving of the product of perpendicular diameters. In both human leukemias and solid tumors, duration of response and/or host survival represents the best clinical correlate of cell kill.

8. Combinations of chemotherapeutic drugs have been used with substantial success, particularly when each of the drugs used acts on the cancer cells in a different way. Major improvements in the treatment of certain types of cancer have been achieved both by using several of the active drugs simultaneously and by the use of different drugs in sequence.

9. The cumulative results of cancer treatment research have brought the tally of types of cancer that are controllable to the point of being curable to 11 out of the 100 or more different forms.

a. These are acute leukemia in children, Hodgkin's disease, histiocytic lymphoma, skin cancer, testicular carcinoma, rhabdomyosarcoma, Ewing's sarcoma, Wilms' tumor, Burkitt's lymphoma, retinoblastoma, and choriocarcinoma.

b. Eleven additional types of cancer have shown significant improvement in survival. These are ovarian carcinoma, breast carcinoma, adult acute leukemias, multiple myeloma, endometrial carcinoma, prostatic cancer, lymphocytic lymphomas, neuroblastoma, adrenal cortical carcinoma, malignant insulinoma, and osteogenic sarcoma.

CELL KINETICS

1. Cellular reproduction (cell division cycle or cell kinetics) is divided into five phases.

2. These are:

Growth 1 (G1)—postmitotic and takes at least one-half the life cycle of the cell

Synthesis (S)—in which the DNA content is doubled and takes up about 30 per cent of the cell cycle of the cell

Growth 2 (G2)—which occurs just before mitosis and takes up about 20 per cent of the life cycle of the cell

Mitosis (M)—takes up about 1 per cent of the cell cycle

Growth 0 (G0)—is the resting or nondividing phase of the cell. G0 phase is variable and depends upon the type of cancer. The cell is relatively resistant to attack by the anticancer drugs during the resting phase (G0).

3. Studies on cell kinetics reveal that certain anticancer drugs have a more predictable effect on different phases of the cell.

4. Approximately 40 to 80 per cent of the marrow stem cells are in G0 at any given time. When chemotherapeutic agents cause lowering of the white blood cells, the resting marrow cells temporarily enter the cell cycle and proliferate rapidly.

5. Studies have shown that a given dose of drug kills the same percentage of cells that are in cycle, no matter how many are present.

a. For example, the same dose will kill 99 per cent of 100,000 leukemic cells or 99 per cent of 100 cells, whichever number of leukemic cells is present in the animal.

b. Therefore, 1,000,000 cells can be reduced to 10,000 and 10,000 reduced to 100, and 100 to 10 or less, and then 10 cells to 0.

c. By instituting an intermittent schedule to allow for recovery of normal cells, cures can be produced if the dose is large enough so that the percentage of cell population killed outpaces the multiplication of surviving cancer cells.

d. If the anticancer chemotherapy does not reduce the cell population at least 75 per cent, each day's multiplication of surviving cancer cells will outpace the inhibiting effect of the drug and will soon kill the animal.

6. Cancer-cell population studies have concluded that each tumor cell divides into two cells once each generation time, i.e., the time for one entire division cycle.

a. The time required for this cycle is about the same for all cells in a given population of cells.

b. Since each tumor cell divides into two cells at each generation time it is evident that by ten generations, a single cell proliferates into 1,000 (10^3) cells. Therefore, the growth of many cells following this pattern of growth will result in a thousandfold increase every ten generations.

c. The growth pattern is referred to as exponential or logarithmic.

d. By charting the log cells against time the pattern is charted as a smooth curve.

7. In order to be detected, a tumor must have a volume of at least 1 cubic centimeter consisting of about 10^9 cells (one billion, or 1,000,000,000).

8. The volume of cells necessary to kill a patient (critical volume) is $10 \times 10 \times 10$ cm., or about 10^{12} cells (one trillion).

9. Since these values are a thousandfold (10^3) apart, their separation in time represents ten generations of growth.

10. If treatment reduces the cell population from 10^{12} to 10^6 in acute lymphatic leukemia, the patient is in remission but is not cured.

11. The goal of anticancer chemotherapy is to reduce the last million cells (10^6) to zero. It is accepted that 100-per-cent cell kill of leukemic cells is necessary to achieve cure.

CHEMISTRY, MECHANISMS OF ACTION, TOXICITY, METHODS OF ADMINISTRATION, AND USES

1. The central dogma of molecular biology deals with the genetic material deoxyribonucleic acid (DNA), the replication of DNA to produce more DNA, the transcription of DNA into ribonucleic acid (messenger RNA), and the translation of RNA into protein (amino acids in the cytoplasm are activated by enzymes, transferred by transfer RNA to a ribosome, at which point the message is read off and the completed protein released).

CALCULATION OF DOSES ON BODY SURFACE AREA

There is increasing evidence that calculation of doses based on body surface is important in relating tolerated and effective doses in animals to those in man. Calculating by the body surface area helps to minimize the apparent dose differences between children and adults. Nomograms, from which body surface areas can be calculated when height and body weight are known, are available (Ca - A Cancer Journal for Clinicians, May/June 1977, vol. 27). When doses are expressed in mg./kg., the following formula can be used to convert roughly to mg./m.^{2}, that is, mg./kg. $\times$ 40 = mg./m.^{2} Depending on the drug, there may be an upper limit to the single dose given to patients weighing more than 70 kg.

A brief outline is given of the principal groups of anticancer drugs used in practice.

PRINCIPAL GROUPS OF ANTICANCER DRUGS USED IN PRACTICE

ANTIMETABOLITES

Folic Acid Antagonists

Chemistry

1. Derivatives of folic acid

2. The component parts of the folic acid molecule are:
   a. Plexidine nucleus
   b. *p*-Aminobenzoic acid
   c. Glutamic acid

3. Folinic acid is the formyl-containing analogue of reduced folic acid. It is called synthetic citrovorum factor of leucovorin.

Mechanism of Action

1. Blocks folic and reductase to prevent availability of single carbon fragment. This blocks purine ring biosynthesis.

2. By a lesser action it inhibits methylation of deoxyuridylic acid to thymidylic acid, blocking pyrimidine synthesis.

Toxicity

1. Mouth lesions
2. Ulceration of the gastrointestinal tract
3. Bone marrow depression
4. Susceptibility to infection
5. Alopecia
6. Hyperpigmentation
7. Teratogenic properties
8. Toxicity enhanced by impaired kidney function

Method of Administration and Dosage

1. 4 Amino-N^{10}-methylpteroylglutamic acid. Oral 2.5–5.0 mg./day
2. Amethopterin,methotrexate
   I.V. or I.M. 5–25 mg./day for 5 days

Uses

1. Choriocarcinoma
2. Cancer of the ovary
3. Cancer of the breast
4. In combination with other anticancer drugs for treating cancer of the cervix

PURINE ANTIMETABOLITES

Chemistry

1. 6-Mercaptopurine (6 MP) Purinethol

Mechanism of Action

1. Blocks purine ring biosynthesis
2. Inhibits interconversion of purines

Toxicity

1. Leukopenia
2. Thombocytopenia
3. Stomatitis
4. Nausea and vomiting (about 25% of adults)

Method of Administration

Usual dose: 2.0–2.5 mg./kg./day orally or 500 mg./m.^{2}/day intravenously for 5 days every 10 to 14 days.

Uses

1. Acute lymphatic leukemia
2. Acute granulocytic leukemia
3. Chronic granulocytic leukemia
4. Occasionally in choriocarcinomas

PYRIMIDINE ANTIMETABOLITE

Fluorouracil (5-FU)

Mechanism of Action

1. Blocks thymidylate synthetase
2. Inhibits methylation of deoxyuridylic to thymidylic acid blocking pyrimidine synthesis

Toxicity

1. Myelosuppression
2. Stomatitis
3. Gastrointestinal ulceration
4. Nausea and vomiting
5. Alopecia
6. Cerebellar ataxia (uncommon)
7. Diarrhea
8. Dermatitis
9. Skin hyperpigmentation

Method of Administration

1. 12 mg./kg./day × 3
2. Smaller dose, 1–2 times weekly for maintenance.

Uses

1. Bladder carcinoma
2. Breast carcinoma
3. Colorectal carcinoma
4. Gastric carcinoma
5. Hepatoma adenocarcinoma
6. Ovarian carcinoma
7. Pancreatic adenocarcinoma

GLUTAMINE ANTAGONISTS

Azaserine (0-diazoacetyl-1-serine)
DON (6-diazo-5-oxo-1-norleucine)

Chemistry

1. Diazo compounds, closely related in structure to glutamine
2. Derived from both filtrates of a streptomyces

Mechanism of Action

1. Interference of the donation of an amino group by glutamine to various biochemical needs in the body, thereby blocking the conversion of formyl glycineamide ribonucleotide (FGAR) to formyl glycineamidine ribonucleotide (FGAM)
2. A step in purine biosynthesis in which glutamine acts as an amine donor under the influence of an amidotransferase

Toxicity

1. Mouth lesions
2. Gastrointestinal tract disturbances
3. Leukopenia
4. Thrombocytopenia
5. Liver damage

Methods of Administration and Dosage

1. Azaserine
   I.V. 5–10 mg./kg./day
   Oral × 10 or more
2. DON
   I.V. 0.2 mg./kg./day

Uses

1. Choriocarcinoma (rarely now)
2. Childhood acute leukemia

POLYFUNCTIONAL ALKYLATING AGENTS

Chemistry

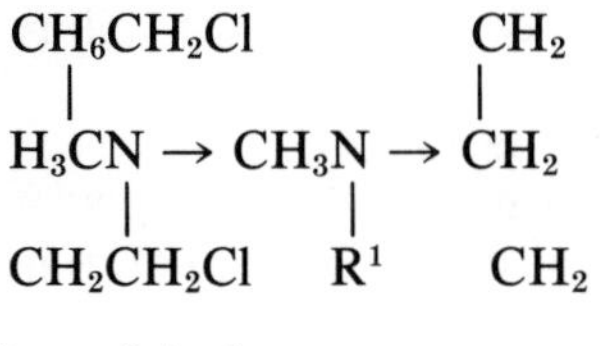

Mechanism of Action

1. Important sites of action appear to be on the nucleic acids, probably within the nucleus; this is suggested by the following observations:
   a. They are mutagenic.
   b. They are carcinogenic.
   c. Preferentially deactivate DNA-containing viruses
   d. Inactivate the pneumococcal and *H. influenzae* transforming principles
2. Alkylation (insertion of an alkyl group) may interfere with synthesis of cross-linking in a number of places. Prevents H bonding between chains of DNA
3. A monofunctional compound produces nuclear energy by a sheet mass effect
   a. Has only one active alkyl group
4. Polyfunctional agents are 50 to 100 times more active than the monofunctional group
   a. They are cross-linking agents
   b. Reactive atoms bridge across two chromosomal strands or react at two points on a chromosome

Toxicity

1. Delayed deaths may occur 3 to 7 days after exposure to LD50
2. Decrease in antibody production
3. Increased susceptibility to infection
4. Diarrhea
5. Ulceration of the gastrointestinal tract
6. Hemorrhagic cystitis
7. Involution in size of lymph nodes, thymus, and spleen
8. Progressive fall in the leukocytes and platelets in the peripheral blood
9. Decrease in spermatogenesis
10. Teratogenic effect

Methods of Administration and Dosage

1. Mechlorethamine HCl (HN_2CHl, Mustargen)
   I.V. 0.4 mg./kg., single or divided doses
2. Chlorambucil (Leukeran)
   Oral 0.1–0.2 mg./kg./day (6–12 mg./day)
3. Melphalan (Alkeran) (L-phenylalanine mustard, L-PAM) (L-Sarcolysin)
   Oral 0.2 mg./kg/day × 5 2–4 mg./day maintenance
4. Cyclophosphamide (Endoxan, Cytoxan)
   I.V. or Oral 200 mg./day I.V. for 5 days 50 mg./BID orally
5. Triethylenethiophosphoramide (TSPA, Thio-Tepa)
   I.V. 0.2 mg./kg. × 5 days
6. 1,4 Dimethanesulfonyloxybutane (Busulfan, Myleran)
   Oral 2–6 mg./day 150–250 mg./course
7. Nitroso-urea alkylating agents
   a. 1,3-bis (2 chloroethyl)-1-nitrosourea (BCNU)
   I.V. 100 mg./m.^{2} every 6 weeks Next course in 4 to 6 weeks
   b. Chloroethyl-cyclohexyl-nitrosourea (CCNU)
   Oral 120–150 mg./m.^{2} every 6 weeks

Uses

1. Carcinoma of the ovary
2. Hodgkin's disease
3. Lymphomas
4. Burkitt's tumor
5. Multiple myeloma
6. Cancer of the breast
7. Neuroblastoma
8. Carcinoid
9. Leukemias

ANTIBIOTICS

Mechanism of Action

1. Form a complex with DNA involving selective binding at the guaninecystosine segments, with a specific block in the DNA-dependent RNA synthesis (inhibits formation of messenger RNA [mRNA]).

Toxicity

1. Damage to bone marrow and intestinal epithelium
2. Nausea and vomiting
3. Diarrhea
4. Skin eruption

Methods of Administration and Dosage

1. Actinomycin D or Dactinomycin (Cosmegen)
   I.V. 0.01 mg./kg./day × 5 days or 0.04 mg./kg. weekly
2. Daunomycin
   I.V. 0.8–1.0 mg./kg./day × 3 to 6 days; total dose never to exceed 25 mg./kg.
3. Mitomycin C (Mutamycin)
   I.V. 0.06 mg./kg. × 2 weekly if blood counts permit
4. Adriamycin
   I.V. 50–75 mg./m.^{2} in single or divided doses every 2 weeks
5. Mitramycin
   I.V. 25 μg/kg. every other day × 3–4 days

Uses

1. Lymphomas
2. Leukemias
3. Solid tumors
4. Embryonal tumors
5. Trophoblastic disease
6. Carcinoid
7. Lower calcium level (Mithramycin)

ADRIAMYCIN (ADRIA)

Adriablastina, Doxorubicin

Toxicity

1. Gastrointestinal
2. Hematologic
3. Cardiac
   a. Electrocardiogram changes may occur, such as sinus tachycardia, T wave flattening, ST segment depression, voltage reduction and arrhythmias. These are indications to stop or defer treatment.
   b. Congestive heart failure secondary to cardiomyopathy.
4. Alopecia
5. Dermatitis
6. Red urine (not hematuria)

Administration

1. 60 to 75 mg./m.^{2} I.V., single dose q3 weeks
2. 30 mg./m.^{2} I.V., single dose for 3 days every 4 weeks. Administer through running I.V. infusion.
3. Avoid giving to patients with significant heart disease; reduce dosage in patients with impaired hepatic function.
4. The total cumulative dose of adriamycin should not exceed 550 to 600 mg./m.^{2} since the risk of congestive failure increases markedly above this level. A smaller cumulative dose (500 mg./m.^{2}) should be used when multiple drugs are included in the therapy. It is important to follow for EKG abnormalities and signs of heart failure.

Uses

1. Ovarian cancer
2. Embryonal tumors
3. Sarcomas
4. Breast carcinoma

MITOTIC INHIBITORS

Vinka Alkaloids

Chemistry

1. Dimeric indole-dihydroindole alkaloids
2. Periwinkle plant

MAJORS SCIENTIFIC BOOKS, INC.

6632 S. MAIN • HOUSTON, TEXAS 77030

TEL. 522-1361

CASH SALE RECEIPT

No. 49229

Customer's Order No. ______ Date 2/18 19 81

Name ______

Address ______

SOLD BY	CASH	C.O.D.	CHARGE	ON ACCT.	MDSE. RETD.	PAID OUT
BR	✓					

QUAN.	DESCRIPTION	PRICE	AMOUNT	
1	BARBER — QUICK REF., OB GYN	L	17	50
			17	50
		TAX	1	05
		TOTAL	18	55

All claims and returned goods MUST be accompanied by this bill.

RECEIVED BY ______

Mechanism of Action

1. Arrest of mitosis in metaphase by destruction of spindles

Toxicity

1. Nausea and vomiting
2. Diarrhea
3. Leukopenia
4. Neurotoxic paresthesias
5. Palsies
6. Peripheral neuritis
7. Alopecia
8. Ileus

Methods of Administration and Dosage

1. Vinblastine (Velban)
   I.V. 0.1–0.15 mg./kg. weekly
2. Vincristine (Oncovin)
   I.V. 0.03–0.075 mg./kg./weekly

Uses

1. Choriocarcinoma
2. Lymphoma
3. Leukemia
4. Hodgkin's disease

ENZYMES

L-asparaginase

1. Normal cells can synthesize their own supply of asparagine. It appears that asparagine-dependent cells lack an enzyme, asparagine synthetase, which in normal cells converts aspartic acid to asparagine. Certain types of leukemia (such as acute lymphoblastic) have an asparagine dependence. This provides an explanation for the effect of L-asparaginase. The tumor activity of L-asparaginase is also found with transplanted rat tumors and with primary dog lymphosarcoma. The final indications for the use of the enzyme in the treatment of malignancy remain to be determined.

Method of Administration and Dosage

1. L-asparaginase

I.V. 50–200 I.U./kg./day or 200–1,000 I.U./kg. 3–7 days each week for 28 days

Uses

1. Acute lymphoblastic leukemia

NONALKYLATING AGENT THERAPY

Hexamethylmelamine (HMM, HXM)

Mechanism of Action

Although hexamethylmelamine structurally resembles triethylenemelamine (TEM), a known alkylating agent, it is not thought to act as an alkylating agent at first but more like an antimetabolite.

Toxicity

1. Gastrointestinal
2. Myelosuppression
3. Neurologic
4. Alopecia
5. Dermatitis

Dose

8 mg./kg./day, P.O.

Cis-Platinum Dianmine Dichloride (CPDD)

Mechanism of Action

Upon loss of chlorine atom, the drug binds to DNA, high molecular weight RNA, and transfer RNA. The resulting inhibition of DNA synthesis is persistent for several days following administration of the drug. It is a cell cycle nonspecific agent.

Toxicity

1. Nephrotoxicity
2. Tinnitus and hearing loss
3. Nausea and vomiting
4. Myelosuppression

Dose

1. 50 mg./m.^{2}, I.V., $\times$ 3 every 28 days with mannitol diuresis

NEW AGENTS AND OTHER AGENTS THAT HAVE NOT BEEN EVALUATED IN OVARIAN CANCER

1. Cytembena
2. Porfiromycin
3. Porcarbazine
4. F Torafur
5. Bleomycin
6. Streptozotocin
7. DTIC

Traditionally the treatment for ovarian cancer has been surgery followed by x-ray therapy. Chemotherapy was reserved for the far-advanced and recurrent ovarian cancers. The results from this treatment have been poor.

The chemotherapeutic treatment for each gynecologic organ system is discussed in Chapter 29.

Index

Numerals in italics indicate figures; a "t" after a numeral indicates a table.

Clinical OB & GYN
MED DEPT HARPER + ROW PUBL INC
2350 VIRGINIA AVE
HAGERSTOWN MARYLAND
21740 $32.50/YR

FRIEDMAN LABOUR